Drugs of Abuse

DATE DUE			

Drugs of Abuse

Second edition

Simon Wills

PhD, MSc, MRPharmS

Head of Wessex Drug and Medicines Information Centre
Southampton University Hospitals Trust, UK

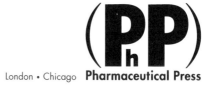

London • Chicago **Pharmaceutical Press**

Published by the Pharmaceutical Press
Publications division of the Royal Pharmaceutical Society of Great Britain

1 Lambeth High Street, London SE1 7JN, UK
100 South Atkinson Road, Suite 206, Grayslake, IL 60030-7820, USA

© Pharmaceutical Press 2005

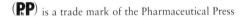 is a trade mark of the Pharmaceutical Press

First edition published 1997
Second edition published 2005

Typeset by Photoprint, Torquay, Devon
Printed in Great Britain by TJ International, Padstow, Cornwall

ISBN 0 85369 582 2

A catalogue record for this book is available from the British Library

To Little B
Mum and Dad, Richard and Charlie
and, of course, all the Donuts

Contents

Preface

Whether we approve of drug abuse wholly, selectively or not at all, it has been with the human race since before the dawn of written history and is here to stay. This book aims to be a detailed guide for the health-care professional who works with drug users or who wants to know more about the subject in an easily digestible form. I have tried to be concise but clear, so that the book is small, relevant, easy to read and relatively cheap. I want the book above all to be useful – as an educational tool, a clinical resource, or a reference.

I have found writing the second edition even harder than writing the first. Fortunately, readers and colleagues have been kind enough to give me suggestions about new material to include and, for this advice, I would like to express my thanks. Wherever possible, I have taken these ideas on board. This edition has been comprehensively revised, and many chapters have been completely rewritten. In general, I have now included more detail about side-effects throughout the book and the problems they may create for patients with particular medical conditions. I have provided more information on the prevalence of drug use, and have been as comprehensive as space allows in identifying substances that may be abused and their variants. Each of the illicit drug chapters now includes information about interactions between illicit drugs and medicines, and there are new chapters on gamma hydroxy-butyrate and on the use of the Internet as an information resource.

Simon Wills
October 2004

Acknowledgements

Perhaps the nicest part about writing a book is this page, where I have the opportunity to thank everyone. As with the first edition, the biggest problem I had when writing this book was finding the time to write. In this respect, I owe an enormous debt to all those close to me for understanding how limited my time had become and how important the book was to me. I want to say how grateful I am to them all for putting up with me being so antisocial. They are: Mum and Dad; Jonathan and Shirley; Richard and Charlie; Mike, Annie, Lucy and Ben; Jonathan, Catherine, Oscar and Fergus; Aileen, Leighton, James, Evelyn and Izzie; Tabitha and Rob; Nick, Kate, Beccy and Will; Jeremy, Leigh and Lauren; Jake, Martin and Laura; Andy and Jane. I have probably forgotten some important people, but I hope not.

I would also like to thank the team at the Pharmaceutical Press for making the book possible, and for not sticking too closely to deadlines, and the UK Medicines Information network and the Pharmacy Misuse Advisory Group (PharMAG) for their unstinting support. There are too many people to single out all of them individually, but I would particular likely to thank Andi Barrett, who has been very kind.

I am very grateful to two of my colleagues, who devoted much time to carefully reviewing my manuscript. I would like to thank Kay Roberts (Lead Pharmacist, Royal College of General Practitioners National Drug Misuse Training Programme, Glasgow) and Janie Sheridan (Associate Professor of Pharmacy Practice, The University of Auckland) for their most valuable input.

Finally, I would like to thank my own team at the Wessex Drug and Medicines Information Centre – they really are a terrific group of people and although I hope they do not think I take them for granted I am sure that I do not say thank you to them enough. They are Jill, Ang, Jon, Anne, Jennie, Nicola, Meghna, Kate, Margie and Gill. I like working with you, and thanks for putting up with me.

About the author

Simon Wills studied for a degree at King's College, London University, and qualified as a pharmacist in 1988. For ten years, he ran the Drug Information Service in Portsmouth, UK, becoming a founder member of the Pharmacy Misuse Advisory Group (PharMAG). During this time, he also completed a PhD. This research involved an analysis of drug- and medicine-related attendances at a hospital Accident and Emergency unit. In 2000, he moved to Southampton to manage the Wessex Regional Drug and Medicines Information Centre, based in Southampton University Hospitals NHS Trust. The clinical information team employed at the Centre advise health professionals on all aspects of the use of drugs and medicines. The Wessex Centre is also well known for its creative publications in a wide variety of fields, including the national evaluation of new medicines prior to UK launch, evidence-based health promotion resources, assessments of complementary medicines, and a range of national education and training materials.

Apart from substance abuse, his other professional interests include the ethics of healthcare information provision, research, critical appraisal and drug interactions. He is also a keen gardener, has an avid interest in Roman history, and has been mad enough to become a season ticket holder for Southampton Football Club.

1

Introduction

> *'Where shall I begin, please your Majesty?' he asked.*
> *'Begin at the beginning' the King said, gravely, 'and go on till you come*
> *to the end: then stop.'*
> Lewis Carroll, 'Alice's Adventures in Wonderland'

The global problem

Patterns of drug abuse around the world are constantly changing. They vary considerably on a geographical basis – from country to country, and from region to region within the same country. At the time of writing, the spread of metamfetamine (methamphetamine) abuse, for example, is causing concern in the USA, Australasia and South-East Asia, but has had less impact in northern Europe. Similarly, tobacco smoking has been slowly declining in the Western world since the 1950s as its long-term negative health consequences have been exposed, but at the same time, use is still increasing in underdeveloped countries. The popularity of individual drugs also varies with time. For example, compared to their heyday, the abuse of ether, barbiturates and phencyclidine is in long-term decline whereas alcohol, cocaine and ecstasy abuse generally seems to be increasing.

It was estimated by the World Health Organization (WHO) that there were about 185 million global consumers of illicit drugs in 2000, 2 billion users of alcohol and 1.3 billion smokers (Figure 1.1). As a proportion of disease burden, illicit drugs have the greatest impact in developed countries – western and northern Europe, North America and Australasia.[1] They have the least impact in central and southern Africa. The annual prevalence of individual illicit drugs as a proportion of the total users is shown in Figure 1.2.

The WHO has approximated the number of deaths worldwide attributable to a selected number of leading risk factors. Some of these figures are reproduced in Table 1.1. It is a surprising – even shocking – list.

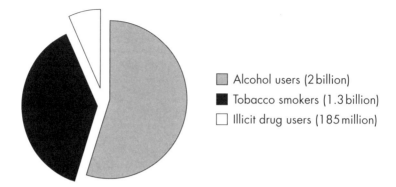

Figure 1.1 World extent of psychoactive substance abuse in 2000.[2] Adapted from reference 2.

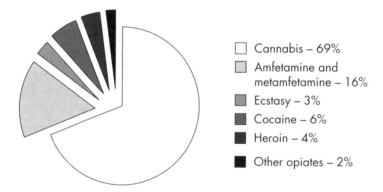

Figure 1.2 Annual prevalence of illicit drug abuse by drug over the period 1998 to 2001.[1] Adapted from reference 1.

From this information two key points emerge that are particularly relevant to this book. Firstly, although illicit drugs can harm individuals and society in a wide range of ways, the number of deaths globally per year is small in comparison to many of the other preventable and treatable factors identified by the WHO. The 0.2 million annual deaths in 2000 was 0.4% of all global deaths. Secondly, the number of people who die because of the effects of tobacco and alcohol – which are legal substances in most countries – far exceeds those killed by illegal drugs. Deaths caused by tobacco and alcohol represented 8.8% and 3.2% of global deaths respectively. The body count is not the only means by which the impact on the population of a serious health-related problem should be measured, but it is perhaps the ultimate measure. To this extent, it is only reasonable to put the importance of drug abuse as a world health problem into perspective.

Table 1.1 Global deaths in 2000 attributable to selected leading risk factors[3]

Risk factor	Deaths (millions)
Blood pressure	7.1
Tobacco	4.9
Cholesterol	4.4
Underweight	3.8
Unsafe sex	2.9
Fruit and vegetable intake	2.7
High body-mass index	2.6
Physical inactivity	1.9
Alcohol	1.8
Unsafe water, sanitation and hygiene	1.7
Indoor smoke from solid fuels	1.6
Iron deficiency	0.8
Urban air pollution	0.8
Zinc deficiency	0.8
Vitamin A deficiency	0.8
Unsafe healthcare injections	0.5
Occupational risk factors for injury	0.3
Illicit drugs	0.2

Interestingly, about 80% of the global deaths due to illicit drug use are in men. Men predominate to a similar extent in the global deaths due to tobacco smoking and alcohol.

The remainder of this chapter introduces some of the terms and concepts used in this book, discusses drug withdrawal, explains the methods of drug administration and the environments in which drugs are used, and describes the legal implications of drug abuse.

Concepts

Abuse

The term 'abuse' is typically used to describe the non-medical self-administration of a substance to produce psychoactive effects, intoxication or altered body image, and usually despite knowledge of the risks involved. This is the definition used in this book. The term is widely applied to situations in which illicit drugs are taken, whether or not the individual involved has actually suffered adverse consequences.

In the USA, the *Diagnostic and Statistical Manual of Mental Disorders* (DSM) has attempted to define criteria for diagnosing abuse.[4]

The criteria specify that the individual must satisfy at least one of the following signs recurrently because of drug usage:

- Failure to fulfil important personal commitments.
- Abuse of drug in physically hazardous situations.
- Legal problems related to abuse.
- Problems in relating to other people due to abuse.

This rather rigid classification concentrates on individuals who are already suffering adverse consequences from their behaviour. The DSM criteria focus on the social consequences for the individual rather than the purpose of abuse and they can only apply to those who use a drug repeatedly. In addition, according to the DSM criteria, the term 'abuse' cannot be applied to tobacco, because smokers do not suffer the specific consequences listed, or to the majority of people who regularly or occasionally use drugs such as cannabis, LSD (lysergide) or ecstasy, most of whom do not experience the consequences described. As a result, this definition has limited value.

The term 'drug abuse' is viewed by some as inappropriate because it can be seen as judgemental. However, alternatives are not very satisfactory. 'Drug use' is bland and fails to separate medicinal agent from recreational drug. 'Drug misuse' tends to imply that a drug has a proper use and is being employed for an incorrect purpose. For many illicit substances there are no legitimate medical uses – their sole use is as a psychoactive drug. Most dictionaries make little distinction between the definitions of abuse and misuse, and when applied to illicit drugs both terms are commonly used.

Dependence

Dependence is an inappropriate compulsion to take a substance regularly, which may cause physical, mental and/or behavioural impairment. The drug is taken to make the user feel good or more usually to avoid withdrawal, but in either case it is clear that the user has lost control over their behaviour, and gives the drug greater priority over other behaviours that previously were more important. It is equivalent to the older term 'addiction', but dependence is now the more widely used term. According to the DSM criteria,[4] at least three of the following must be satisfied over a 12-month period to qualify as true dependence:

1. The user shows tolerance.
2. The user suffers withdrawal – the withdrawal syndrome appears or there is clear evidence of negative reinforcement.

3. The quantity taken and/or the duration of the habit exceed the initial expectations of the user.
4. The user consistently wishes to reduce or control substance use and may have already tried to, unsuccessfully.
5. Drug-seeking behaviour, drug administration and/or post-exposure recovery take up a significant amount of the user's time.
6. Important personal activities are given little time or are abandoned.
7. Use of the substance continues despite the user experiencing physical or psychological harm from it.

The DSM suggests that the term physiological (or physical) dependence be used to describe situations where the user meets three of these criteria, including one or both of the first two criteria. However, the WHO recommends that the terms physiological (physical) and psychological dependence be avoided because in clinical practice it is difficult to distinguish between them, and because all drug effects should be potentially explainable in biological terms.[5] It is also notable that the DSM criteria for diagnosing do not incorporate craving for the drug as a diagnostic criterion, and yet this is an almost universal feature of dependence.

At a biochemical level, a variety of neurotransmitters are potentially involved in triggering dependence, but dopamine seems to have a pre-eminent influence, and increased levels of dopamine are seen in the brains of patients abusing most drugs with a psychotropic effect. It is involved in central nervous systems (CNSs) associated with pleasure, elation and reward.

Designer drugs

This term was originally introduced in the USA to describe analogues of street drugs that were manufactured in order to circumvent the law in the 1970s and early 1980s.[6] Ecstasy and other amfetamine analogues were being synthesised and used legally in the USA because their structures were not specified as illicit substances in the legislation of the time.

The term has now acquired a different meaning because current legal specifications for illicit substances in the USA and many other countries are so detailed that circumventing the law is very difficult. A designer drug, in the most popular use of the term, is an analogue of an existing well-known street drug, with similar pharmacological properties but a different chemical structure.[7] It is therefore a very imprecise term. Substances referred to as designer drugs include analogues of fentanyl, metamfetamine, pethidine and phencyclidine.

The term 'designer drug' should not be taken to imply that an analogue can be synthesised or prepared to meet an individual's requirement. This is not possible.

Drug-seeking behaviour

Those with a compulsion to take an abusable substance may go to great lengths to obtain further supplies. This may include regularly buying the drug, registering with several doctors in order to obtain supplies, theft (of the drug, or money to buy it), forgery of prescriptions, feigning medical illness to obtain prescribed drugs, selling valuable possessions in order to obtain drugs, travelling long distances, and prioritising drug-seeking above other more urgent matters. In some cases, the life of an individual can become totally dominated by the various activities necessary to secure a continued supply.

Harm reduction

The principle of harm reduction accepts that illicit drug use will always happen and that minimising the dangers to individuals, communities and society as a whole is a more realistic approach than simply condemning it. Harm reduction describes the measures used to achieve this despite continued use of illicit substances. Abstinence can be a goal for individual users, but it is not the only acceptable outcome – attention to quality of life issues and prevention of both short- and long-term health consequences of abuse are at least equally important. Harm reduction includes measures such as needle exchange schemes and prescribing of substitute drugs to prevent withdrawal. This is discussed in more detail in Chapter 2.

Intoxication

This is a characteristic transient pattern of behavioural, mental and physical changes caused by the administration of a psychoactive drug. The DSM criteria[4] describe the changes induced by intoxication as 'maladaptive', i.e. inappropriate to the social or environmental setting, and may place the individual at risk of harm. Examples of common changes wrought by intoxication include:

- Mental and behavioural changes – emotional lability, impaired judgement, risk-taking, impaired social functioning, delusions.

- Perceptual distortions – illusions, hallucinations.
- Changed level of consciousness – stimulation, sedation.
- Psychomotor changes – ataxia, disorientation.

Broadly, the nature of intoxication is similar in individuals who ingest the same drug; the detailed effects differ depending on a variety of factors. Some of the most important factors are dose, tolerance, method of administration, state of mind, the environment, and the rate of drug clearance. Intoxication abates gradually as a drug is eliminated.

Polydrug use

In recent years, it has become more common for individuals to abuse or be dependent upon more than one illicit drug simultaneously. Drugs may or may not be actually administered at the same time. For example, a common occurrence is for individuals who mainly abuse stimulant drugs (e.g. amfetamine, cocaine) to use sedative drugs (e.g. benzodiazepines, opioids, alcohol) to counteract undesirable stimulant effects such as insomnia or anxiety. Sometimes users claim novel psychotropic effects from taking two drugs together (e.g. cyclizine with opioids). It should also not be forgotten that use of alcohol and tobacco is common in those who use illicit substances. Healthcare professionals should be careful to take a full drug history from patients who are suspected of abuse or dependence, even if the identity of one drug is known.

Psychoactive drugs

The adjectives 'psychoactive' or 'psychotropic' are generic ones that can be applied to drugs that affect the mind or behaviour. The effects that they produce include illusions (perceptual distortions), delusions (false beliefs), hallucinations (sensory events without a real sensory stimulus), sedation, intoxication, mental stimulation, emotional reactions, disinhibition, disrupted thinking, increased creativity, mystic experiences and dissociation (mental isolation from the environment).

The term 'psychedelic' tends to be applied to drugs that cause primarily illusions (especially visual) and hallucinations and it is classically applied to LSD. 'Psychotomimetic' is a rather old-fashioned term applied to drugs that produce symptoms such as hallucinations, perceptual distortions and bizarre behaviour that are similar to psychotic conditions such as schizophrenia.

Reinforcement

Both positive and negative reinforcement exist. When the pleasurable effects of drug-taking are the main cause of repeat administration, this is termed positive reinforcement. Each time a dose is taken, the desired effects are produced, reinforcing the desire to take more drug.

When the main drive behind repeated administration is the desire to avoid or reverse a withdrawal reaction, this is called negative reinforcement. Whenever the drug is taken, the individual manages to stave off the unpleasantness of withdrawal for a bit longer.

Tolerance

This occurs when repeated administration of a drug eventually produces a reduced effect, such that larger doses are required to achieve the same response. The escalation of dose that often results may lead an individual to take amounts that would be fatal in a naïve user. The extent to which tolerance occurs and the speed with which it reverses varies considerably between drugs.

Withdrawal

The withdrawal reaction to a drug comprises a collection of signs and symptoms, and hence is known as a withdrawal syndrome. It occurs if the chronic use of a drug is stopped abruptly, if an antagonist is given, or if the dose is reduced suddenly. Sustained heavy administration of a drug on a regular basis for a number of weeks is usually required before such a state can be precipitated. The reaction has a finite duration, although the timescale and exact symptomatology varies widely between individuals. There may be a relatively brief (days) acute phase that occurs shortly after dosage reduction or cessation, and a chronic phase that succeeds this and lasts much longer (months). Both acute and chronic phases may be associated with craving for the drug. For all drugs that are known to be capable of causing a withdrawal syndrome, there are always some individuals that do not appear to experience it, despite pursuing a pattern of administration that would be expected to cause such a reaction.

Note that although the existence of a withdrawal reaction is one potential sign of dependence, withdrawal alone is not sufficient evidence to classify an affected individual as dependent.

Withdrawing drugs in dependence

It is important to understand that withdrawal from a drug is not necessarily the only successful endpoint in managing drug dependence. In some circumstances, there are other legitimate aims such as stabilisation of drug use (e.g. substitute prescribing of methadone for those dependent on heroin), or harm reduction (e.g. needle exchange schemes).

However, where withdrawal is a potentially achievable option, there are three basic approaches, all of which should ideally be assisted by counselling, professional support and behavioural therapy:

1. *Unmedicated cessation ('cold turkey').* In those who are highly motivated, it may be acceptable to simply stop the drug in question abruptly, without any pharmacological support. Personal motivation and the support of others are important determinants of a positive outcome, but success rates are low. In those smoking tobacco for example, only about 1 in 30 attempts like this are successful. Most chronic drug dependents attempt withdrawal unsuccessfully several times and dependency should be viewed as a chronic relapsing condition.

2. *Support medication.* For some drugs, the best option may be to stop abruptly, but with agreed support medication. For example, in those dependent upon cocaine or amfetamine, an antidepressant may be prescribed to counteract the intense depression that often follows abrupt withdrawal. Similarly, benzodiazepines are used to cover the acute period of alcohol withdrawal, and acamprosate or naltrexone may assist with the succeeding phase of chronic withdrawal. These support medications do not prevent withdrawal reactions, but they can make them more bearable.

3. *Gradual withdrawal.* For drugs such as benzodiazepines and opioids, a gradual tapering of the daily dose may help to wean the patient off. Often, a substitute long-acting alternative is prescribed instead of the original drug (e.g. methadone in heroin dependents, and diazepam in benzodiazepine dependents). This can make the withdrawal reaction less intense, but it also prolongs withdrawal. The drug, or substitute drug, can be withdrawn via a fixed reduction regimen, or a more flexible approach determined by the patient's tolerance of withdrawal symptoms.

When withdrawal is attempted, managing the withdrawal reaction can be difficult. However, three factors in particular are likely to increase the chances of success:

1. *Patient commitment.* Without a belief that their dependency is a problem, the patient or client is not committed to success. For example, he or she may continue to take the offending drug clandestinely, may not comply with the directions from a clinician, or may fake/overdramatise

withdrawal reactions, thus ensuring that the attempt at withdrawal fails. It is vital that the patient and the clinician agree that withdrawal is necessary for long-term success. Attempts at imposing withdrawal generally fail. Both parties must be honest with each other and establish a trust. On a practical level, note that an inadequate dose of substitute medication may also encourage the continued use of illicit drugs, especially early in treatment.

2. *A planned approach*. Clinician and patient need to agree a plan for withdrawal in advance. An informed discussion of available options is necessary. The plan should cover such factors as the method of withdrawal, speed of withdrawal, what to do if withdrawal reactions become unbearable, and the likely total duration of the withdrawal period. As part of this process of planning, it is helpful to establish the details of previous attempts by the patient and look at the reasons why these may have failed. This may enable patient and clinician to build safeguards into a withdrawal attempt to improve the chances of success.

3. *Anticipate the reaction*. Both clinician and patient need to know what the withdrawal reaction looks like. This allows the patient to anticipate likely problems and the clinician to medicate against them if necessary. If a reducing-dose technique is employed, withdrawal tends to be easier for the patient at the beginning than at the end – so reducing from, say, 22 tablets per day to 15 may not be too difficult, but going from six to zero is likely to be harder. In this situation, it may be advisable to be more flexible/slower in the reduction regimen towards the end.

Methods of administration

The method of administration of a drug plays an important part in determining the speed of onset and intensity of desired or toxic effects. Routes that give rise to rapid, high blood levels of a drug are more likely to result in escalating usage and dependence.[4]

There are three basic methods by which drugs of abuse are taken into the body: by injection, by mouth and via the airways.

Injection

Many drugs are commonly given by intravenous injection, including cocaine hydrochloride, heroin, amfetamine and temazepam. The intravenous route affords rapid access to the circulation and then to the brain, allowing fast onset of intense psychoactive effects. However, bypassing the body's normal defence mechanisms in the gut carries great risks to health. This topic is addressed more fully in Chapter 2.

The subcutaneous or intramuscular routes are alternatives that are occasionally used if the intravenous route is not available. Intra-arterial injections are usually only given by mistake when a needle misses a vein. The intramuscular route is only used commonly for anabolic steroids.

Oral administration

For some drugs, the oral route is preferred for convenience – ecstasy, LSD and alcohol are all usually taken in this way. In addition, many of the plants, smart drugs and abused medicines discussed in this book are administered by mouth. Nearly all drugs can be taken orally, but many drugs are absorbed from the gut unpredictably, and compared to administration by injection or via airways, psychotropic effects can take a long time to develop and/or can be blunted when drugs are given by mouth. Testosterone, methylphenidate, alkyl nitrites and fentanyl are examples of drugs with particularly poor oral bioavailability.

Administration via airways

The human airways offer a large surface area for absorption, and there are several methods for exploiting this when administering drugs. Certain solvents, propellants and fuels can be inhaled directly into the lungs by those engaged in volatile substance abuse. Alkyl nitrites are also volatile and can be inhaled directly. Other compounds need to be heated before inhalation is possible. This is called vaporisation. Examples include heroin ('chasing the dragon'), crack cocaine, cannabis resin ('hot knifing') and metamfetamine. Smoking has a similar net effect but the drug – or drug plus an inflammable vehicle – is set alight first. Tobacco, heroin, phencyclidine and cannabis can be smoked. Some examples of homemade smoking apparatus are shown in Figure 1.3.

Dry powdered drug can be inhaled into the nose, a procedure known as 'snorting'. Amfetamine and cocaine hydrochloride are classically taken by this route.

Drug abuse environments

Substance abuse and dependence is more common amongst men. Within the developed world, however, there are certain specific situations or environments in which substance abuse can be more common. These are described below.

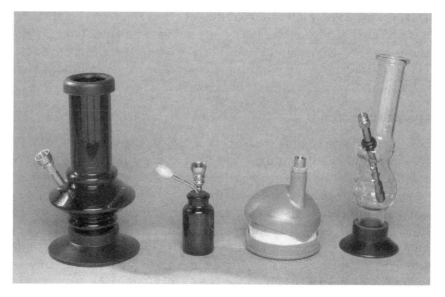

Figure 1.3 Apparatus used for smoking street drugs (Photo courtesy of Multimedia Research Partners Ltd).

Clubs and raves

Raves are all-night dance parties staged at large private venues and attended mainly by adolescents and young adults. They first appeared in the mid to late 1980s and promoted a blend of music, dance, drugs and a specific culture ('peace, love, unity and respect'). These concepts have gradually been adopted by more mainstream nightclubs and bars and so certain drugs used in these venues are referred to as club drugs or rave drugs; typical examples include ecstasy, ketamine, gamma hydroxy-butyrate, and metamfetamine. However, other drugs are also widely used, including cannabis, alkyl nitrites, amfetamine and cocaine.

Mental health disorders

Patients with serious psychiatric illness may be more likely to abuse drugs than most other sectors of the population. They may continue to do so even after being admitted to hospital. This has led to the concept of 'dual diagnosis'. This term refers to the common situation where substance abuse or dependence occurs in a patient with a psychiatric disorder (especially schizophrenia and related conditions). Sometimes this problem is also called 'comorbidity'. Alcohol and many illicit drugs can cause psychiatric conditions, but it is also clear that many patients with existing mental illness are attracted to using these substances. Consequently, it is rarely clear whether substance abuse/dependence has preceded mental illness (and maybe caused or triggered it), or developed after the illness has started (and maybe is contributing to symptoms and social care needs).

Mysticism

The psychedelic and dissociative effects of certain drugs have given them a mystical quality that attracts some individuals to experiment with them for the purpose of self-exploration or revelation. Notable examples include ecstasy, LSD and several plant species.

Prisons

As the extent of substance abuse is increasing, it is not surprising that more offenders enter prison with a serious substance abuse or dependency problem. This is one factor that makes it difficult to control drug abuse amongst the prison population. In the UK, about 55% of persons entering prison have a substance misuse problem, with 80% having some history of it; up to 80% test positive for opioids on admission at some prisons. However, once in prison, the rate of positive testing for drugs declines: in the UK in 2004, this was an average of 12.3%.[8] Popular drugs include cannabis, opioids and benzodiazepines.

Sports

Substance abuse in international athletics and sports is commonly reported when individuals fail random tests for banned substances. However, during the past two or three decades substance abuse has progressively extended to private gymnasia and sports clubs. Individuals use drugs in order to develop strength, endurance and musculature. Drugs involved include anabolic steroids, stimulants and a variety of prescription medicines (see Chapter 11).

Drug-facilitated sexual assault

This is also known as 'date rape'. Male or female victims are subjected to sexual acts without their consent after being rendered unconscious or intoxicated by drugs. Although drugs such as flunitrazepam, gamma hydroxybutyrate (GHB) and ketamine have been used and have gained media notoriety, alcohol is probably the most widely employed agent. The non-alcohol drugs are sometimes called 'predatory' drugs. They are typically added to a drink without the victim's knowledge and, because the effects of these drugs may take some time to wear off, the victim may not realise an assault has occurred for several hours. Flunitrazepam and GHB can also cause amnesia, so the memory of events may be partially or completely erased.

Legalisation

The arguments surrounding the legalisation of any one, or all, of the currently illicit substances are very interesting; not least the debate over what form legalisation might take. These could include allowing the sale of substances via registered premises only; decriminalising personal possession if the individual has no intent to supply; legalising possession and supply of substances manufactured under government licence only and not those from illicit sources; permitting wider supply via drug dependency clinics to registered users; and limiting legalisation to certain drugs only. The legal status of commonly abused substances in the UK is given in Appendix B.

Without targeting a specific drug, what are the reasons for and against legalising a currently illegal substance? Some of the arguments commonly used on both sides are summarised below.

Arguments in favour of legalisation

Freedom of choice.   Any individual should have the right to take any pharmacologically active agent that he or she chooses. Alcohol, tobacco and caffeine are legal substances that can have potentially harmful effects – why should other psychoactive substances not be freely available in a similar way? Many substances are thought to be considerably less harmful than tobacco or alcohol. Use of some of them is tolerated in certain countries (e.g. cannabis in the Netherlands), and others, although now illegal, have been legal in the past (e.g. opium in the UK until 1868).

Quality control.   Legalisation opens the door to quality control of abusable substances. This would prevent the involvement of potentially harmful contaminants, avoid accidental overdoses due to lack of knowledge of concentration and enable an individual to know exactly what he or she was taking. Injectable drugs could be supplied, correctly formulated, in sterilised ampoules, reducing the risk of injection site infection and other adverse consequences of injection (see Chapter 2). Needles and syringes would be supplied to cut down the spread of HIV (human immunodeficiency virus) and other infections from the sharing of injection equipment.

Reduced crime.   Thefts and assaults to obtain money to buy drugs would be drastically reduced if drugs were legalised and available to purchase at modest cost from agreed outlets.

Reduced profits for criminal organisations.   A number of large criminal organisations generate vast sums of money by manufacturing and supplying illegal substances. All street drugs are very cheap to mass produce and are not intrinsically costly; their illegal status currently keeps street prices high. Legalisation would remove a vital source of income for criminal organisations and, with reduced revenue, this might in turn reduce their activity and influence in other areas.

Decreased workload for law enforcers.   Drug abuse currently forms a large part of the workload of the police, customs, lawyers and courts. Legalising a drug reduces public expenditure in these areas and frees public servants for other duties.

Laws have not worked.   Drug abuse is widespread, so the current legal controls have not worked. People who really want to abuse drugs will do so whether they are illegal or not. It is time to be more liberal in our approach and stop wasting effort on enforcing a system that has not worked.

Arguments against legalisation

The unknown.   Legalisation is largely a voyage into the unknown. Arguments in favour of legalisation are rather theoretical and based on conjecture. We cannot foresee what might happen to individuals and to our society if a drug is legalised. It is not appropriate to guess what may happen in the UK based on what has happened in our own past or in other countries because each culture and era is different. It would be difficult to reverse a decision to legalise a drug if we found the effects of legalisation were not to our liking. Tobacco and alcohol do have harmful effects but they are legal substances for historical reasons;

rendering both of these illegal would be extraordinarily difficult because large sections of the population that would not have taken them were they illegal would now resist criminalisation.

Adverse effects. The abusable substances that are currently illicit have never been subjected to formal clinical trials so there is insufficient information on human safety. There is little information on long-term safety for most drugs of abuse, especially with regard to CNS toxicity and psychiatric effects. Many drugs produce dependence, which can have great personal costs. However, it is not just the direct toxicity to the individual which can be a problem, it is the indirect effects arising from intoxication such as accidents, violence and crime. The legalisation of drugs of abuse would lead to increased usage and consequently increased health problems. Alcohol and tobacco are bad enough in terms of the health and social problems they cause. Health campaigns do warn of the dangers of tobacco and alcohol but if other abusable substances were legalised this would add to the problem.

Control. The current legal framework for controlling drug abuse is not perfect, but it does at least allow some control to be exerted over individuals. If new drugs of abuse were freely available, this could result in vastly increased usage and anarchy, and it might be uncontrollable.

Society's protective role. Society has a duty to protect the vulnerable, who might be swept up in the use of new abusable substances. People who are young, suffering from psychiatric illness, poorly educated or in financial difficulty could all suffer disproportionately as a result of legalisation.

Cost. The expense of regulation, quality control and potentially increased health costs could be very great.

Philosophy of life. Individuals should not need to resort to pharmacological methods in order to enjoy life. We should try to find happiness in real life experiences.

References

1.   World Health Organization. Other psychoactive substances. http://www.who.int/substance_abuse/en (accessed 16 November 2004).
2.   World Health Organization. The global burden. http://www.who.int/substance_abuse/en (accessed 16 November 2004).

3. World Health Organization. World deaths in 2000 attributable to selected leading risk factors (ref WHR 2002). http://www.who.int/substance_abuse/en (accessed 16 November 2004).

4. American Psychiatric Association. *DSM-IV, Diagnostic and Statistical Manual of Mental Disorders*. Washington, DC: APA, 1994: 175–184.

5. World Health Organization. *WHO Expert Committee on Drug Dependence, 28th report* (WHO Technical Report Series No. 273). Geneva: WHO, 1993.

6. Buchanan J F, Brown C F. 'Designer drugs' – a problem in clinical toxicology. *Med Toxicol* 1988; 3: 1–17.

7. Anonymous. Designer drugs. *NIDA Capsule (CAP10)*. Bethesda, MD: National Institute on Drug Abuse, 1993, pp. 1–4.

8. Wheatley P. *HM Prison Service (Public Sector Prisons) Annual Report and Accounts. April 2003–March 2004*. London: HM Prison Service (Public Sector Prisons), 2004.

2

Injection of drugs

Hypodermic injections should be prepared extemporaneously. In most cases they are plain solutions of alkaloidal or other salts in water. All utensils used should be sterilised by thorough washing and drying in an oven at 220 degrees Fahrenheit. The distilled water must also be sterilised by boiling.
Instructions for preparation of injections, in
'Pharmaceutical Formulas', 1911

Heroin, cocaine and amfetamine are drugs that are commonly administered intravenously. The majority of injectors begin by taking other non-parenteral psychotropic drugs, or by taking their first intravenous drug in a non-parenteral form. Many chronic drug users eventually prefer to inject rather than administer by other routes and there are a number of reasons for this. Intravenous administration provides the quickest access to the circulation, resulting in rapid passage of the drug to the brain. This produces the fastest possible onset of intoxication, and usually a 'rush' or 'buzz' of initial euphoria occurs when a bolus of drug reaches the brain. This effect is particularly sought after. Other methods of administration generally provide a slower onset and a less intense 'rush'. Non-parenteral methods often involve a degree of wastage as well: when given orally a proportion of the dose may not be absorbed or may be metabolised by the liver before reaching the brain; smoking or vaporisation usually destroys some of the drug; nasal inhalation wastes the percentage of the drug that passes down the throat to be absorbed more slowly later.

Apart from these considerations, injecting forms an important ritual for many individuals and, for those who become dependent, abandoning the ritual of preparation and administration is often a difficult part of stopping. The process of injecting may also be tied to a particular social setting, environment or time. The importance of ritual is seen in other areas of substance dependence – for example, tobacco smokers may prefer to smoke at specific times of the day, or to use particular techniques for preparation, and feel discontent if unable to do this.

Injection equipment (needle and syringe) is often referred to at street level by terms such as 'works' and the process of injection is called 'mainlining', 'fixing' or 'shooting up'. The typical sites chosen for injection in the beginning are the veins of the forearms, but users may switch to the lower leg, back of the hand, groin or neck if forearm veins are difficult to access. If intravenous access is severely restricted (as may occur in chronic users because of venous damage), the subcutaneous or intramuscular routes may be employed. Some users may actually prefer these routes.

Despite the many problems connected with injecting drugs at street level, most injectors generally do not seek medical assistance. A study of 112 injectors in Glasgow identified 107 with current injection-related medical problems.[1] There was a mean of 2.3 problems per patient. However, 73% of subjects had not sought medical assistance, mainly because such problems were perceived as normal or not serious. The remainder had had unpleasant previous experiences with healthcare professionals, feared discrimination, or did not want to be seen as wasting healthcare resources.

The dangers arising from the process of intravenous injection of street drugs are discussed below.

Infection

Injecting drug users arc prone to infections from bacteria, viruses and fungi. The most serious infections associated with intravenous drug abuse arise from the transfer of blood-borne infections between individuals as a result of the sharing of needles, syringes and filters. These infections include human immunodeficiency virus (HIV) and viral hepatitis (see below).

However, the drugs themselves and the process of administering them can also give rise to infections. Street drug injections are usually prepared by dissolving a non-sterile powder or crushed tablet in tap water, as illustrated in Figure 2.1. Occasionally other sources of non-sterile water are used, such as bottled mineral water. The preparation may be prepared in a spoon or bottle cap. When injecting heroin in countries where the drug is supplied as base heroin (e.g. Europe), intravenous drug users commonly heat the mixture and use citric, ascorbic or other weak acids to aid heroin dissolution (see Chapter 3); sometimes readily available acidic liquids are used such as vinegar or lemon juice. Oral liquid preparations such as methadone mixture are also injected but this is rare in countries such as the UK where a viscous dilute formulation is used. Once a solution has been prepared, a filter may then be

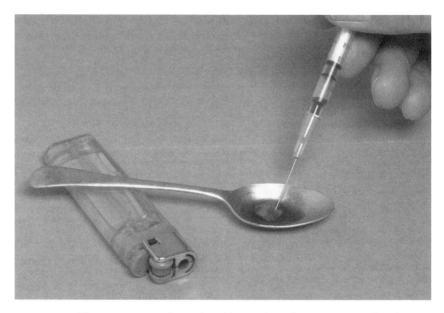

Figure 2.1 The preparation of powdered heroin base for injection involves heating the powder with water and a weak acid to create a solution of a heroin salt. In countries where heroin is supplied as the hydrochloride, the drug is freely soluble and neither heating nor a weak acid are required (Photo courtesy of Multimedia Research Partners Ltd).

used to remove any solid particles. Although in certain countries sterile medical filters are supplied via needle exchange schemes, at street level a variety of non-sterile filters are commonly used, such as cigarette filters, or a piece of permeable fabric, cotton wool or blotting paper.

Finally, the preparation is injected with a needle and syringe through the skin and into a vein. The injection equipment may be shared with another person, or used by the same individual on numerous occasions, and may or may not be washed between injections. Even if washing does take place it is impossible to guarantee that this will prevent contamination.

All of these steps in the injection process are clearly a potential source of contamination with pathogenic organisms: the drug itself and anything non-sterile added to it, the solvent, the receptacle it is made up in, the needle and syringe if not sterile, the filter, and the skin of the patient. By conveying a contaminated solution directly into the bloodstream, the individual bypasses all of the body's normal safeguards against the entry of micro-organisms. For this reason, the infections seen in intravenous drug users are frequently well-known conditions but with atypical pathogens, or they may occur in unusual body locations.

The likelihood of infection occurring, and of atypical organisms being responsible for them, is further increased if the individual is also suffering immunodeficiency due to HIV/AIDS (human immunodeficiency virus/acquired immunodeficiency syndrome).

Infections can be difficult to diagnose, because of the wide range of micro-organisms that are potentially responsible. However, not all fevers or infections in injecting drug users are caused by the injection of contaminated drug solutions. Many (but by no means all) users have generally poor health due to inadequate nutrition, unsuitable living conditions and deficient personal hygiene, amongst other considerations. In this environment, certain infections are likely to be more common anyway, for example chest infections, 'coughs and colds' and urinary tract infections. Tuberculosis and other contagious infections can be spread by affected individuals associating with others. Another important point is that withdrawal from some drugs, most notably opioids, can cause fever without any underlying infection.

Attempts at harm reduction include methadone maintenance programmes, counselling, supplying clean equipment, and educating users to try to minimise the risk of infection. Harm reduction in all its forms seeks to reduce the risk of infection, but it does not eliminate it. Needle and syringe exchange schemes aim primarily to prevent users sharing injection equipment or using the same equipment more than once themselves. In countries such as the USA, which have been slow to introduce needle exchange schemes, injecting drug users represent a comparatively high proportion of HIV/AIDS cases compared to countries such as the UK, where needle exchange schemes were implemented at an early stage. The supply of sterile needles and syringes also gives the drug user the opportunity to return used equipment for safe disposal and to interact with a healthcare professional. An extension of the idea of opportunistic interactions with a professional is to provide supervised injecting rooms where intravenous drug users can inject safely, knowing that medical assistance is available in case of overdose, accident or side-effects, and that advice can be offered on injection technique.[2,3]

Other materials can be issued with needles and syringes via formalised programmes.[4] Sterile alcoholic swabs enable users to clean the injection site immediately before drug administration to decrease the likelihood of skin commensal bacteria being injected into the body. Sterile water may be supplied as an alternative to the tap water that is typically used. Those injecting base heroin, 'crack' cocaine or crystal metamfetamine may be supplied with sachets of weak acids (e.g. citric acid). These acids convert the base form of the drug to a more soluble salt, enabling preparation of a solution for injection. Supplying an acid prevents use of more inappropriate alternatives such as lemon juice (see below). Sterile containers for mixing drugs, and filters, can also be made available. If all of these materials are supplied and used appropriately, the principal remaining source of infection is the street drug itself. While widespread prescribing of sterile pharmaceutical heroin (diamorphine injection) to dependent users has not been advocated, prescribing for those who have failed first-line treatments has been evaluated within supervised injectable maintenance clinics.[3,5]

A variety of specific infections can occur in injecting drug users and some of these are discussed in more detail below.

Skin and injection site infections

The skin is a common source of pathogenic bacteria in intravenous drug users, and so the risk of causing superficial infections is increased when injections are given without first cleaning the surface of the skin with an alcohol swab. The risk is further increased when injection occurs through parts of the skin that carry a particularly high population of commensal bacteria (e.g. groin) and when injections are deliberately given subcutaneously or intramuscularly. Nonetheless, infection is a common complication after repeated non-sterile injection by any route and tends to initially occur local to the sites of injection. Abscesses and cellulitis are the most frequently recognised presentations.

In one US study of 242 consecutive injection drug users presenting to an emergency department with soft tissue infections, 72% suffered from abscesses, and 23% had cellulitis.[6] For the total cohort, the median length of time for which participants had tolerated symptoms before seeking medical attention was 4 days; by the time they were seen in the emergency department 40% required hospital admission. Infections were most frequently seen on the arms (50%), legs (23%), buttocks (20%) and deltoid area (14%). Several studies suggest that skin and soft tissue infections are the most common reason for injecting drug users to be admitted to hospital.[7]

The organism most commonly identified as causing skin infections is *Staphylococcus aureus*, reflecting its widespread presence on the surface of the skin itself. *Streptococcus* species are probably the next most common. However, polymicrobial infection or the involvement of atypical pathogens is well known. These skin infections can develop into more severe local infections (e.g. cervical abscess, necrotising fasciitis or myonecrosis), but can also metastasise to other areas (e.g. bone, heart valves, septicaemia). The importance of local infection as a potential source of more serious harm is illustrated by an outbreak of infections with *Clostridium novyi* and other *Clostridium* species in Scotland, England and Ireland in injecting drug users in 2000.[8,9] It is believed that initial clostridium infection at injection sites, perhaps facilitated by soft tissue damage secondary to use of citric acid, enabled the spread of infection and the release of bacterial toxins, which led to the death of many injectors. Clostridia are anaerobic species and infections in injecting drug users may arise due to heroin contamination with soil or faeces.

Infected ulcers occur as a consequence of impaired blood flow in the limbs of chronic injectors.[4,7] The lower leg is the most common site. They may initially arise due to infection at the site of a venous injury caused by injecting, or they can develop from minor trauma sustained by other means that becomes infected. The fact that local veins have become occluded leads to a reduced blood supply, which in turn hinders healing of these small wounds. From this beginning the damage may increase to form deeper and larger ulcers, which are painful and difficult to heal.

Endocarditis

In the USA, the incidence of infective endocarditis in intravenous drug users has been quoted as 2–5% per year, and is responsible for up to 20% of hospital admissions and 5–10% deaths in this patient group.[10] More than half of the intravenous drug users presenting with this condition are found to have *Staphylococcus aureus* endocarditis. It is assumed that this organism is derived largely from skin infections. Most infections are of the tricuspid valve (i.e. right side of the heart), especially in HIV-positive patients.[10,11] However, *Streptococcus viridans* and other *Streptococcus* species, enterococci, or fungal micro-organisms (especially *Candida* species) are more likely to be responsible if the endocarditis affects the left-hand side of the heart. A variety of theories have sought to explain why the right side of the heart seems more prone to endocarditis in injecting drug users.[12] It has been suggested that insoluble particles in injected drugs or the drugs themselves could damage heart valves, enabling them to act as a focus for the adherence of platelets and then micro-organisms, and because venous blood drains to the right side of the heart first it would be exposed to a more concentrated effect. Another theory suggests that after intravenous injection any blood contaminated with micro-organisms will drain into the right side of the heart first, predisposing it to infection. However, neither of these theories alone, or others that have been put forward, seem to adequately explain the phenomenon, which may be caused by a number of factors acting in concert.[12]

There are many other organisms that have caused endocarditis in intravenous drug users, including other *Staphylococcus* species, *Pseudomonas* species, *Serratia*, respiratory organisms and anaerobes. A particular micro-organism can predominate in a specific geographical location, and at a specific time.[13] This is most often linked to the fact that non-staphylococcal endocarditis is likely to be caused by contaminants of the drug itself. Polymicrobial infection can occur in an estimated 2–5% of cases.[10]

Infective endocarditis often responds favourably to antimicrobials once the causative organism has been identified. However, long courses of treatment (4–6 weeks) are often needed and prognosis is worst for patients with left-sided infection, certain infective micro-organisms (e.g. *Candida*), and severe immunosuppression due to HIV/AIDS.[10,11]

Viral infection

When injecting street drugs intravenously, it is common practice to pull on the plunger of the syringe during injection to check that the needle has entered a vein. This results in blood being drawn into the syringe, together with any micro-organisms. If the injection equipment is then shared, the second user will inject any pathogenic organisms in the blood of the donor directly into his or her own bloodstream. This is a very important method by which blood-borne viruses are transferred from one person to another – especially HIV and hepatitis B and C.

HIV can remain viable inside blood-contaminated needles and syringes for more than 4 weeks.[14] However, the tip of the needle is contaminated whether or not the individual actually draws blood into the barrel of the syringe, so any sharing of injection equipment should be discouraged. Once an injecting drug user has become HIV-positive, the infection can spread beyond the injecting community via sexual contacts of the injector. A full discussion of the implications of HIV status is outside the scope of this book, but those who become immunocompromised as a result of their HIV status are more prone to a whole range of other infections, some of which are diagnostic for AIDS, e.g. *Pneumocystis carinii* pneumonia.

Injecting drug users should be encouraged to seek vaccination against the hepatitis B virus, which is thereby a preventable infection.

Unfortunately there is no hepatitis C vaccine. Hepatitis C infection, like HIV infection, can remain largely asymptomatic for many years so persons carrying the disease can pass it on to others before becoming ill themselves. Some carriers seem never to develop overt liver disease, but about a quarter develop serious chronic liver disease (including cirrhosis and liver cancer).

Fungal infections

One review has estimated that fungal infections represent 5–50% of serious infections in intravenous drug users.[15] *Candida* species are most commonly involved, causing disseminated candidiasis, endocarditis, CNS infections and endophthalmitis. In the 1980s, an outbreak of severe candida infections in Australia and Europe was found to have arisen because of the use of lemon juice to dissolve heroin before injection. This is a known growth medium for fungi.[16] Aspergillosis and mucormycosis have also been described in the injecting population.

Bacterial septicaemia

This usually occurs secondary to wider dissemination of an infection from elsewhere (e.g. the skin). *Streptococcus* species are typically responsible. Tetanus has only rarely been encountered since the widespread adoption of prophylactic vaccination.

Joint and bone infections

Septic arthritis and osteomyelitis have been described in intravenous drug users. In 1987, a study of 37 heroin users with septic arthritis revealed that the joints involved were somewhat atypical. In 39% of patients sacroiliac joints were affected and in 37% chondrosternocostal unions.[17] Diagnosis can be difficult because infection has an insidious onset, the joint is often painless, and there may be no systemic signs of infection.[18] However, without prompt treatment, chronic incurable infection may result.

Irritant effects

Most drugs that are injected are not themselves irritant. Temazepam and dextropropoxyphene are notable exceptions as they both cause irritation of tissues or veins after injection, leading to abscesses, tissue necrosis, venous fibrosis and phlebitis.[19-21] These areas of damaged tissue can then act as foci for infection or thrombosis.

Irritant reactions such as phlebitis from most other injectable preparations may be attributed to adulterants or additives, local infection, or other forms of poor injection technique. Areas of phlebitis are sometimes called 'track marks' when they appear as inflamed red lines on the surface of the skin following a vein. Base forms of heroin, cocaine or metamfetamine are often deliberately mixed with acidic substances such as citric acid to aid dissolution; this can be irritant and cause local tissue damage (so-called citric acid 'burns'). It has also been reported that ammonia may contaminate 'crack' or 'freebase' cocaine as a result of the manufacturing procedure. This can be very caustic if injected.[22] Other potentially irritant adulterants in street drugs include quinine and sodium bicarbonate. Clearly, irritant effects local to the injection site are more likely to occur if the offending preparation is administered subcutaneously[23] or if there is extravasation during venous injection. Those who inject cocaine may be at particular risk because this drug has local anaesthetic properties that can mask the pain of impending damage.

The repeated intravenous administration of injections at the same location eventually destroys the normal pliable nature of the vein because of the accumulated effects of fibrosis around numerous puncture marks, episodes of phlebitis, local thrombosis, irritation and swelling, venous collapse, infection and the actions of impurities. Veins may block temporarily or permanently, but once scar tissue forms it tends to be irreversible. This requires injectors to seek alternative intravenous access sites and eventually, sometimes, to use subcutaneous or intramuscular injection instead.

Emboli, blood vessel occlusion and thrombosis

Most injections given at street level are prepared by mixing an impure powder, or a crushed tablet, with water. Consequently, injectors typically attempt primitive filtration to try to remove non-soluble particles, with varying degrees of success. Those that are not removed, or which arise from the filter itself, will become microemboli in the bloodstream. In some cases the drug itself may form microemboli if it is very insoluble in plasma (e.g. temazepam[20]). When injected intravenously, these particles can form granulomas in the lung that may impair gaseous diffusion across alveoli (pulmonary granulomatosus), ultimately giving rise to dyspnoea, hypoxia, pulmonary hypertension or emphysema. Microembolisation of temazepam to the lungs causing death has been reported.[24]

Embolisation of insoluble particles can also cause retinopathy. This has been particularly reported in those injecting crushed methylphenidate tablets, but other crushed tablets and heroin have also been cited as potential causes. In many cases visual acuity is not affected, despite the obvious accumulation of obstructive particles in retinal blood vessels. However, impairment of sight can occur. In one study, five out of 23 patients with retinopathy had reduced visual acuity.[25]

Occlusion of veins as a direct result of particulate contamination may occur, but embolisation to other parts of the body is frequently undetected because it is asymptomatic. In many cases particulate emboli probably dissolve over a period of time leaving no trace.

Certain risk factors increase the chance of venous blockage by blood clots. These include the presence of phlebitis (see above), injecting into the groin, lack of exercise, smoking, and taking oral contraceptives. Subsequent to the development of a deep vein thrombosis (DVT), thromboembolism may also occur, giving rise, for example, to pulmonary embolus (PE). DVTs are reported quite commonly in the injecting population and those injecting temazepam in any form may be more at risk because of the irritant nature of the drug. Moreover, in response to the widespread abuse of temazepam liquid-filled capsules, a gel-filled capsule was introduced with the intention of making injection more difficult. However, injectors learned to heat the gel and/or mix it with water to enable injection. This had the unfortunate consequence of causing DVTs, probably as a result of the gel solidifying within veins.[21,26]

Intra-arterial injection is particularly likely to give rise to serious forms of blood vessel occlusion. For example, the intra-arterial injection of temazepam has been widely reported as it can result in severe damage to many parts of the body. Often the femoral artery or a forearm artery is involved, the patient having missed a vein and punctured an artery by mistake. As with intravenous administration, the gel capsule formulation may solidify in blood vessels after injection causing ischaemia. The irritant nature of temazepam might also cause arteries to go into spasm, or damage the arterial wall (e.g. vasculitis) and so act as a focus for thrombus formation. Temazepam itself is very insoluble and solid particles of it may cause vascular blockade downstream of the injection site via microembolism;[20] the common practice of filtration through a cigarette filter may introduce further microemboli. The gel capsule formulation in particular can cause severe tissue damage distal to the site of intra-arterial injection, especially muscle necrosis, necessitating fasciotomy or limb/digit amputation.[26–30] Rhabdomyolysis and renal failure may subsequently ensue, as may secondary DVT or PE.

The injection of temazepam represents an extreme example of the potential consequences of intra-arterial injection of irritant substances or those containing solid particles. Similar effects have been reported after intra-arterial administration of most other parenteral street drugs.[31–34] The general symptoms are swelling distal to the injection site, pain, discolouration, and sensory and/or motor deficit. The subsequent pattern of events will depend on the site of injection and the tissues affected. Muscle ischaemia will cause rhabdomyolysis and its sequelae. Vasculitis is common and this can result in thrombosis leading to gangrene and amputation; it can also trigger secondary thromboembolism, which may manifest as DVT or PE. Gangrene may occur if blood supply to an area is blocked by restrictive jewellery during swelling, or if a tight tourniquet is inadvertently left *in situ* by an injecting drug user for very long periods.

In long-term injectors the cumulative effects of blood vessel occlusion, venous irritation and damage, and infections commonly results in impaired blood flow to the legs. This is called chronic venous insufficiency and can reduce mobility.[35] Symptoms include swelling, pain, an itching or burning sensation, changes to skin colour, dermatitis, and persistent ulcers.

Air embolus is a potential hazard when large volumes are injected intravenously. A substantial amount of air in the heart causes blood to froth in the chambers during pumping, leading to inefficiency and heart failure. It has been estimated that 10 mL of air would be required in the heart to cause failure;[36] this would be very difficult to achieve after injection with a hand-held syringe and is unlikely to occur at street level.

Pharmacological effects

Compared to oral administration, the pharmacological effects of street drugs appear much more rapidly after intravenous injection. The effects may in some cases also be more dramatic. For example, large doses of intravenous opioids are known to cause sudden respiratory depression and death. Usually this occurs because a sample of heroin is more potent than the user anticipated, or because of a lowering of tolerance due to a reduction in heroin usage (e.g. those leaving prison and returning to illicit drug use). Fentanyl analogues are particularly powerful drugs that are known to have caused death so rapidly that individuals have died with the needle still in place (see Chapter 3).

One reasonably common reaction that can occur after intravenous administration of most street drugs is fainting. In one study of 13 methylphenidate users, 12 reported fainting immediately after injection;[37] in a study of 23 temazepam users, 12 reported 'blackouts' after injection.[21]

Adulterants, diluents and impurities

At street level no drugs are pure; even prescription medicines that are injected, such as tablets, contain excipients.

A variety of cheap, inert or pharmacologically active adulterants are used to dilute or bulk out ('cut') illicit drugs, including glucose, paracetamol, mannitol and lactose. The active adulterants are often those considered appropriate to the illicit drug in question. For example, amfetamine and cocaine powders may include other stimulants such as amfetamine derivatives, pseudoephedrine and caffeine. Cocaine may be adulterated with other local anaesthetics.[38] The pharmacological effects of adulterants may be important. Thrombocytopenia has been reported in intravenous heroin users and is believed to be an immune reaction to an unknown toxin.[39,40] Thrombocytopenia explicitly caused by quinine in street drugs has been identified.[41] Quinine can also be a venous and dermal irritant. Two deaths associated with strychnine contamination of street drugs have been described.[42] Strychnine has been found in heroin and cocaine. Arsenic can be an adulterant of opium in some areas.[43] Finally hyoscine (scopolamine) has been included in some batches of cocaine and heroin in sufficient quantities to require emergency hospital admission for antimuscarinic poisoning.[44,45]

It should be noted that a wide range of chemicals are used to synthesise, transform and purify street drugs, and data are often lacking on the effects in humans of these chemicals and of the intermediate products that arise from the various manufacturing processes.

'Stigmata'

Repeated intravenous injection over a prolonged period frequently results in certain characteristic changes around veins that mark the individual as an intravenous drug user. These are most frequently seen in the forearm. These may include needle marks, scarring caused by abscesses, phlebitis, granulomas, bruising, and discolouration of the skin along the line of veins due to insoluble particles accumulating within the skin.

References

1. Morrison A, Elliott L, Gruer L. Injecting-related harm and treatment-seeking behaviour among injecting drug users. *Addiction* 1997; 92: 1349–1352.
2. Wright N M J, Tompkins C N E. Supervised injecting centres. *BMJ* 2004; 328: 100–102.
3. Strang J, Fortson R. Commentary: supervised fixing rooms, supervised injectable maintenance clinics – understanding the difference. *BMJ* 2004; 328: 102–103.
4. Derricott J, Preston A, Hunt N. *The Safer Injecting Briefing*. Liverpool: HIT Publications, 1999.
5. van den Brink W, Hendriks V M, Blanken P, *et al*. Medical prescription of heroin to treatment resistant heroin addicts: two randomized controlled trials. *BMJ* 2003; 327: 310–315.
6. Takahashi T A, Merrill J O, Boyko E J, *et al*. Type and location of injection drug use-related soft tissue infections predict hospitalisation. *J Urban Health* 2003; 80: 127–136.
7. Ebright J R, Pieper B. Skin and soft tissue infections in injection drug users. *Infect Dis Clin North Am* 2002; 16: 697–712.
8. Bonn D. *Clostridium novyi* revealed as heroin contaminant. *Lancet* 2000; 355: 2230.
9. McGuigan C C, Penrice G M, Gruer L, *et al*. Lethal outbreak of infection with *Clostridium novyi* type A and other spore-forming organisms in Scottish injecting drug users. *J Med Microbiol* 2002; 51: 971–977.
10. Miro J M, Del-Rio A, Mestres C A. Infective endocarditis in intravenous drug abusers and HIV-1 infected patients. *Infect Dis Clin North Am* 2002; 16: 273–295.
11. Robera E, Miro J M, Cortes E, *et al*. Influence of human immunodeficiency virus 1 infection and degree of immunosuppression in the clinical characteristics and outcome of infective endocarditis in intravenous drug users. *Arch Intern Med* 1998; 158: 2043–2050.
12. Frontera J A, Gradon J D. Right-side endocarditis in injection drug users: review of proposed mechanisms of pathogenesis. *Clin Infect Dis* 2000; 30: 374–379.
13. Cherubin C E, Sapira J D. The medical complications of drug addiction and the medical assessment of the intravenous drug user: 25 years later. *Ann Intern Med* 1993; 119: 1017–1028.
14. Abdala N, Stephens P C, Griffith B P, *et al*. Survival of HIV-1 in syringes. *J Acquir Immune Defic Syndr Hum Retrovirol* 1999; 20: 73–80.
15. Leen C L S, Brettle R P. Fungal infections in drug users. *J Antimicrob Chemother* 1991; 28(A): 83–96.
16. Newton-John H F, Wise K, Looke D F M. Role of the lemon in disseminated candidiasis of heroin abusers. *Med J Aust* 1984; 140: 780–781.

17. Lopez-Longo F J, Menard H A, Carreno L, *et al*. Primary septic arthritis in heroin users: early diagnosis by radioisotopic imaging and geographic variations in the causative agents. *J Rheumatol* 1987; 14: 991–994.

18. Kak V, Chandrasekar P H. Bone and joint infections in injection drug users. *Infect Dis Clin North Am* 2002; 16: 681–695.

19. Tennant F S. Complications of propoxyphene abuse. *Arch Intern Med* 1973; 132: 191–194.

20. Launchbury A P, Drake J, Seager H. Misuse of temazepam. *BMJ* 1992; 305: 252–253.

21. Ruben S M, Morrison C L. Temazepam misuse in a group of injecting drug users. *Br J Addiction* 1992; 87: 1387–1392.

22. Pickering H, Donoghoe M, Green A, *et al*. Crack injection. *Druglink* 1993; 8: 12.

23. Thomas W O, Almand J D, Stark G B, *et al*. Hand injuries secondary to subcutaneous illicit drug injections. *Ann Plast Surg* 1995; 34: 27–31.

24. Vella E J, Edwards C W. Death from pulmonary microembolisation after intravenous injection of temazepam. *BMJ* 1993; 307: 26.

25. Tse D T, Ober R R. Talc retinopathy. *Am J Ophthalmol* 1980; 90: 624–640.

26. Fox R, Beeching N J, Morrison C, *et al*. Misuse of temazepam. *BMJ* 1992; 305: 253.

27. Scott R N, Woodburn K R, Reid D B, *et al*. Intra-arterial temazepam [letter]. *BMJ* 1992; 304: 1630.

28. Adiseshiah M, Jones D A, Round J M. Intra-arterial temazepam [letter]. *BMJ* 1992; 304: 1630.

29. Blair S D, Holcombe C, Coombes E N, *et al*. Leg ischaemia secondary to non-medical injection of temazepam. *Lancet* 1991; 338: 1393–1394.

30. Dodd T J, Scott R N, Woodburn K R, *et al*. Limb ischaemia after intra-arterial injection of temazepam gel: histology of nine cases. *J Clin Pathol* 1994; 47: 512–514.

31. Begg E J, McGrath M A, Wade D N. Inadvertent intra-arterial injection. *Med J Aust* 1980; 2: 561–563.

32. Borrero E. Treatment of 'trash hand' following intra-arterial injection of drugs in addicts – case studies. *Vasc Surg* 1995; 29: 71–75.

33. Stueber K. The treatment of intra-arterial pentazocine injection injuries with intra-arterial reserpine. *Ann Plast Surg* 1987; 18: 41–46.

34. Samuel I, Bishop C C R, Jamieson C W. Accidental intra-arterial drug injection successfully treated with Iloprost. *Eur J Vasc Surg* 1993; 7: 93–94.

35. Pieper B, Templin T. Lower extremity changes, pain, and function in injection drug users. *J Subst Abuse Treat* 2003; 25: 91–97.

36. Gunson H H, Martlew V J. Blood replacement. In: Huth, E J. *Oxford Textbook of Medicine*. Oxford: Oxford University Press, 1996: 3687–3696.

37. Parran T V, Jasinski D R. Intravenous methylphenidate abuse – prototype for prescription drug abuse. *Arch Intern Med* 1991; 151: 781–783.

38. Shannon M. Clinical toxicity of cocaine adulterants. *Ann Emerg Med* 1988; 17: 1243–1247.

39. Adams W H, Rufo R A, Talarico L, *et al*. Thrombocytopenia and intravenous heroin use. *Ann Intern Med* 1978; 89: 207–211.

40. Warkenstein T E. Thrombocytopenia and illicit drug use. *Ann Intern Med* 1994; 120: 693.

41. Christie D J, Walker R H, Kolins M D, *et al.* Quinine-induced thrombocytopenia following intravenous use of heroin. *Ann Intern Med* 1983; 143: 1174–1175.

42. Decker W J, Baker H E, Tamulinas S H, *et al.* Two deaths resulting from apparent parenteral injection of strychnine. *Vet Hum Toxicol* 1982; 24: 86.

43. Wijesekera A R L, Henry K D, Ranasighe P, *et al.* The detection and estimation of (A) arsenic in opium, and (B) strychnine in opium and heroin, as a means of identification of their respective sources. *Forensic Sci Int* 1988; 36: 193–209.

44. Nogue S, Sanz P, Munne P, *et al.* Acute scopolamine poisoning after sniffing adulterated cocaine. *Drug Alcohol Depend* 1991; 27: 115–116.

45. Centers for Disease Control and Prevention. Scopolamine poisoning among heroin users – New York City, Newark, Philadelphia, and Baltimore, 1995 and 1996. *JAMA* 1996; 276: 92–93.

3

Opioids

*If opium-eating be a sensual pleasure, and if I am bound to confess that
I have indulged in it to an excess not yet recorded of any other man, it
is no less true that I have struggled against this fascination with a
fervent zeal, and have at length accomplished what I never yet heard
attributed to any other man, have untwisted, almost to its final links,
the chain which fettered me.*
Thomas de Quincy, 'Confessions of an English Opium Eater', 1821

History

This group of drugs was originally only available from the opium poppy
(*Papaver somniferum*), native to Asia Minor (Figure 3.1). The active
constituents can be found in the latex that exudes from incisions in the
unripe capsule of the flowering head. The alkaloids that occur in the
poppy include morphine, noscapine, codeine, papaverine and thebaine.
Morphine is responsible for most of the psychotropic activity and comprises some 9–17% of the weight of dried opium but is usually about
10%. Strictly speaking, alkaloids derived from the opium poppy that
have morphine-like actions are termed opiates, whereas opioids are synthetic derivatives, e.g. methadone. However, in recent times the term
opioid has been understood to encompass opiates.

Opium itself has been used by humans for thousands of years,
both as a medicine and as an intoxicant. It was cultivated in many
places in Neolithic Europe, where it may have been burned to produce
an intoxicating smoke. However, in most cultures, opium was usually
taken orally. It is not known when opioids were first used therapeutically, but the Romans and the Greeks were well aware of the medicinal
properties of opium.

Smoking of opium using an individual pipe probably originated in
China in the 17th century and a huge population of dependent individuals began to develop there. Opium was subsequently the cause of two
wars between Britain and China in the 19th century, when the British
continued to sell opium to the Chinese people despite a decree from the
Emperor outlawing the use of it.

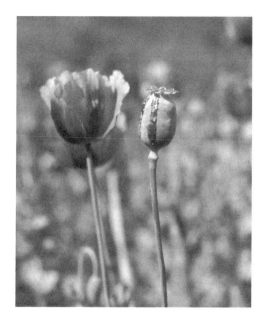

Figure 3.1 Heads of opium poppies (Photo courtesy of Multimedia Research Partners Ltd).

In the USA, the widescale use of opium as an analgesic during the Civil War created many thousands of 'addicts'. In both the USA and Europe, opium purchased for 'medicinal purposes' and sold overtly to produce intoxication caused serious social problems in the 19th century. Many medicines that were freely sold over-the-counter (OTC) for coughs, gastrointestinal complaints, sleep disorders and so forth contained appreciable quantities of opium. The extent of this problem was not officially recognised for many years, but it abated to some extent following legislation rendering opium an illegal substance. However, the problem of opioid abuse has remained ever since, in one form or another.

Morphine was first isolated in 1806 by a pharmacist, Wilhelm Sertürner, and named after the Greek god of dreams, Morpheus. Diacetylmorphine (or diamorphine), a simple derivative of morphine, was initially marketed in 1898 as a treatment for coughs under the brand name Heroin. The manufacturer's confidence in the drug is reflected in the choice of brand name – derived from the Greek word 'hero', which refers to beings half-god and half-human who possess extraordinary powers. Like many products since, heroin was seen as a 'less addictive' form of an existing drug and only later was its true dependence potential realised.

Opium has originated from much the same parts of the world for hundreds of years. The area of Afghanistan, Iran and Pakistan where opium poppies are grown is traditionally known as the 'Golden Crescent'; the corresponding area of Myanmar, Laos and Thailand is called the 'Golden Triangle'. In 2002, the worldwide production of illicit opium was approximately 4500 tonnes, and the United Nations estimated that there were about 10 million heroin users and 5 million opium users in the world in 2000–2001.[1] In 2002, 76% of world illicit opium came from Afghanistan, 18% from Myanmar, 2% from Laos and 1% from Colombia.

In 2003, about two-thirds of patients demanding treatment for an illicit substance abuse problem in Europe, Asia and Australia had a problem with opioids. In North America this was about a quarter. Table 3.1 gives data on population prevalence of opioid abuse in Australia, England/Wales and the USA.

Table 3.1 Opioid use amongst the population in national surveys

Country (year)	Heroin	Methadone	Other opioids	Ref.
Australia (2001)	1.6% of the adult population have abused at least once; 0.2% in the last year.	0.3% of the adult population have abused at least once; 0.1% in the last year.	1.2% of the adult population have abused at least once; 0.3% in the last year.	2
England + Wales (2002)	0.2% of the adult population have abused in the last year. 1% of children aged 11–15 have abused in the last year.	0.1% of the adult population have abused in the last year.	–	3, 4
USA (2002/3)	1.6% of the adult population have abused at least once; 0.2% in the last year in 2002. 1.5% of 16-year-olds have abused at least once in 2003.	–	13.2% of 16-year-olds had abused non-heroin opioids in 2003.	5, 6

Effects sought

When heroin is injected the user commonly experiences a rapid feeling of intense pleasure. This euphoria is replaced by a feeling of warmth (resulting from peripheral vasodilation), relaxation and happiness – although some people experience stimulatory effects. Unlike various other central nervous system (CNS) depressants, doses sufficient to cause euphoria do not impair movement (ataxia) or intellectual ability. Larger doses produce sedation or a pleasant light sleep. The individual is able to feel detached from the ongoing concerns and pressures of real life. With chronic administration, however, the user becomes tolerant to the psychotropic effects that were the original purpose of abuse. The object of each 'fix' then effectively becomes to avoid withdrawal symptoms (negative reinforcement).

Smoking, vaporising or 'snorting' heroin produces a milder 'rush' than intravenous injection. Non-heroin opioids produce similar but usually less intense effects, because of reduced CNS penetration and potency. The oral route does not produce a 'rush' and is therefore not popular for illicit opioids.

Administration

Opioids involved

The heroin abused on the street is made illegally in small-scale laboratories around the world, and very little is diverted from legitimate medical sources. However, all of the opioids available medicinally have been abused to some extent and supplies of these are largely obtained through abuse of pharmaceutical products. Examples of prescription opioids that are abused include:

Buprenorphine	Methadone
Codeine	Morphine
Dihydrocodeine	Nalbuphine
Dextropropoxyphene	Oxycodone
Diamorphine (heroin)	Pentazocine
Dipipanone	Pethidine
Fentanyl	Tramadol

Heroin is the most widely used opioid because of its potency, availability, solubility in water, and high biological lipophilicity, which affords rapid brain access. It is known as 'junk', 'H', 'smack', 'skag' or 'horse' and is usually supplied as a brown or off-white powder, depending on the purity and the manufacturing process. It is always adulterated with other substances when bought at street level. The drug is progressively diluted (or 'cut') as it moves down the line from manufacturer through various dealers to the end user. Diluents include almost any powder (e.g. sugars, paracetamol) and adulterants are typically drugs with CNS depressant actions (e.g. other opioids, diazepam). A typical dealer's preparation slab is shown in Figure 3.2. Note that two different forms of heroin are sold around the world: base heroin and the hydrochloride salt. The heroin used in Australia, for example, is largely derived from the Golden Crescent and is supplied as the hydrochloride salt. It is readily soluble in cold water. Heroin sold in western Europe is derived from the Golden Triangle and is supplied as base heroin; in order to be made soluble enough for injection it must be heated in an acidic solution (e.g. using citric acid).

The **methadone** and **buprenorphine** encountered at street level has usually been diverted from healthcare sources (e.g. prescribed methadone, thefts) where these drugs are prescribed mainly as a substitute for street opioids in dependent individuals (see below), but also as analgesics. Methadone is supplied most commonly as a liquid

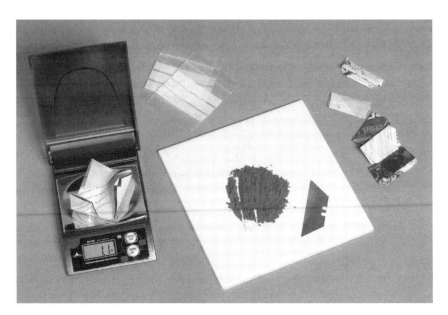

Figure 3.2 A heroin dealer's slab. Powdered heroin is 'cut' with an inert powder on a smooth surface, such as a mirror, using a razor blade. Resultant powders are sold in small bags or card 'wraps', as here (Photo courtesy of Multimedia Research Partners Ltd).

formulation. Depending on the nature of the formulation it may or may not allow injection: viscous dilute formulations as used in the UK tend to preclude injection, whereas the concentrated watery formulations used in some countries (e.g. Australia) may make injection an option. Buprenorphine, a partial opioid agonist, was initially claimed to have low dependency potential and to produce only mild symptoms upon withdrawal. However, perhaps predictably, buprenorphine abuse eventually became so widespread that many countries were obliged to reclassify the drug into a higher legal category to try to prevent diversion. The tablets are designed to be soluble in water because buprenorphine is administered sublingually; hence preparing an injection is easy. High-dose buprenorphine tablets may also be crushed and snorted.

The potent opioid **oxycodone** has attracted increasing levels of abuse in the USA, often as a substitute for heroin.[7] The modified-release tablet formulation of oxycodone is taken orally and chewed, or crushed and inhaled nasally as a powder. The tablets may also be injected: after removal of the coating, they are ground into a powder, and then heated on a spoon with water to encourage dissolution.

Fentanyl is another potent opioid that is abused: this is of concern because it is many times more potent than heroin and inexperienced users risk death from opioid overdose. It is available in a variety of non-oral formulations but, increasingly, abuse of fentanyl transdermal patches has been reported – the contents of patches being injected, taken orally or vaporised for inhalation, often with fatal consequences.[8–13] Patches may be stolen from patients or healthcare facilities, but discarded 'used' patches also contain appreciable quantities of fentanyl. In the USA, illicit derivatives of fentanyl have had surges in popularity.[14] As a group, the fentanyl-derived opioids are often sold under the name of 'synthetic heroin'. The most well-known example is alpha-methyl-fentanyl, known on the street as 'China white'; another example is 3-methylfentanyl ('3MF' or 'TMF'). These and other analogues can be over 1000 times more potent than heroin and have a short duration of action (typically 30–90 minutes). The two properties combined dramatically increase the positive reinforcement potential and therefore the risk of dependence occurring after only a few doses. They are usually injected but smoking or nasal inhalation is also common. The drugs produce intense opioid effects with a very rapid onset and they can cause dramatic, sudden respiratory depression and death. Many deaths have been reported in the USA – in some cases death was so quick that injectors have been found with the needle still *in situ*.[15] Unfortunately, fentanyl derivatives are not detected by all routine immunoassay screening tests for opioids and so their abuse may not always be identified.[16]

Dextropropoxyphene, dihydrocodeine and **codeine** are less popular at street level because they are weak opioids and because most pharmaceutical formulations are not very convenient from the abuse standpoint. For example, many of them also contain paracetamol or aspirin so it is difficult to take enough of the opioid for intoxication without risking potentially fatal paracetamol/aspirin overdose, although separation is sometimes attempted. OTC liquid formulations of codeine are popular but have the disadvantage to the user of a low concentration, such that the large volume required for intoxication prevents injection. If pure opioid tablets are available, these may be crushed and injected. Dextropropoxyphene, dihydrocodeine and codeine are often taken when more potent alternatives are not available. Nonetheless, they are still abused in their own right, taken to stave off withdrawal, or even used to synthesise more powerful opioids. These and other aspects of OTC opioid abuse are discussed in more detail in Chapter 13. **Tramadol** is another weaker opioid that has been subject to abuse.[17]

Abuse of **pethidine** analogues has also been reported from the USA – one in particular has come to public attention: 1-methyl-4-phenyl-4-propionoxypiperidine (MPPP). Several batches of illicitly produced MPPP were contaminated with MPTP (1-methyl-4-phenyl-1,2,3,6-tetrahydropyridine), a very potent neurotoxin that causes irreversible brain damage with Parkinson-like symptoms.[15]

Dipipanone has been widely abused because some branded products (e.g. Diconal) contain cyclizine as well as dipipanone, both of which are psychoactive. The abuse potential of this antihistamine is discussed in Chapter 13. **Nalbuphine** is abused particularly by sportsmen and bodybuilders and is discussed in more detail in Chapter 11.

Opium itself is still used, particularly in eastern and southern Asia, and is traditionally smoked.

Method of administration

Most of the opioids can be administered orally, but the CNS effects are slow to develop and are blunted after administration by this route. In addition, all opioids are subject to some presystemic metabolism – for example the bioavailability of oral buprenorphine is only 16%, whereas for morphine it is 40–50%. Many users prefer the intravenous route as this produces an intense 'rush' of euphoria that does not occur following oral ingestion. A variety of non-sterile preparations are injected (or 'fixed'), including heroin powder bought on the street, crushed opioid-containing tablets and liquid medicinal preparations. For the purpose of injecting, base heroin is typically mixed by the user with simple organic acids (e.g. ascorbic acid, citric acid) to increase heroin solubility and facilitate its extraction from the mixture of inactive diluents and adulterants; occasionally lemon juice or vinegar is used. Lemon juice carries particular infection risks (see Chapter 2). The hydrochloride salt of heroin does not require treatment with acids and is freely soluble in water. Persistent injection of non-sterile solutions that are contaminated with particles eventually causes blood vessel damage, which, in turn, severely restricts venous access (see Chapter 2). If this occurs, users may sometimes resort to subcutaneous injection.

Heroin can be inhaled nasally ('snorted'), and the base form can be smoked in cigarettes ('reefers') or heated on foil and the vapour inhaled ('chasing the dragon' or 'skagging'). Non-injection forms of administration offer an alternative method of administration that may produce an acceptable 'rush' without the infection risks associated with intravenous injection.

Pharmacokinetics and pharmacology

Opioid receptors in the CNS mediate the actions of endogenous peptides such as enkephalins and dynorphins, which probably initiate or control a range of behaviours and moods. There are three types of opioid receptor in humans that have become firmly established – μ (mu), κ (kappa), and δ (delta) – but there are others that are less well characterised. The euphoria and physical dependence attributable to opioids are thought to be mediated through μ receptors in the brain. Receptors outside the CNS facilitate some of the peripheral side-effects of opioids, e.g. constipation and effects on renal blood flow.

The commonly abused opioids are all metabolised principally in the liver and the metabolites are then excreted renally. Heroin is unusual in that the molecule itself has no intrinsic actions at opioid receptors, all of its actions are due to its two main metabolites: 6-monoacetylmorphine and morphine. Heroin is rapidly deacetylated in the liver, kidney, blood, brain and other tissues to form these metabolites, such that it has an average half-life of only 3 minutes; 6-monoacetylmorphine has a similarly short half-life. Morphine is converted to a range of metabolites in the liver and has an average half-life of about 3 hours. The two most important metabolites are formed by conjugation: morphine-3-glucuronide and morphine-6-glucuronide. The latter only comprises about 5% of metabolites, but is a much more potent opioid agonist than morphine. All the morphine metabolites are excreted renally.

Adverse effects

The adverse effects associated with opioid abuse fall into four distinct categories: adverse-effects of opioid drugs seen at normal doses, effects of overdose, adverse consequences of the abuse process/dependence, and withdrawal symptoms. The adverse effects of opioids outside the overdose setting are well known and are listed in Table 3.2.

Intoxication with opioids may increase the chance of the individual causing or being exposed to accidents. Disinhibition and subjectively enhanced sexual performance (especially in the early stages of heroin use) can result in increased sexual activity and therefore increased risk of HIV (human immunodeficiency virus), viral hepatitis, other sexually transmitted diseases or unwanted pregnancies.

The effects of overdose are given in Table 3.3. Many of these may be reversed with the opioid antagonist naloxone, but at the risk of precipitating acute opioid withdrawal. The dose of naloxone needs to be repeated because it has a shorter half-life than most opioids. Some

Table 3.2   Adverse effects of opioids (non-overdose)

Common
- Nausea, vomiting, constipation
- Drowsiness, mental confusion
- Libido may be enhanced during initial abuse, but chronic administration tends to depress sexual desire and performance
- Sweating (especially in long-term methadone recipients)

Infrequent
- Facial flushing, pruritus
- Dry mouth
- Hallucinations, dysphoria
- Urinary retention
- Headache

Rare
- Thrombocytopenia – may be an immune-based reaction to adulterants, and quinine has been identified as the cause in at least one case[18,19]
- Rashes, urticaria
- Vertigo
- Palpitations, postural hypotension

Table 3.3 Signs and symptoms of opioid overdose

- Dysphoria, hallucinations, heavy sedation
- Miosis
- Hypothermia
- Respiratory depression, pulmonary oedema, coma
- Hypotension, bradycardia, arrhythmias, cardiac arrest
- Convulsions (dextropropoxyphene and pethidine only)

drugs, such as dextropropoxyphene, methadone and buprenorphine, have particularly long half-lives and prolonged naloxone administration may therefore be required after overdose with these substances (up to 72 hours with methadone). Opioid overdose may occur with the intention of committing suicide, but it may arise by accident as a result of the unexpected potency of a sample purchased at street level or after a period of abstinence during which tolerance has decreased. The incidence of overdose amongst heroin users was estimated at about one-quarter of the affected population in a London study,[20] but two-thirds of the population in Sydney, Australia.[21] Consequently it has been proposed that the opioid antagonist naloxone be supplied to street users of opioids[22] and paramedics in many countries now carry it routinely.

Adverse effects arising from the abuse process include the harmful consequences of injection, which are discussed in Chapter 2. There are also a large number of adverse social effects resulting from opioid dependence, including increased likelihood of criminal activity, general poor health and diet, antisocial behaviour, and disrupted relationships.

Opioid dependence

Opioid dependence is a well-established and clearly defined phenomenon. It is common and becomes more likely as the dose and duration of administration increase. Those who abuse opioids regularly become tolerant to the pleasurable psychotropic effects quite rapidly. The dose is increased in an attempt to regain the lost experience. This is effective for a time, but tolerance redevelops and the dose is then progressively increased to a maximum, often determined by drug affordability. At this level there is permanent tolerance to most of the effects of opioids, including euphoria, although complete tolerance to constipation, miosis and sweating does not seem to occur. The drive to continue drug administration becomes the desire to avoid a withdrawal reaction (negative reinforcement) rather than the pleasure of the experience (positive reinforcement). Cross-tolerance exists between all the opioid drugs and so those dependent on an illicit opioid such as heroin may seek an alternative in an attempt to stave off withdrawal when it is not available. OTC opioids in particular can be used for this purpose in countries where they are available.

The opioid withdrawal syndrome is characterised by a range of symptoms (Table 3.4). When a person dependent on an opioid attempts to cease administration abruptly, without medical support, he or she is said to be doing 'cold turkey'. This is believed to originate from the gooseflesh appearance of the skin that is commonly seen in this situation. The symptoms of withdrawal manifest as the reverse of normal opioid action on the body, i.e. they are suggestive of CNS hyperactivity rather than depression. Although subjectively very unpleasant, these effects are not life-threatening, and the subject remains relatively lucid throughout.

Signs of acute heroin withdrawal commence within 6–12 hours of abstinence, but the peak effects are seen after 36–72 hours, followed by gradual abatement over the subsequent 5–10 days. The acute phase of methadone withdrawal starts within 1–3 days of the last dose, peaks at 3–6 days and lasts for 14 days or more. If opioid dependents are given naloxone, withdrawal may develop almost instantly.

The acute phase of withdrawal is followed by a period of relatively chronic symptoms usually characterised by a craving for opioids and accompanied by anxiety, emotional lability, depression, fatigue, malaise

Table 3.4 Symptoms of acute opioid withdrawal

Initial symptoms
- Anxiety, restlessness, insomnia
- Mild tachypnoea, yawning, coughing, sneezing
- Craving for drug
- Lacrimation, perspiration, rhinorrhoea

Later symptoms
- Tremors, myalgia, arthralgia, muscle twitching
- Chills, piloerection (gooseflesh), hot flushes
- Anorexia, abdominal pains
- Mydriasis
- Insomnia, headache

Severe cases
- Tachycardia, hypertension
- Nausea, vomiting, diarrhoea
- Fever, dehydration
- Severe or persistent tachypnoea
- Agitation

or insomnia. These persistent effects can take months to abate, are very hard to ignore, and may encourage a return to opioid abuse.

Research in animals has helped to elucidate the mechanisms of opioid withdrawal. The locus coeruleus in the brain seems to play a particularly important part in mediating the physical signs of opioid withdrawal. Furthermore, the existence of anti-opioid peptides has been postulated.[23] These peptides may be released in the CNS as a response to chronic exogenous opioid administration and therefore help to mediate tolerance. The excess anti-opioid peptides that remain following opioid discontinuation may at least be partly responsible for causing the symptoms of withdrawal.

Treatment of dependence and withdrawal

Opioid dependence should not be seen as a hopeless cause. A 22-year follow-up of 128 heroin injectors from London in 1996 revealed that 50% of them had stopped using opioids (this included seven non-users who had died from natural causes unrelated to drug use).[24] The initial aims of healthcare professionals when they come into contact with those injecting opioids in some countries include general harm minimisation measures, which are discussed briefly in Chapter 2. However, dependence itself can be treated by a variety of means. Figure 3.3 summarises some of the pharmacological approaches available; in practice these are often supported by a range of non-pharmacological means (counselling, etc.) but a discussion of these options is beyond the scope of this book.

Substitute-opioid prescribing

The substitute opioids used include methadone, high-dose buprenorphine, pharmaceutical diamorphine, levacetylmethadol and dihydrocodeine. The substitute is prescribed to users in a dose sufficient to prevent withdrawal symptoms; larger doses of some prescribed opioid agonists may be used to saturate receptors such that top-up doses of street opioids do not produce psychotropic effects. Prescribing regular maintenance doses may allow those dependent on an opioid such as heroin to lead comparatively normal lives unperturbed by cravings for heroin, drug-seeking behaviour and all the concomitant unhealthy aspects of the regular street drug user's lifestyle. Some people may receive daily maintenance doses of medication indefinitely. This is a legitimate endpoint of treatment with these objectives:

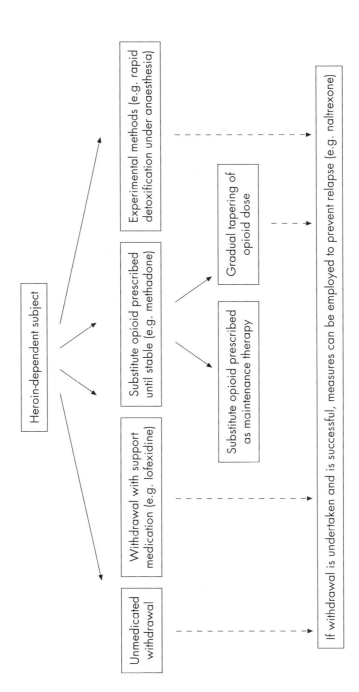

Figure 3.3 Summary of pharmacological methods of assisting with heroin dependence.

- Reduced use of injection drugs with all the harms these pose to the individual, and to society from the spread of blood-borne viral diseases (see Chapter 2).
- Reduced risk of illicit drug side-effects, suicide and overdose.
- Improved psychological and social functioning; improved relationships.
- Reduced criminal activity to fund illicit drug abuse.
- Sustained contact with healthcare services allowing the opportunity for other interventions.

The substitute may offer a convenient 'bridge' between an old drug culture lifestyle and the prospect of a drug-free existence. Once stabilised upon a suitable dose, some patients can begin a structured withdrawal programme, involving gradual dosage reduction over a period of weeks or months.

The substitute opioid most commonly used is **methadone**. It is usually supplied as an oral liquid formulation; intravenous methadone has a very limited clinical place (e.g. for patients who repeatedly fail on oral methadone or who cannot take it orally).[25] However, injection should be the rare exception rather than the rule, and the number of prescriptions for methadone injection in the UK (about 9% of the total in 1995) has been criticised.[26] Note that methadone tablets are also likely to be crushed and injected and should not normally be prescribed.

If the abused opioid is of a pharmaceutical origin, then a dose of methadone of equivalent potency can be given. However, for street heroin it is impossible to reliably determine an equivalent methadone dose because it is very impure and the potency varies from location to location, from dealer to dealer, and from batch to batch. Furthermore, drug users may not be honest about the quantities of heroin they take, or may be unable to express it accurately. In this case, the methadone dose must be titrated up to relieve symptoms of withdrawal. The lethal dose of methadone for a non-tolerant adult can be as little as 40–50 mg, so it has been suggested that this dose not normally be exceeded in the first 24 hours, especially because cumulative toxicity can develop over the first few days.[25,27] Initial doses are normally even less than this. In practice the dose chosen for an individual will depend upon a variety of factors including the severity of withdrawal symptoms, and the degree of likely existing opioid tolerance. The dose on subsequent days is then adjusted by small increments.[25] Methadone has a long half-life, allowing once-daily administration when used chronically.

It is important to realise that supply of methadone itself is not all that is required. If true social rehabilitation is to occur, full counselling and psychosocial support is necessary to prevent a return to old habits.

Some subjects may use prescribed methadone to provide a baseline plasma level on which 'top-ups' of street drugs are superimposed. Clearly this defeats an important objective of treatment. It can be identified by random urine tests during clinic visits. An analysis of published studies suggests that prescribing larger daily doses of methadone may help to counteract this problem.[28] Daily doses of 60–100 mg are more effective than lower doses at retaining patients in treatment programmes and in reducing the use of heroin. These high doses of methadone are believed to induce such a level of opioid tolerance that 'top-up' doses of street heroin have no effects. However, in the presence of liver disease, extreme care with larger doses is advisable, as methadone is cleared hepatically. Ten deaths were reported from Australia in 1990 in patients with hepatitis who died within 2–6 days of starting an average of 60 mg of methadone per day.[29] This was a larger starting dose than is normally recommended. It is possible that methadone accumulated to toxic levels. High doses of methadone have also been linked to torsade de pointes via prolongation of the QTc interval.[30]

Methadone must be supplied with care, because it is clearly a substance that might itself be abused. The nature of the oral liquid formulation of methadone determines how widely it is injected: viscous, low concentration formulations need to be diluted with large volumes of water in order to be drawn up into a syringe and the subsequent volume after dilution tends to discourage injection; conversely, high-concentration non-viscous formulations of methadone liquid can be injected more easily. The drug does appear on the street because those prescribed it may swap their methadone for other drugs of abuse or simply sell it, and healthcare supplies are stolen. Deaths may occur when non-tolerant individuals ingest this very potent drug.[31] There have also been a number of accidental ingestions of methadone (some fatal) reported in young children who have gained access to it because family members prescribed the drug have stored it carelessly.[32]

Other opioids have been used as maintenance treatment or to aid withdrawal. Most notable among these is high-dose **buprenorphine**. This differs from methadone in that it is a partial opioid agonist – it will give some rewarding opioid-like CNS effects but it may also antagonise the psychotropic effects of any heroin taken surreptitiously while on a treatment programme. It is given as a sublingual tablet. As with methadone, a lower dose is given initially, which can be increased according to the patient's response. The first dose must be given at least 4 hours after the last use of heroin because the partial agonist properties of buprenorphine may otherwise effectively result in varying degrees of withdrawal-like symptoms. The dose is usually given daily, but once the patient is stable the daily dose may be doubled and given on alternate days. Three-times-weekly regimens are also sometimes used. Despite its partial agonist activity, the intravenous abuse of buprenorphine tablets can still be a potential problem. In some countries buprenorphine is combined with the opioid antagonist naloxone to discourage intravenous abuse: naloxone has negligible actions via the sublingual route due to poor absorption but acts as an opioid antagonist if the tablets are given intravenously.

Levacetylmethadol (levomethadyl acetate, LAAM), is a potent opioid with a duration of action of some 72 hours. The long half-life of the parent drug and its metabolites allows administration three times weekly.[33] Although it has been widely used in the USA as an alternative to methadone, in Europe its marketing authorisation was suspended in 2001 by the European Medicines Agency (EMEA) because of a link with life-threatening cardiac disorders.[34] Specifically, it prolongs the QTc interval and has been associated with torsade de pointes, other arryhthmias, and cardiac arrest. The EMEA states that it has a greater pro-arrhythmic potential than methadone. LAAM itself is believed to be largely responsible for the pro-arrhythmic effect, whereas its metabolites have the therapeutic effect. The enzyme that metabolises LAAM is CYP3A4, and inhibitors of this enzyme might increase the pro-arrhythmic effect.

Several studies in Europe have assessed the role for prescribed intravenous, smoked or vaporised **diamorphine** in patients resistant to other treatments.[35–38] In some of these studies, it was supplied in addition to a baseline daily dose of methadone and had to be used on the premises. In theory supplying diamorphine should lessen the need for street heroin and should help to retain users in treatment, so it could act as a harm reduction measure. However, although the authors of the various studies conclude that employment of prescribed diamorphine is valuable, its exact place in therapy remains to be clarified and this practice has not been widely adopted.

Dihydrocodeine and **codeine** are sometimes used for maintenance therapy, but the evidence to support their value is exceedingly weak, being mainly anecdotal.[25,39] The abuse potential of codeine is discussed in Chapter 13, but there are also significant concerns with dihydrocodeine. In Scotland for example there is increasing evidence for the involvement of dihydrocodeine in the deaths of drug users,[40] and some clinicians have recommended that dihydrocodeine be used to assist with opioid withdrawal only in the short term, because of the dangers of abuse.[41] Dihydrocodeine is usually supplied as tablets, which can easily be injected.

Individuals maintained on any prescribed 'maintenance' opioids commonly require antidepressants and laxatives as additional medication.

Opioid withdrawal

Withdrawal from opioids can be achieved in one of three ways:

1. without any support medication ('cold turkey')
2. with support medication such as lofexidine
3. by substitution of another opioid for the abused substance and then withdrawing this slowly.

Unsupported abrupt withdrawal usually occurs when those who are dependent on opioids decide to stop on their own initiative or if supplies of opioid are interrupted for any length of time, so forcing the user into withdrawal (e.g. imprisonment, hospitalisation). Those who are dependent upon illicit opioids typically make many unsuccessful attempts to stop on their own before seeking medical assistance. Heroin withdrawal starts within 6–12 hours of the last dose.

Abrupt withdrawal can also take place with the use of medication to ameliorate symptoms. Overactivity of central noradrenergic neurones is thought to mediate many of the effects of withdrawal and this activity is suppressed by drugs such as **lofexidine** and **clonidine**. These are pre-synaptic alpha-2 adrenergic agonists that inhibit neurotransmitter release. A short course (7–10 days) of either drug is useful for suppressing the noradrenergic signs of acute opioid withdrawal, although they do not prevent the more chronic symptoms that develop after the acute phase such as craving for opioids, which is the most significant cause of relapse. Side-effects may include sedation, dry mouth and hypotension, although hypotension is more common with clonidine. Compared with a reducing dose of methadone (see below), clonidine and lofexidine seem to be equally effective at treating the acute phase of opioid withdrawal but treatment duration is shorter, and withdrawal symptoms appear earlier and resolve more quickly.[42] Subjects taking methadone suffer fewer side-effects, at least compared to clonidine.[42]

Withdrawal can also be accomplished by gradually tapering the dose of a prescribed opioid. Most commonly this is methadone or buprenorphine. Signs of methadone or buprenorphine withdrawal can take up to 72 hours to develop after the last dose or dosage reduction because both drugs have a long half-life of about a day during chronic administration. The duration of the withdrawal programme is highly variable and is best individualised according to the subject's response and circumstances. As mentioned above, complete detoxification may not be appropriate or desirable for everyone. Another advantage of the long half-life is that although withdrawal symptoms tend to be more sustained than those associated with heroin, they are also milder. Sometimes lofexidine is prescribed as a short course on a 'when required' basis to help manage any breakthrough withdrawal symptoms during a period of opioid dose reduction. Some clinicians may swap patients over to dihydrocodeine during the final stages of methadone withdrawal because it is a shorter-acting opioid with allegedly a more mild withdrawal.[25] However, there is inadequate published evidence to justify this course of action, and the dangers of dihydrocodeine abuse have already been described.

Rapid opioid detoxification techniques are advocated by some practitioners. These involve the opioid-dependent patient being sedated and then monitored while opioid antagonists are given. The details of the technique vary between practitioners. The sedative used may vary from a minimal one such as a benzodiazepine to a full general anaesthetic. The evidence to support the efficacy of such techniques is limited. In particular the details of methods used are not standardised and although they may allow the patient to negotiate the acute phase of withdrawal it is not clear how effective they are in securing medium- to long-term abstinence compared to other approaches.[43,44] There are also significant safety concerns (e.g. vomiting while sedated), which require continuous intense supervision of the patient, and a number of deaths have been reported in association with techniques that use heavy sedation or anaesthesia.[43]

The experimental drug **ibogaine** is claimed to halt the craving for opioids that occurs in those who are attempting abstinence.[45] It is derived from an African shrub, *Tabernanthe iboga*. There has been concern over the potential toxicity of ibogaine and some deaths have been associated with its use. At the time of writing, the drug had not been systematically studied in a large controlled clinical trial – the only information on efficacy is from animal studies, human case series, and anecdotal reports. The drug is itself psychoactive and those who use it experience a 'trip' after one dose, lasting 24–36 hours. Individuals are purported to emerge from this state free from opioid craving. There is inadequate published evidence regarding the safety or efficacy of ibogaine to recommend its use.

Relapse prevention

Naltrexone is an orally active opioid antagonist. It has no agonist effects and blocks the effect of opioids without the reward of an opioid 'buzz'. Naltrexone has been advocated as a means to prevent relapse in highly motivated people who have successfully negotiated acute opioid withdrawal because it not only prevents positive reinforcement but can diminish craving. However, the methodological quality of published clinical trials is generally poor and does not allow definite conclusions to be drawn concerning its effectiveness as maintenance therapy.[46] If used, naltrexone must be given to patients who have completed the acute phase of opioid withdrawal, otherwise it will precipitate an acute withdrawal reaction. It is a long-acting drug and can be given daily, or three times weekly by mouth. Naltrexone implants are also available.

Tolerance to opioids diminishes as they are withdrawn. Hence those who have withdrawn from chronic opioids for a reasonable length of time are at risk of overdose if they suddenly return to drug use at doses similar to those used before withdrawal was initiated.

Interactions with medicines

Compared to most other street drugs, there are more data on the potential interactions between opioids and conventional medicines because opioids are so widely used therapeutically. A full medication and substance abuse history is necessary before investigating drug interactions in an individual patient. Factors that may predispose opioids to interact include:

- All of them are CNS depressants and so will have at least additive effects with medicines that have this property.
- Methadone and buprenorphine are both metabolised by the enzyme CYP3A4.
- The enzyme CYP2D6 is occasionally important in interactions. For example, it is responsible for the metabolism of oxycodone, and for the transformation of codeine and tramadol into active metabolites. Methadone inhibits CYP2D6.

Some interactions are highlighted in the text below. It is not the intention to present a comprehensive list of all potential interactions here and the reader is referred to other sources providing a more complete list.[25,47,48]

Medicines with sedative side-effects

The CNS depression wrought by opioids is likely to be increased by medicines that also do this. Example groups of medicines that may be affected include other opioids, benzodiazepines, many tricyclic anti-depressants, many neuroleptics, and older antihistamines.

Increased buprenorphine or methadone levels

Some medicines inhibit the enzyme CYP3A4 and so could increase buprenorphine or methadone levels, potentially causing increased opioid side-effects. Examples include:

- cimetidine
- ciprofloxacin
- erythromycin and clarithromycin
- fluconazole and ketoconazole
- fluvoxamine and possibly other selective serotonin reuptake inhibitors (SSRIs).

Decreased buprenorphine or methadone levels

Some medicines induce the enzyme CYP3A4 and so could be expected to decrease buprenorphine or methadone levels, potentially causing withdrawal symptoms. Examples include:

- anticonvulsants (e.g. barbiturates, carbamazepine, phenytoin)
- HIV medicines (e.g. efavirenz, nevirapine)
- rifampicin
- spironolactone
- St John's Wort.

Other interactions

1. *Buprenorphine and opioid agonists.* Because buprenorphine has some antagonist actions at opioid receptors it can cause opioid withdrawal symptoms if given to patients stabilised on chronic opioids.
2. *Medicines affecting QT intervals.* Some medicines can prolong the QTc interval or cause torsade de pointes. They should be used cautiously with methadone because of its ability to cause arrhythmias. Examples include tricyclic antidepressants.

3. *Urine pH.* Methadone is excreted more rapidly if there is an acidic urine and more slowly if it is alkaline. Medicines that alter urine pH (e.g. vitamin C, sodium bicarbonate) may thus affect methadone activity.

Use and concurrent illness

Asthma

Opioids are respiratory depressants and should be used with care in patients with asthma. Overdose of intravenous opioids can cause bronchospasm, respiratory arrest and pulmonary oedema. However in the absence of overdose, heroin has been associated with bronchospasm when injected[49] or vaporised.[50,51] The process of smoking or vaporising any drug can cause respiratory symptoms.

Diabetes

The balance of food intake and dose of hypoglycaemic drug can be disrupted by vomiting, which is a recognised side-effect of opioids, particularly when first used. The apathy and poor motivation engendered in some individuals by chronic drug dependence may mitigate against adequate control of blood glucose in established diabetes. Non-compliance with diet, failure to administer medication correctly or inadequate monitoring could result. Intoxication may prevent a diabetic recognising and/or dealing with a hypoglycaemic episode. The hypoglycaemic episode can also resemble intoxication, so bystanders may not seek medical attention.

Epilepsy

Heroin abuse is associated with fitting,[52,53] as are other opioids when used in high dose therapeutically. However, this effect of therapeutic opioids has been attributed to accumulation of preservatives[54] or to the misdiagnosis of intense opioid-induced muscular rigidity.[55] Opioid withdrawal is not associated with convulsions in adults but seizures have been occasionally described in neonates undergoing withdrawal due to *in utero* exposure. Overdose with dextropropoxyphene or pethidine is particularly linked to drug-induced fitting. Use of pethidine or pethidine analogues in patients with renal failure has also been associated with convulsions due to accumulation of a neurotoxic metabolite, norpethidine.

Hepatic disease

Reports of significant opioid-induced hepatic damage are extremely rare. Liver biopsies have shown that those who inject heroin may have sinusoidal dilatation, and sinusoidal and hepatic vein inflammation. In ex-users this inflammation is largely replaced by fibrosis.[56] However, the functional significance of these changes is unclear. Studies using cultured human hepatocytes have suggested that alcohol may potentiate the cytotoxic actions of heroin and methadone.[57]

Most opioids are metabolised via the liver, so hepatic failure may allow them to accumulate to a greater or lesser extent. Smaller doses and greater dosage intervals are therefore usually recommended in this situation. Note that the constipating actions of opioids may be particularly undesirable in patients with severe liver disease.

Hypertension

Opioids are not known to worsen existing hypertension; in fact, opioids tend to cause hypotension. Some patients may develop an elevated blood pressure during withdrawal.

Immunity impairment

The prospect of certain drugs of abuse altering immunity is an important consideration for many users, not least those who are HIV-positive or who have AIDS (acquired immunodeficiency syndrome). A study in San Francisco, in which HIV-infected individuals were followed for 6 years, revealed that none of the drugs of abuse taken was associated with increased likelihood of progression to AIDS.[58] These drugs included opioids. This contrasts with a Scottish study suggesting that although other drugs of abuse had no effects, heroin might hasten progression to AIDS.[59]

The potential for opioids to affect immunity has been studied in some detail. Endogenous opioids seem to have an immunoregulatory function in many species, including humans,[60] and the administration of exogenous opioid may disrupt this process. The addition of morphine to cells infected with HIV and cultured *in vitro* results in increased replication of the virus.[61] A variety of signs of impaired immunity have been detected in both HIV-negative and HIV-positive patients taking methadone, including alterations in lymphocyte phenotype, suppressed lymphocyte function and reduced cytotoxic function of certain lymphocytes.[62] An analysis of the immunocompetence of 220 patients receiving daily methadone as maintenance treatment also revealed detrimental effects upon immunity regardless of HIV status. Specifically, the ratio of CD4 lymphocytes, which bolster immunity, to CD8 lymphocytes, which have a suppressor function, was reduced, apparently because of relatively increased CD8 numbers.[63] Animal and *in vitro* work suggest that a major mechanism by which opioids might exert these immunosuppressive effects is by hastening the death of lymphocytes.[64]

Renal disease

Intra-arterial opioids or prolonged unconsciousness secondary to intoxication can lead to rhabdomyolysis. This can in turn cause acute renal failure. Acute renal failure may also occur subsequent to hypotension caused by overdoses of intravenous heroin. This usually resolves quickly. Heroin-associated nephropathy has been described but this now seems to be more rare than previously thought. It has been suggested that this is because the condition might have been caused by heroin adulteration in the past and the drug is now much more pure at street level.[65] Septicaemia can also cause acute renal failure. It can occur secondary to non-sterile injections.

Morphine and heroin (which is converted to morphine), are metabolised to morphine-6-glucuronide which, although only produced in small quantities, is a very potent opioid agonist. It is known to accumulate in patients with renal failure, with potentially serious consequences, and so heroin should be used with extreme caution in renal disease. A varying proportion of methadone and buprenorphine is eliminated renally, so a deterioration in renal function may also encourage their accumulation. Pethidine is metabolised to a neurotoxic derivative, norpethidine, which is eliminated renally. This metabolite accumulates in renal failure and causes excitation of the CNS and even convulsions. Fentanyl is eliminated hepatically, and with inactive metabolites, so should not, therefore, accumulate in renal impairment. However, the overall situation is complicated by the fact that patients with renal failure typically become more sensitive to the CNS effects of many drugs, including opioids, probably because of the accumulation of urea.

Pregnancy and breastfeeding

Pregnancy

Opioids are perhaps second only to cocaine as the most extensively studied drugs of abuse in human pregnancy. They are not thought to cause congenital abnormalities, but the administration of heroin or methadone during pregnancy is associated with increased rates of prematurity, low birth weight and small neonatal size.

Withdrawal reactions are common in neonates exposed to opioids throughout the third trimester. The typical symptoms are similar to those experienced in adults undergoing withdrawal (Table 3.5). Withdrawal symptoms may be present at birth but if not, onset may occur within 24–48 hours for babies born of heroin-dependent mothers and within 2–7 days for babies exposed to methadone. Sometimes the peak intensity of symptoms can be delayed by as much as 10–14 days. The acute symptoms may persist for several weeks but usually these abate within 3 weeks for those exposed to heroin; the time course of methadone's effects is much more variable. Sub-acute symptoms such as sleeping problems, irritability and poor feeding may last for months in some cases. The intensity of neonatal withdrawal symptoms is not necessarily related to maternal opioid dose.

Preschool children who were exposed to opioids in the womb may exhibit a range of cognitive or behavioural problems. It is not clear whether these are caused by drug exposure or other factors.

Table 3.5   Withdrawal symptoms in the newborn after *in utero* exposure to opioids

- Hypertonia, hyper-reflexia, tremor, convulsions
- Hyperactivity, irritability, poor sleeping pattern, decreased sleep
- Diarrhoea, vomiting
- Tachypnoea, rhinorrhoea, yawning, hiccups, sneezing, apnoea, high-pitched cry
- Poor feeding, weight loss or failure to gain weight
- Fever
- Hypertension, tachycardia
- Lacrimation

Breastfeeding

The effects of heroin abuse in breastfeeding have not been investigated recently. Morphine does pass into breast milk in small amounts and the results of single-dose studies suggest that when given for therapeutic effect, small doses are probably not a significant problem in breastfeeding. Morphine in breast milk would be subject to the baby's first-pass liver metabolism which, although not studied in this age group, is quite extensive in adults. However, the effects on the breastfed baby of maternal chronic administration of large doses of opioids is not known.

One study has suggested that quite small doses of morphine may inhibit the secretion of oxytocin and this might theoretically impair the ability of patients to breastfeed successfully.[66]

Neonates are notoriously sensitive to opioids and metabolise them very slowly, so accumulation is possible. Methadone, which has a long half-life in adults, could be particularly liable to accumulate in babies in theory but the concentration in milk is less than that in maternal plasma,[67] probably because methadone is quite highly bound to plasma proteins. The amount ingested by the baby appears to be very small.

Opioids are administered therapeutically to babies from time to time in very small doses and can cause CNS depression and constipation. In overdose, excessive sedation and respiratory depression can occur. In practical terms, if a woman taking or abusing opioids wished to breastfeed it would be sensible to monitor the baby for signs of sedation. Furthermore, when breastfeeding stops the baby might experience withdrawal symptoms.[68]

References

1.   United Nations Office on Drugs and Crime. *Global Illicit Drug Trends 2003*. Vienna: UNODC, 2004 (available from http://www.unodc.org/pdf/trends2003_www_E.pdf; accessed 17 November 2004).
2.   *Statistics on Drug Use in Australia 2002. Drug Statistics Series No. 12*. Cat no. PHE 43. Canberra: Australian Institute of Health and Welfare, February 2003.
3.   Aust R, Sharp C, Goulden C. *Prevalence of Drug Use: Key Findings from the 2001/02 British Crime Survey*. Home Office Research Study 182. London: Home Office, 2002.
4.   National Centre for Social Research/National Foundation for Educational Research. *Drug Use, Smoking and Drinking among Young People in England in 2003: headline figures*. London: Department of Health, 2004.
5.   *National Survey on Drug Use and Health*, Substance Abuse and Mental Health Services Administration (SAMHSA), Report ref. 30415. Rockville, MD: Office of Applied Studies, 2002.
6.   Johnston L D, O'Malley P M, Bachman J G, *et al. Ecstasy Use Falls for Second Year in a Row, Overall Teen Drug Use Drops*. National press release, University of Michigan News and Information Services, Ann Arbor, 19 December 2003.
7.   *OxyContin: Pharmaceutical Diversion*. DEA Drug Intelligence Brief. Washington, DC: US Drug Enforcement Administration, March 2002.
8.   Gualtieri J F, Roe S J, Schmidt C L. Lethal consequences following oral abuse of a fentanyl transdermal patch. Proceedings of the 20th International Congress of the European Association of Poisons Centres and Clinical Toxicologists. Amsterdam, the Netherlands, 2–5 May 2000. Abstract 105.

9. Arvanitis M L, Satonik R C. Transdermal fentanyl abuse and misuse. *Am J Emerg Med* 2002; 20: 58–59.

10. Flannagan L M, Butts J D, Anderson W H. Fentanyl patches left on dead bodies – potential source of drug for abusers. *J Forensic Sci* 1996; 41: 320–321.

11. Purucker M, Swann W. Potential for Duragesic patch abuse. *Ann Emerg Med* 2000; 35: 314.

12. Marquardt K A, Tharratt R S. Inhalation abuse of fentanyl patch. *J Toxicol Clin Toxicol* 1994; 32: 75–78.

13. Reeves M D, Ginifer C J. Fatal intravenous misuse of transdermal fentanyl. *Med J Aust* 2002; 177: 552–553.

14. Hibbs J, Perper J, Winek C L. An outbreak of designer drug-related deaths in Pennsylvania. *JAMA* 1991; 265: 1011–1013.

15. Buchanan J F, Brown C F. 'Designer drugs' – a problem in clinical toxicology. *Med Toxicol* 1988; 3: 1–17.

16. Beren A I L, Voets A J, Demedts P. Illicit fentanyl in Europe. *Lancet* 1996; 347: 1334–1335.

17. Withdrawal syndrome and dependence: tramadol too. *Prescrire Int* 2003; 12: 99–100.

18. Adams W H, Rufo R A, Talarico L, *et al*. Thrombocytopenia and intravenous heroin use. *Ann Intern Med* 1978; 89: 207–211.

19. Christie D J, Walker R H, Kolins M D, *et al*. Quinine-induced thrombocytopenia following intravenous use of heroin. *Ann Intern Med* 1983; 143: 1174–1175.

20. Gossop M, Griffiths P, Powis B, *et al*. Frequency of non-fatal heroin overdose: survey of heroin users recruited in non-clinical settings. *BMJ* 1996; 313: 402.

21. Darke S, Ross J, Hall W. Overdose among heroin users in Sydney, Australia, I. Prevalates and correlates of non-fatal overdose. *Addiction* 1995; 91: 405–411.

22. Strang J, Darke S, Hall W, *et al*. Heroin overdose: the case for take-home naloxone. *BMJ* 1996; 312: 1435–1436.

23. Rothman R B. A review of the role of anti-opioid peptides in morphine tolerance and dependence. *Synapse* 1992; 12: 129–138.

24. Tobutt C, Oppenheimer E, Laranjeira R. Health of cohort of heroin addicts from London clinics: 22 year follow-up. *BMJ* 1996; 312: 1458.

25. Department of Health UK, Scottish Office Department of Health, Welsh Office, Department of Health and Social Services Northern Ireland. *Drug Misuse and Dependence – Guidelines on Clinical Management*. London: The Stationery Office, 1999.

26. Strang J, Sheridan J, Barber N. Prescribing injectable and oral methadone to opiate addicts: results from the 1995 national postal survey of community pharmacies in England and Wales. *BMJ* 1996; 313: 270–272.

27. Preston A. *The Methadone Briefing*. London: Island Press, 1996.

28. Faggiano F, Vigna-Taglianti F, Versino E, *et al*. Methadone maintenance at different dosages for opioid dependence (Cochrane review). In: *The Cochrane Library*, Issue 1, 2004. Chichester, UK: John Wiley & Sons Ltd.

29. Drummer O H, Syrjanen M, Opeskin K, *et al*. Deaths of heroin addicts starting on a methadone maintenance programme. *Lancet* 1990; 335: 108.

30. Krantz M J, Kutinsky I B, Robertson A D, *et al*. Dose-related effects of methadone on QT prolongation in a series of patients with torsade de pointes. *Pharmacotherapy* 2003; 23: 802–805.

31. Harding-Pink D. Opioid toxicity – methadone: one person's maintenance dose is another's poison. *Lancet* 1993; 341: 665–666.

32. Binchy J M, Molyneux E M, Manning J. Accidental ingestion of methadone by children in Merseyside. *BMJ* 1994; 308: 1335–1336.

33. Eissenberg T, Bigelow G E, Strain E C, *et al*. Dose-related efficacy of levo-methadyl acetate for treatment of opioid dependence: a randomized clinical trial. *JAMA* 1997; 277: 1945–1951.

34. The European Agency for the Authorisation of Medicinal Products. *EMEA Public Statement on the Recommendations to Suspend the Marketing Authorisation for Orlaam (Levacetylmethadol) in the European Union.* London: EMEA, 19 April 2001. EMEA/8776/01.

35. Farrell M, Hall W. The Swiss heroin trials: testing alternative approaches. *BMJ* 1998; 316: 639.

36. van den Brink W, Hendriks V M, Blanken P, *et al*. Medical prescription of heroin to treatment resistant heroin addicts: two randomized controlled trials. *BMJ* 2003; 327: 310–315.

37. Rehm J, Gschwend P, Steffen T, *et al*. Feasibility, safety, and efficacy of injectable heroin prescription for refractory opioid addicts: a follow-up study. *Lancet* 2001; 358: 1417–1420.

38. Marks J A, Palombella A. Prescribing smokable drugs. *Lancet* 1990; 335: 864.

39. Krausz M, Verthein U, Degkwitz P, *et al*. Maintenance treatment of opiate addicts with codeine – results of a follow-up study. *Addiction* 1998; 93: 1161–1167.

40. Seymour A, Black M, Jay J, *et al*. The role of dihydrocodeine in causing death among drug users in the west of Scotland. *Scott Med J* 2001; 46: 143–146.

41. Banbery J, Wolff K, Raistrick D, *et al*. Dihydrocodeine: a useful tool in the detoxification of methadone-maintained patients. *J Subst Abuse Treat* 2000; 19: 301–305.

42. Gowing L, Farrell M, Ali R, *et al*. Alpha2 adrenergic agonists for the management of opioid withdrawal (Cochrane review). In: *The Cochrane Library*, Issue 1, 2004. Chichester, UK: John Wiley & Sons Ltd.

43. Gowing L, Ali R, White J. Opioid antagonists with minimal sedation for opioid withdrawal (Cochrane review). In: *The Cochrane Library*, Issue 1, 2004. Chichester, UK: John Wiley & Sons Ltd.

44. Gowing L, Ali R, White J. Opioid antagonists under heavy sedation or anaesthesia for opioid withdrawal (Cochrane review). In: *The Cochrane Library*, Issue 1, 2004. Chichester, UK: John Wiley & Sons Ltd.

45. Alper K R, Lotsof H S, Frenken G M N, *et al*. Treatment of acute opioid withdrawal with ibogaine. *Am J Addict* 1999; 8: 234–242.

46. Kirchmayer U, Davoli M, Verster A. Naltrexone maintenance treatment for opioid dependence (Cochrane review). In: *The Cochrane Library*, Issue 1, 2004. Chichester, UK: John Wiley & Sons Ltd.

47. Leavitt S B. Methadone–drug interactions. *Addict Treat Forum* Jan 2004; 1–6.

48. Stockley I H (ed). *Stockley's Drug Interactions*, 6th edn. London: Pharmaceutical Press, 2002.
49. Anderson K. Bronchospasm and intravenous street heroin. *Lancet* 1986; i: 1208.
50. Oliver R M. Bronchospasm and heroin inhalation. *Lancet* 1986; i: 915.
51. Gaeta T J, Hammock R, Spevack T A, *et al*. Association between substance abuse and acute exacerbation of bronchial asthma. *Acad Emerg Med* 1996; 3: 1170–1172.
52. Alldredge B K, Lowenstein D H, Simon R P. Seizures associated with recreational drug abuse. *Neurology* 1989; 39: 1037–1039.
53. Ng S K C, Brust J C M, Hauser W A, *et al*. Illicit drug use and the risk of new-onset seizures. *Am J Epidemiol* 1990; 132: 47–57.
54. Gregory R E, Grossman S, Sheidler V R. Grand mal seizures associated with high-dose intravenous morphine infusions: incidence and possible etiology. *Pain* 1992; 51: 255–258.
55. Smith N T, Benthuysen J L, Bickford R G, *et al*. Seizures during opioid anesthetic induction – are they opioid-induced rigidity? *Anesthesiology* 1989; 71: 852–862.
56. Trigueiro de Araujo M S, Gerard F, Chossegros P, *et al*. Vascular hepatotoxicity related to heroin addiction. *Pathol Anat Histopathol* 1990; 417: 497–503.
57. Jover R, Ponsoda X, Gomez-Lechon M J, *et al*. Potentiation of heroin and methadone hepatotoxicity by ethanol: an *in vitro* study using cultured human hepatocytes. *Xenobiotica* 1992; 22: 471–478.
58. DiFranco M J, Sheppard H W, Hunter D J, *et al*. The lack of association of marijuana and other recreational drugs with progression to AIDS in the San Francisco men's health study. *Ann Epidemiol* 1996; 6: 283–289.
59. Ronald P J M, Robertson J R, Elton R A. Continued drug use and other co-factors for progression to AIDS among injecting drug users. *AIDS* 1994; 8: 339–343.
60. Stefano G B, Scharrer B, Smith E M, *et al*. Opioid and opiate immuno-regulatory processes. *Crit Rev Immunol* 1996; 16: 109–144.
61. Schweitzer C, Keller F, Schmitt F, *et al*. Morphine stimulates HIV replication in primary cultures of human Kupffer cells. *Res Virol* 1991; 142: 189–195.
62. Klimas N G, Blaney N T, Morgan R O, *et al*. Immune function and anti-HTLV-I/II status in anti-HIV-I-negative intravenous drug users receiving methadone. *Am J Med* 1991; 90: 163–170.
63. Carballo-Dieguez A, Sahs J, Goetz R, *et al*. The effect of methadone on immunological parameters among HIV-positive and HIV-negative drug users. *Am J Drug Alcohol Abuse* 1994; 20: 317–329.
64. Yin D, Mufson R A, Wang R, *et al*. Fas-mediated cell death promoted by opioids. *Nature* 1999; 397: 218.
65. Bakir A A, Dunes G. Drugs of abuse and renal disease. *Curr Opin Nephrol Hypertens* 1996; 5: 122–126.
66. Lindow S W, Hendricks M S, Nugent F A, *et al*. Morphine suppresses the oxytocin response in breast-feeding women. *Gynecol Obstet Invest* 1999; 48: 33–37.

67. Begg E J, Malpas T J, Hackett L P, *et al*. Distribution of R- and S-methadone into human milk during multiple, medium to high oral dosing. *Br J Clin Pharmacol* 2001; 52: 681–685.
68. Malpas T J, Darlow B A. Neonatal abstinence syndrome following abrupt cessation of breastfeeding. *N Z Med J* 1999; 112: 12–13.

4

Cannabis

When you return to this mundane sphere from your visionary world,
you would seem to leave a Neapolitan spring for a Lapland winter – to
quit paradise for earth – heaven for hell! Taste the hashish, guest of
mine – taste the hashish!
Alexandre Dumas, 'The Count of Monte Cristo', 1844

History

The term 'cannabis' actually refers to a variety of preparations derived from the Indian hemp, *Cannabis sativa* (Figure 4.1). This dioecious, bushy plant was originally native to India, Bangladesh and Pakistan, but is now much more widely distributed, mainly because of man's intervention. Cannabis has been an important plant historically, with three major uses:

- It has been used for thousands of years as a source of fibre for making rope and textiles.
- The seeds are a source of food and of oil for lamps.
- The resin has been used as a medicine and as an intoxicant.

Cannabis has a long association with humans.[1] It was known to the ancient Chinese at least 5000 years ago and it is mentioned in an Egyptian papyrus dated to 1600 BC. The Greeks and Romans also made use of the cannabis plant. Interestingly, there are no records of these four early civilisations using cannabis intentionally to produce intoxication for pleasure, despite the popularity of alcohol for this purpose. By contrast, there is a relatively long tradition of this practice in eastern Europe, India and 'Arabia'. The taking of cannabis for pleasure in western Europe and the USA began in the mid-19th century, but only became a widespread practice from the 1960s onwards.

Glandular hairs (trichomes), which secrete the resin, are most abundant in the flowering heads and surrounding leaves. The major pharmacologically active constituents of the resin are called cannabinoids. There are over 60 of these but the most important psychoactive compound is delta-9-tetrahydrocannabinol (THC). Cannabidiol and

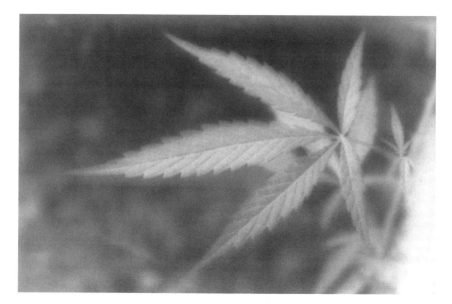

Figure 4.1 The distinctive leaf of *Cannabis sativa*, the Indian hemp.

cannabinol are other constituents that have been extensively investigated for pharmacological activity. The amount of resin secreted is strongly influenced by weather conditions during growth, the sex of the plant (females produce more) and the time of harvest. Cannabis plants are commonly grown outside of their native climate in anticipation of producing a cheap supply of homegrown drug. However, unless grown under specially controlled conditions these plants have a low resin yield because of the particular environmental conditions required by wild strains of the plant for resin production.

Cannabis has several potential medical uses (Table 4.1). Historically, the resin has been used to treat a huge variety of inappropriate conditions and many claims have been made for therapeutic efficacy with little or no evidence to support them. Several synthetic cannabinoids have been investigated for therapeutic efficacy. However, only nabilone and dronabinol are still used medicinally in the West. Dronabinol is structurally identical to naturally occurring THC.

Cannabis is the most commonly used, widely cultivated, and extensively trafficked illicit drug in the world. Population surveys in various countries show that it is widely used (Table 4.2). The United Nations estimated that about 163 million people per year in the world consumed cannabis during 2000–2001.[10] This figure was 2.7% of the world population at the time. In 2003, less than 15% of patients

Table 4.1 Uses of cannabis or cannabinoids

Established uses

Examples of current approved uses for cannabis:

- Chemotherapy-induced nausea and vomiting (e.g. nabilone, dronabinol)
- Appetite stimulation (dronabinol, a synthetic THC, is licensed as an appetite stimulant in patients with AIDS [acquired immunodeficiency syndrome] in the USA)
- Fibre to produce paper, textiles and rope*
- Hempseed oil is used in cosmetics, emollients and some foods*

Medical uses

There is limited evidence of benefit in the following areas, although increasingly the evidence suggests that cannabis is unlikely to have a major therapeutic role:

- Glaucoma (despite some initial enthusiasm cannabis may not be useful in practice[2])
- Pain (gradually accumulating evidence has cast doubt on a clinically useful analgesic role[3,4])
- Multiple sclerosis (research suggests cannabis is not very effective in alleviating symptoms, but some sufferers claim that it can be effective[5–7])
- Epilepsy (cannabidiol might be of some benefit, but early work has not been followed up[8])
- Anxiety (cannabis may have anxiolytic actions, but again old research has not been developed[9])

Historical uses

The following are defunct indications for use, which are no longer considered appropriate:

- Hysteria, depression, 'insanity', dementia
- Jaundice
- Venereal diseases
- Menorrhagia, dysmenorrhoea, difficult labour
- Gut spasm, flatulence, dysentery, cholera
- Tetanus, chorea, Parkinson's disease
- Cough
- Opioid withdrawal
- Aphrodisiac
- General anaesthetic
- Anthelminthic

---

*Varieties with a poor ability to produce resin are cultivated for these purposes.

demanding treatment for an illicit substance abuse problem in Europe, Asia and Australasia had a problem with cannabis; in the American continents this was about 23%, yet in Africa cannabis was the single most common reason for presenting for treatment, affecting over 60% of patients asking for medical help.[10]

The frequency of cannabis use varies. In a large household survey from Australia in 2001 for example, 16% of recent users administered

Table 4.2   Cannabis use amongst the population in national household surveys

Country (year)	% ever used cannabis	% used cannabis in past year	Use in young people	Ref.
Australia (2001)	33	13	34% of 14- to 19-year-olds and 59% of 20- to 29-year-olds had used cannabis at least once.	11
England + Wales (2002)	27	11	44% of 16- to 24-year-olds and 16% of 11- to 15-year-olds had used cannabis at least once.	12, 13
USA (2002)	40	11	In 2003, 18% of 12-year-olds, 36% of 14-year-olds, and 46% of 16-year-olds had used cannabis at least once.	14, 15

cannabis daily, 23% used it at least once per week and 13% about once per month.[11] The remainder used the drug less often. Although daily users were a minority of the recent users, the numbers involved still equate to 2% of the population of Australia.

Effects sought

In general, the desired effects of cannabis start within a few minutes of smoking and within 1–3 hours if ingested (depending on whether food is consumed at the same time). The duration of intoxication is determined by the dose and route. A small dose smoked may give effects lasting for only an hour, whereas larger doses may last up to 4 hours. After oral administration the effects are more persistent and can last 8 hours. As with most other drugs of abuse, the experience is to some extent determined by the surroundings, and the mood, character and expectations of the user.

Cannabis commonly evokes elation (the 'high') and merriment in the initial stages, followed by relaxation, disinhibition and sociability. However, some first-time users report little or no effect. This may be due to inadequate dosage but there is also a high placebo response to cannabis. Regular users claim that one must know what to expect. Cannabis may produce heightened sensory awareness and enhanced imagination: colours and sounds may appear more intense. During intoxication, time may seem to pass more slowly. Only at high dosage will profound illusions or hallucinations appear – these are only rarely reported. As the effects wear off, users often feel drowsy and may sleep.

Administration

The various forms of cannabis have different names, and these are sometimes used interchangeably, causing confusion over their precise meaning. They also vary considerably in their potency. Work in the USA has demonstrated that the concentration of THC in cannabis sold at street level increased by a factor of almost three over the period 1980 to 1997.[16] This is mainly due to carefully controlled growing conditions, selective cultivation of plants with high resin yields, and improved methods of harvesting and preparation. It is important to be aware of this because the side-effects of cannabis are mainly dose-related. In the 1970s the average 'joint' contained about 10 mg of THC, but by the late 1990s this figure had increased to 60–150 mg or even more.[17] The World Health Organization (WHO) estimates that while 2–3 mg of inhaled THC may be sufficient to produce brief euphoria in an occasional user, a heavy user in Jamaica, smoking several times per day, may consume up to 420 mg THC daily.[18]

The following is a brief guide to the three main types of cannabis sold at street level.

Marijuana

This term usually refers to the grey-green dried and crushed flower heads and small leaves of the cannabis plant (Figure 4.2). 'Marijuana' is actually the Hispanic spelling of the word but in American literature, it is often written 'marihuana'. The derivation is obscure. The term is more popular in the USA and is largely synonymous with slang terms such as 'grass', 'dope', 'blow', 'skunk', 'weed', 'pot', 'hemp', 'bhang' and 'ganja'. Marijuana is sometimes used to describe the cannabis plant itself; the alternative is 'hash plant'. Cannabis herb prepared for use in this way contains up to 5% THC.

Hashish

The name hashish typically refers to the cannabis resin alone, after removal from the plant; it is also known as hash (Figure 4.3). The term is derived from the Arabic 'hashish al kief' (dried herb of pleasure). The colour and texture of the resin varies according to the geographical

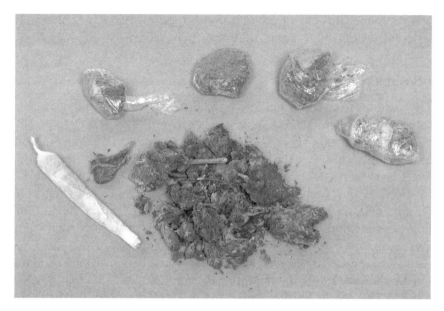

Figure 4.2 Dried cannabis herb (Photo courtesy of Multimedia Research Partners Ltd).

source and purity – it can be soft and putty-like, friable or hard, and red, yellow, brown or black in colour. It is typically brown with a toffee-like texture when pure. Hashish can contain up to 20% THC. Sinsemilla is the strongest variety of hashish, being derived from unfertilised female plants.

Hash oil

Hash oil is a concentrated resin extract and the most potent form of cannabis used. The greenish-black viscous liquid can comprise 60% or more THC.

In Europe, Australia and the Americas, cannabis is nearly always smoked. Marijuana herb can be rolled into pure cigarettes or mixed with tobacco. These are called 'spliffs', 'joints' or 'reefers'. Hashish or hash oil is usually mixed with tobacco first because the amount needed to produce intoxication is quite small. The tobacco acts as a bulking agent and helps the cannabis to burn. Cannabis can also be smoked in a pipe. 'Hot knifing' is another method of burning the pure resin. A hot knife is passed through a block of resin so that some of it sticks and vaporises. The knife is then held under the nose so that the fumes can

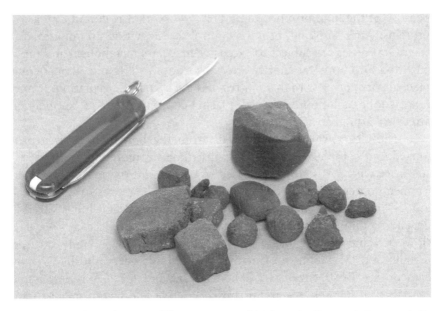

Figure 4.3 Cannabis resin (Photo courtesy of Multimedia Research Partners Ltd).

be inhaled. Bongs or water pipes are commonly used for smoking. Bongs are sealed containers part-filled with water. Cannabis is ignited in a separate container and the smoke is drawn through the water in the bong before the user inhales it via a pipe system connected to the bong. The water cools the smoke and many users believe that some of the carcinogens in the smoke dissolve in the water, providing some measure of protection to the lungs.

Cannabis is also active when eaten or prepared as an infusion to drink. It has been a tradition for centuries in India, the Middle East and North Africa to take cannabis orally. The cannabis drink or confection must be flavoured to disguise the unpleasant taste of the crude resin. Oral administration has not been popular elsewhere because psychoactive effects are slow to begin, unpredictable, can be blunted and are often of long duration.

Pharmacokinetics and pharmacology

After entering the lungs, THC dissolves quickly in pulmonary surfactant, enabling rapid passage into the bloodstream. The high lipophilicity also facilitates quick penetration of the central nervous system (CNS) but the proportion of a dose that crosses the blood–brain barrier is low because of the high proportion of THC (97%) that is bound to plasma proteins. After smoking, peak CNS levels occur within 10 minutes.

Oral doses are subject to extensive first-pass metabolism and rapid partition into body fat shortly after absorption, so despite almost complete absorption, less than 15% reaches the systemic circulation. It may take as long as 6 hours for peak plasma concentrations to be obtained after oral administration.

The clearance of cannabinoids from the human body is a prolonged and complex process. THC distributes rapidly into adipose tissue from where it is slowly released over time. Furthermore, THC and its metabolites are subject to significant tubular reabsorption at the kidney and to enterohepatic recycling. The terminal half-life is variable depending upon circumstances, but is very long and reflects a process of slow clearance as the drug is gradually released from body fat and metabolised. Metabolism of many cannabinoids occurs in the liver by cytochrome P450 enzymes of the CYP2C and CYP3A series. Some cannabinoid metabolites are also psychoactive and have similarly long half-lives to their parent molecules.

The key factors that influence how long it takes for a urine test to become negative after cessation of cannabis intake are the amount and frequency of cannabis use, and the sensitivity and specificity of the detection technique. It may take several weeks for cannabis to be completely eliminated from the body – this clearance time being greater in regular users. For example in one study of 86 supervised long-term regular heavy smokers of cannabis, urine tests were intermittently positive for up to 77 days,[19] although the average time to a negative urine screen was 31.5 days. One case report describes a patient who demonstrated a positive urine test for cannabis after 95 days of supervised abstinence.[20] Yet in those who use cannabis infrequently, the drug is eliminated more quickly; it may still take a few weeks but clearance from urine in as little as 1–3 days has been observed.[19,21,22] It is not clear whether the delayed clearance of cannabis in regular heavy users causes any persistence of, perhaps subtle, biological effects. However, subjectively a cannabis 'trip' only lasts for 1–4 hours after smoking.

The mode of action of cannabis is not clear. There are a large number of cannabinoids and there may consequently be a range of different receptor types within the body. Two apparent receptor subtypes for THC have been located, one in the CNS and certain peripheral tissues ('CB1') and one that seems to be concentrated in the immune system ('CB2'). Endogenous ligands for the CNS receptor have also been identified – anandamide (arachidonylethanolamide), 2-arachidonylglycerol and palmitylethanolamide.[23] These endogenous cannabinoids ('endo-cannabinoids') may have a role in central control of muscle movement, the sensing of pain, appetite, memory, vomiting and anxiety regulation. They also inhibit the secretion of follicle-stimulating hormone and pro-lactin, as does THC.

Adverse effects

The adverse effects of cannabis are summarised in Table 4.3. The **gastrointestinal** effects of cannabis are generally mild. A certain degree of gastrointestinal discomfort is not uncommon, but occasionally there may be frank abdominal pains or nausea and vomiting. During intoxi-cation, cannabis users may become very hungry or thirsty. A desire to eat food during or immediately after intoxication is known as the 'munchies'.

The likelihood of **psychiatric** and **cognitive** adverse effects is deter-mined by a variety of factors, including the dose taken, the route of administration, the expectations of the user, the environment at the time of use, the concomitant use of other drugs, the user's emotional state and whether the individual is suffering from any psychiatric illness. The likelihood of all adverse mental effects generally increases as the dose increases.

Table 4.3 Adverse effects of cannabis

Acute effects
- Anxiety, confusion, drowsiness, panic reactions, dysphoria, psychosis, hallucinations
- Psychomotor impairment, ataxia, impaired judgement, impaired attention and ability to learn, memory loss
- Tachycardia, palpitations, postural hypotension, flushing
- Coughing, sore throat, bronchospasm in people with asthma
- Abdominal pain, delayed gastric emptying, nausea, vomiting, dry mouth, increased appetite
- Red eyes

Effects from long-term use
- Bronchitis
- Cancer of head, neck and lungs especially if smoked with tobacco
- Oligospermia, gynaecomastia, decreased libido (both sexes)
- Insomnia, depression, anxiety, 'flashbacks', social withdrawal, decreased mental performance, reduced drive
- Dependence, withdrawal symptoms on cessation

Cannabis intoxication can give rise to anxiety, dysphoria and confusion. Panic reactions and sedation can also occur. First-time users, in particular, may be especially prone to adverse mental effects, perhaps due to a lack of experience in dealing with the psychotropic actions of the drug. All of these effects on the CNS could increase the chance of accidents or risk-taking behaviour. Impaired judgement, incoordination, slowed reaction times, reduced ability to concentrate and other effects lead cannabis to impair psychomotor performance, which has serious implications for the undertaking of complex tasks (e.g. driving a vehicle). Many studies show a link between positive blood and urine tests for cannabis and road accidents, but disentangling the effects of cannabis from that of other drugs or alcohol that may have been taken at the same time is not easy. In addition, positive urine tests for cannabis can persist for weeks after the acute intoxicating effects have dissipated (see above). Nonetheless, the acute effects of cannabis should be seen as incompatible with driving – the WHO has supported the association between cannabis intoxication and an increased risk of motor vehicle accidents.[18] Whether these effects persist beyond the period of acute intoxication is not clear. Obviously, these ill effects are likely to be exacerbated by the co-ingestion of alcohol, and potentially by use of other psychotropic drugs.

Impairment of short-term memory and ability to concentrate and learn occurs while intoxicated, as occurs with other inebriants such as alcohol.[24–26] However, this effect may persist for some time beyond the period of acute intoxication – one study suggested the effect is reversible within 4 weeks of abstinence;[26] another suggested minimal improvement after 6 weeks of abstinence.[24] The mechanism of this impairment is not understood but it may be caused by damage to neurons in the hippocampus.[27]

Paranoia and acute psychoses are well-known reactions.[28–31] As with many other drugs of abuse it can be very difficult to determine in an individual patient whether cases of psychiatric illness attributed to cannabis are chance associations, true *de novo* drug-induced effects, or whether cannabis has unmasked a latent tendency to such illness. Whatever the mechanism, some individuals without a history of mental illness do experience short-lived, reversible, psychotic reactions lasting for a few days to a few weeks after using cannabis. However, cannabis can also exacerbate symptoms of schizophrenia in people with pre-existing illness who seem to be particularly prone to adverse psychiatric effects from the drug. A link between cannabis use and chronic psychosis has not been proven.

'Flashbacks' have been reported but are rare, and more mild than those observed after using LSD (lysergide) (see Chapter 7). They are, however, sometimes linked to a frightening or unpleasant experience under the influence of cannabis.

The chronic effects of cannabinoids on the CNS are not clearly understood. One early study of ten young male subjects who were chronic heavy cannabis users revealed significant cerebral atrophy.[32] Subsequent studies using more sophisticated techniques (computerised tomography) have not confirmed these findings[33,34] and cannabis is not now thought to cause cerebral damage. Some studies suggest that chronic use may be associated with problems such as depression and anxiety,[35,36] while others do not support this link.[37,38]

Heavy daily abuse of most drugs tends to encourage social isolation and poor personal performance; the same is probably true of cannabis. An 'amotivational syndrome' has been said to exist in some chronic heavy users who seem unable to work towards desirable medium- or long-term objectives. They have a short attention span and can become introverted, apathetic and lacking in drive. These observations may simply reflect the decreased ability to learn as discussed above, but may also represent the effects of ongoing intoxication due to frequent use of cannabis and its persistence in the body. The French poet, Charles Baudelaire, who took the drug himself, wrote a discourse entitled 'The Poem of Hashish' in 1846. In it, he makes the following apposite observation about cannabis:

> But can the drug be said to be truly devoid of side effects when it renders the individual useless to Society and Society unnecessary to the individual?

Cardiovascular side-effects can be important. Tachycardia is commonly reported and patients with ischaemic heart disease may experience an increased frequency of angina symptoms during exercise when using cannabis. Some users experience palpitations but arrhythmias are rare. Postural hypotension is another well-known cardiovascular side-effect, probably caused by dilatation of peripheral veins.[39] The transient cerebral ischaemia which results on assuming an upright position can lead to dizziness and fainting. This may be at least partly caused by impairment of the local regulation of cerebral blood flow.[40] Tachyphylaxis may develop to both orthostatic hypotension and tachycardia after regular administration. Facial flushing may occur in some users. Myocardial infarction (MI) has been reported as an adverse effect in a small number of case reports.[41–44] It is very difficult to know whether cannabis was responsible because of the many other variables that are known to predispose to MI. However, the patients involved were generally younger than the average MI sufferer, and the smoking of cannabis is known to significantly increase cardiac output and decrease the oxygen-carrying capacity of the blood.

Respiratory side-effects are not unexpected from a drug that is primarily administered via smoking, and a chronic productive cough is common in long-term users. Although acute inhalation of smoke containing cannabinoids may produce bronchodilation, the smoke is also irritant and can trigger bronchoconstriction in asthmatics. Chronic use is associated with an increase in airways resistance, an effect caused by an action on large airways.[45] This effect is not seen following tobacco smoking, perhaps because of the way in which the two products are smoked:[46,47]

- The cannabis 'joint' is typically smoked to the very end of the butt, so that the smoke inhaled near the end contains more tar, carbon dioxide and particles, and is also hotter.
- A cannabis cigarette is home-made and so more loosely wrapped than a conventional tobacco cigarette. This may mean that fewer particles and tar are filtered out by the shaft of the cigarette itself. Cannabis cigarettes also do not contain filters.
- Cannabis smokers tend to take longer 'draws' and to inhale more deeply.
- It is common practice to hold the breath for a few seconds after inhaling.

All of these features make the practice potentially more damaging to the airways and allow greater numbers of particles to reach the lower airways. Cannabis cigarettes also produce much more tar than tobacco varieties and, because of the way in which they are smoked, a greater proportion of this tar is retained in the lungs.[46] Consequently, the smoking of three or four cannabis 'joints' per day can produce the same degree of damage to the pulmonary epithelium as 20 or more tobacco cigarettes per day.[48]

Smoking cannabis can cause bronchitis or persistent sore throat, but the link between cannabis smoking and lung cancer is not conclusively proven. This is a difficult subject to study because most users either smoke tobacco as well or use tobacco as a vehicle for smoking cannabis resin. The method of smoking cannabis described above may give any carcinogenic component a greater opportunity to operate on lung tissue because of the increased tissue contact time. The consensus of opinion is that because the risk of tobacco causing lung cancer is dose-related – and qualitatively the tar produced by a cannabis 'joint' is at least as toxic as that from a conventional cigarette – there must be at least some risk of lung cancer from chronic smoking of cannabis. The risk might be thought to be reduced by the fact that most chronic cannabis users actually smoke less often than tobacco smokers, however pre-cancerous changes have been observed in the airways of cannabis smokers and those who only smoke cannabis have higher rates of change than those who only smoke tobacco.[49] Those who smoke both cannabis and tobacco have the highest rates of all.

Cannabis smoking may depress pulmonary defence mechanisms and increase the risk of infection *per se*, but in those with compromised immune function it poses an additional risk that is more specific. Dried cannabis herb can harbour fungal spores that in the immunocompromised patient has been reported to cause infection.[50,51] *Aspergillus* is the genus most likely to be involved. Furthermore, hypersensitivity to this fungus can lead to allergic bronchopulmonary aspergillosis after smoking contaminated drug.[52] The pollen of cannabis plants may also be allergenic – potentially causing significant respiratory symptoms such as asthma exacerbation or allergic rhinitis following inhalation.[53]

The **reproductive** adverse effects have not been researched as thoroughly as might be expected. In one study, men who regularly used cannabis developed decreased testosterone levels and in some this was accompanied by a reduced sperm count.[54] Several other studies have failed to confirm this effect, for reasons that are unclear.[55,56] Even in studies that do show reduced testosterone levels, these are still generally within the normal human range.[55] Studies of decreased sperm count have also not reported infertility.[55,56] However, interestingly, in the 1st century AD, the Roman author Pliny wrote that cannabis could 'dry the seed of procreation'. Chronic use has been claimed to cause gynaecomastia,[57] but very few cases of this effect have been described, leading to speculation that the association may be coincidental.[55,56] Cannabis inhibits ovulation in female animals, but although this effect has been reported in women it is unclear to what extent other confounding variables may have contributed to the observation and how important it is clinically.[56] Effects on pregnancy and breastfeeding are summarised below.

Reddening of the whites of the **eyes** (especially after smoking) is a frequently described reaction, caused by cannabis dilating blood vessels in the cornea.

For some years, there has been controversy over whether cannabis use encourages individuals to take more potent illicit drugs. This is an important question because, of all the illicit drugs, cannabis is the one most likely to be taken first by people under the age of 16. The research in this area has limitations, but large studies, adjusting for many variables and potential confounders, have shown a strong link between the use of cannabis and the subsequent use of, or dependence on, other illicit drugs.[58–60] A novel study from Australia looked at 311 pairs of twins where one twin had used cannabis at an early age (before age 17) and the other had not. Those who used cannabis early had odds for illicit drug use/dependence or alcohol dependence that were 2–5 times higher than in their twin.[61] These studies suggest that for many users of illicit drugs, cannabis is the first illicit drug tried – presumably because it is the most readily available. However, this progression is not inexorable because the vast majority of cannabis users do not subsequently take more potent illicit drugs.

The concept of cannabis as a potential introduction to the use of other drugs of abuse is well established in the minds of the public. In a US telephone survey in 1995, 81% of adolescents interviewed and 64% of adults believed that a young person who used cannabis was more likely to progress to so-called harder drugs.[62]

Dependence

Cannabis is generally considered to be a drug with low dependence potential, and most cannabis users appear to be able to stop taking it easily, without complications. In fact, the majority are occasional rather than regular users. However, dependence can occur following sustained regular exposure that meets the necessary diagnostic criteria for dependence outlined by the American Psychiatric Association (see Chapter 1).[31,63,64]

Furthermore, people who use cannabis regularly at high dose may experience withdrawal symptoms on cessation. These symptoms are mild, but include:

- anxiety, irritability, dysphoria, aggressiveness, restlessness, mood swings
- deranged appetite, weight loss
- stomach pains, nausea, diarrhoea
- tremor
- poor sleep
- hot flushes, sweating, chills
- craving for cannabis.

The time to onset, symptomatic presentation, and prevalence of withdrawal varies considerably between studies that have investigated it.[65] More studies are needed.

Interactions with medicines

Interactions between illicit drugs and conventional medicines have not been systematically studied in humans. Most data are derived from case reports and small-scale laboratory research and so should be interpreted cautiously. It should be noted that many people who use cannabis also smoke tobacco or use other illicit substances and the potential for these substances to interact should not be overlooked. A full medication and substance abuse history is necessary before investigating drug inter-actions in an individual patient. In terms of its potential to interact, cannabis has a range of properties that may make interactions more likely:

• It has sedating actions that would be expected to potentiate the action of other CNS depressants (e.g. benzodiazepines).
• It has other significant side-effects, which may be augmented by concurrent use with medicines that have similar effects (e.g. tachycardia).
• Many cannabis users also smoke tobacco, and this is likely to lead to induction of the enzyme CYP1A2; some evidence suggests that this effect may even occur when cannabis is smoked without tobacco (see theophylline below).
• THC is highly plasma protein bound.
• Cannabinoids are metabolised via cytochrome P450 enzymes (mainly CYP3A and CYP2C).

Some documented interactions involving cannabis and medicines are discussed below.

Atropine

A study of two patients showed that one cannabis cigarette or atropine injection 600 mcg both independently increased heart rate by about 20 beats per minute (bpm).[66] When given together, heart rate increased by approximately 50 bpm and remained significantly elevated for 3 hours. This effect might be anticipated to occur with other antimuscarinic medicines and those with antimuscarinic properties (see tricyclic anti-depressants below).

Barbiturates

Oral THC 60–180 mg per day for 14 days increased the average half-life of pentobarbital from about 17 hours to 21 hours in one investi-gation involving eight subjects.[67] Subjective effects of concurrent use were not described, yet in another study, five out of six volunteers experienced intense unpleasant psychotropic effects when given the combination (e.g. hallucinations, anxiety).[68] Similar effects have been described with secobarbital (quinalbarbitone) and THC.[69]

Cocaine

A study of five illicit drug users investigated the effects of smoking cannabis half an hour before nasal inhalation of cocaine.[70] Cannabis led to a faster onset time for cocaine's psychotropic effects (approximately 0.5 min compared to almost 2 minutes) and a near doubling of cocaine plasma levels. The authors attribute these effects to cannabis causing a vasodilatation in the nasal mucosa, increasing the absorption of cocaine.

Disulfiram

A single case report described a patient who on two separate occasions developed hypomania after smoking cannabis while taking disulfiram.[71] He had previously used cannabis alone without ill effect. However, other patients taking the combination have not reported this reaction.[72]

Fluoxetine

One case of mania has been reported in a patient taking fluoxetine who smoked cannabis.[73] This is the only reported case and should be interpreted cautiously because fluoxetine itself can cause mania – indeed the patient described feeling 'hyper' when subsequently taking fluoxetine in isolation. Mania has not been noted in other patients receiving this combination and one case report would seem insufficient reason to withhold selective serotonin reuptake inhibitor (SSRI) antidepressants from cannabis users, especially given the known problems with prescribing tricyclics. Of note is a study in which fluoxetine or placebo was given to 22 alcoholics for 12 weeks. Despite concomitant cannabis use in all 11 patients receiving fluoxetine, no interaction was reported.[74]

HIV (human immunodeficiency virus) medication

Smoked cannabis has been observed to lower the blood concentrations of both indinavir and nelfinavir, which are metabolised by the enzyme CYP3A4.[75] In 11 patients taking nelfinavir chronically, the area under the curve at 8 hours was reduced by an average of 10%, and the maximum plasma concentration by 17%. In 14 patients receiving long-term indinavir the area under the curve at 8 hours was reduced by an average of 15%, and the maximum plasma concentration by 14%. However, only the effects on maximum indinavir plasma concentration were statistically significant, and the authors concluded that these small changes were unlikely to adversely impact on antiretroviral efficacy.

Lithium

The authors of a case report suggest a possible interaction between smoked cannabis and lithium.[76] Lithium levels were significantly raised to toxic levels during a period when cannabis was smoked, but dropped again when cannabis use ceased. However, the patient had a complex psychiatric history with fluctuating lithium levels. Because cannabis and lithium are excreted by completely different mechanisms it seems unlikely that cannabis caused this effect. The authors propose that cannabis might slow gastrointestinal transit and thereby increase lithium absorption. This is not a very likely mechanism because lithium is usually absorbed rapidly and almost completely. No further reports of an interaction have been published.

Neuroleptics

An investigation of 31 patients taking chlorpromazine revealed that smoking either cannabis or tobacco accelerated the rate of clearance.[77] When tobacco and cannabis were both smoked, chlorpromazine clearance was increased by 107%. However, the number of patients taking cannabis was small ($n = 5$), and the population variance in the clearance of chlorpromazine is wide. Given the popularity of illicit substances in patients with psychotic illness this could be a significant problem, yet these results have never been verified by a repeat study. It is also not known whether other phenothiazines interact in a similar way, but the observation that even patients receiving depot neuroleptics for schizophrenia deteriorate when smoking cannabis has led to speculation that cannabis might antagonise their effects.[78] However, as discussed above, cannabis itself can also cause psychotic symptoms.

Because many people who smoke cannabis also smoke tobacco, it is important to note that stopping cannabis/tobacco smoking may lead to increased levels of clozapine and related drugs as smoking induces the activity of CYP1A2, which metabolises these drugs. One patient previously stable on clozapine developed confusion and increased clozapine levels after stopping cannabis/tobacco smoking.[79]

Opioids

In eight volunteers, intravenous THC (up to 0.134 mg/kg) potentiated the sedative and respiratory depressant effects of intravenous oxymorphone (1 mg/70 kg).[68]

Sildenafil

The authors of a case report suggest that the combination of sildenafil and smoked cannabis may have caused MI in a man aged 41 years.[80] They propose that cannabis inhibited the metabolism of sildenafil to potentiate its effects. However, both drugs have independently been linked to episodes of MI and the patient did not develop chest pain until 12 hours after administration of the combination. Thus an interaction seems unlikely based on this evidence alone.

Theophylline and aminophylline

Two studies have assessed the effect of smoked cannabis on the pharmacokinetics of aminophylline and its active metabolite theophylline.[81,82] In the first, 57 subjects were recruited who smoked cannabis, tobacco, both, or neither.[81] Cannabis smokers used the drug at least twice each week for several months. Clearance of theophylline was measured after a standard single dose of oral aminophylline with the following results:

Subjects	Theophylline half-life (hours)	Theophylline clearance (mL/kg/hour)
Non-smokers (*n* = 9)	8.1	52
Smokers of cannabis alone (*n* = 7)	5.9	73
Smokers of tobacco alone (*n* = 24)	5.7	75
Smokers of cannabis plus tobacco (*n* = 7)	4.3	93

In the second study, non-smokers were compared with 'light' cannabis smokers (less than once per week) and 'heavy' smokers (at least twice per week).[82] The results were as below:

Subjects	Theophylline clearance (mL/kg/hour)
Non-smokers (*n* = 177)	56
Infrequent cannabis smokers (*n* = 9)	54
Frequent cannabis smokers (*n* = 14)	83

Regular smoking of cannabis at least twice per week is therefore likely to markedly accelerate the clearance of theophylline from the body, resulting in decreased theophylline efficacy. The co-smoking of tobacco is likely to further increase the rate of clearance. The effect is probably mediated via induction of CYP1A2, the principal enzyme that metabolises theophylline.

Tricyclic antidepressants

Tricyclic antidepressants (TCAs) and cannabis can cause tachycardia, and seven cases reported in the medical literature describe the combination causing a potentially dangerous additive effect.[83–86] None of the patients involved had cardiac conditions and all were 15–21 years old. In five cases the tachycardia was considered alarming (110–130 bpm) and was accompanied by psychotropic side-effects such as confusion, restlessness, mood swings and hallucinations.[83,84] Symptoms resolved within 48 hours.

In one case, tachycardia (160 bpm) was accompanied by tightness in the chest, pain in the throat and extreme agitation, which necessitated treatment in a casualty department with propranolol.[85] The report was also interesting because the patient was exposed to both TCA and cannabis separately without ill effect. In another case, the tachycardia was so extreme (300 bpm) that it failed to respond to intravenous verapamil.[86] The patient was admitted to an intensive care unit for electroconversion, which was successful. This patient had used cannabis uneventfully before starting a TCA, and he had even smoked occasional single 'joints' while taking a TCA, without problems. On the occasion described in the case report he had smoked a greater than normal amount of cannabis while still taking the TCA.

The TCAs involved in these seven cases were desipramine (3 cases: 150–200 mg/day), nortriptyline (2 cases: 30–75 mg/day), amitriptyline (1 case: 25 mg/day) and imipramine (1 case: 50 mg/day). The published details are generally not sufficient to reveal how quickly the ill effects of the combination can begin, although in one case the onset was within an hour of administration.[84] The ability to cause tachycardia is largely related to the antimuscarinic properties of TCAs. It would be anticipated that those with reduced antimuscarinic actions, such as lofepramine, would be less likely to interact in this way, although this specific combination has not been studied.

Abuse and concurrent illness

Cannabis is widely used, and is also believed to have therapeutic utility for various medical conditions (although historically most potential uses have not withstood close scrutiny). These two factors make it particularly likely that patients with common medical conditions may take cannabis. Note that because cannabis can impair short-term memory, this could adversely affect compliance with prescribed medication. The text below outlines some considerations for these patient groups.

Asthma

Acute administration of both smoked cannabis and oral THC cause a short-lived bronchodilation in patients with asthma.[87] However, chronic administration of drugs that are smoked would be expected to cause respiratory symptoms. When smoked, cannabis impairs gaseous exchange, deposits tar in the lungs and can cause bronchitis. The inhalation of smoke particles could trigger an asthma attack either in the smoker or in those subject to passive smoking. Smoking also increases the risk of chest infections. Regular smoking of cannabis results in markedly accelerated metabolism of theophylline, a drug widely used in the treatment of asthma (see above).

Diabetes

After intravenous THC or smoked cannabis in healthy volunteers, plasma glucose may be elevated above that of non-recipients following a glucose tolerance test.[88,89] Away from the specific setting of a glucose tolerance test, cannabis is not known to have adverse effects upon plasma glucose levels in humans.[89,90] However, cannabis can increase appetite and food consumption, especially of carbohydrates, which may disrupt the balance between food intake and dose of hypoglycaemic drug in those with diabetes. Vomiting is an occasional acute side-effect of cannabis which could also affect this balance adversely. The apathy and poor motivation engendered in some individuals by chronic intoxication/dependence may mitigate against adequate control of blood glucose – this could result in non-compliance with diet, failure to administer medication correctly, or inadequate monitoring. Intoxication may prevent a diabetic recognising and/or dealing with a hypoglycaemic episode. The hypoglycaemic episode can also resemble drug intoxication, so that bystanders may not seek medical attention.

Epilepsy

Cannabis smoking has been described as exacerbating seizures in one published case report[91] and a means of preventing them in another.[92] Similarly, in a survey involving 13 patients with epilepsy who used cannabis, one stated that the drug decreased his seizure frequency, while another said that cannabis caused his seizures; the remainder felt that cannabis had no effect.[93] A study comparing cannabis use amongst 308 patients with new onset seizures discovered that cannabis use was significantly less common in this group than in a similar number of control subjects.[94] The authors suggest this provides evidence for cannabis use having a protective effect against new onset seizures. One of the constituents of cannabis, cannabinol, has been used therapeutically as an anticonvulsant.[95]

Hepatic disease

Cannabinoids are metabolised in the liver. Moderate to severe liver failure might therefore impair clearance. Cannabis is not generally recognised as a cause of liver damage.

Hypertension

Cannabis does not cause hypertension. If anything, it tends to lower blood pressure.

Immunity impairment

Cannabis has traditionally been thought to have immunosuppressive properties. However, the evidence for this is equivocal. *In vitro* studies using high doses of cannabis have demonstrated adverse effects upon mammalian immunity, but clinical studies have not demonstrated a convincing link.[96] Studies of HIV-infected individuals have not supported a link between use of cannabis and progression to AIDS.[97,98]

Regular smoking of any drug increases the risk of respiratory tract infections. In some cases contamination of cannabis with fungi has led to the development of fungal chest infections in those with immunodeficiency.[50,51] Those who are immunosuppressed will be more prone to chest infections.

Renal disease

Cannabis is not known to cause or exacerbate impaired renal function. However, moderate to severe renal impairment might delay excretion of cannabis metabolites, although this has not been formally studied. Patients with uraemia can also show increased sensitivity to the CNS effects of drugs.

Pregnancy and breastfeeding

Pregnancy

Cannabis is commonly used in pregnancy and yet the various studies of its effects do not yield consistent results. Some studies have shown that it increases the likelihood of premature delivery, especially in heavy users, but not all studies have confirmed this. Most suggest that this is not likely to be a significant effect when demographic factors are taken into account. It has also been suggested that cannabis can decrease *in utero* growth, leading to small birth-weight babies. However, again, the majority of studies do not seem to support this.

Cannabis has not been definitively identified as teratogenic. There are case reports and small studies in the medical literature suggesting that cannabis might have a teratogenic effect, but the diverse array of adverse fetal effects mitigates against a drug-related effect. In addition, many of these studies did not exclude potentially confounding variables. If cannabis does cause fetal malformations then the effect is probably rare because most large studies do not reveal a teratogenic effect.

A study in 1989 suggested that fetal exposure to cannabis was associated with an increased risk for developing childhood leukaemia.[99] Ten out of 204 exposed cases had leukaemia, compared to only one of 203 controls. The leukaemia developed at a younger age than normal in the cannabis group (at about 38 months). This study requires confirmation.

The effects of *in utero* cannabis exposure upon subsequent development have been studied. Results suggest that children who were exposed to cannabis during their development as a fetus might suffer from subtle ongoing neurobehavioural changes as they grow older, manifested for example by hyperactivity, impulsivity and inattention. More study is needed.

Breastfeeding

THC passes into breast milk after smoking, or when given orally for therapeutic reasons (dronabinol). It may become concentrated in milk compared to plasma during long-term administration.[100] Despite this, two detailed case reports provided no evidence of acute adverse reactions in the infant.[100] Yet given the nature of cannabis and its actions in humans, which are more subtle than many of the other illicit substances, any effects in babies would probably be difficult to identify. As with tobacco, the baby may be exposed to the drug via passive inhalation of smoke as well as via milk, so parents should avoid smoking in the same room as babies. The long-term effects upon infants have not been studied adequately. One study of 27 babies exposed to cannabis via breast milk revealed no mental or physical differences between exposed babies and controls at 1 year.[101] By contrast, another study showed a deficient motor development at 1 year in cannabis-exposed infants.[102]

In animals, cannabis may reduce lactation by suppressing prolactin secretion.[103] A similar effect has been observed in non-breastfeeding women,[104] but this has not been studied in lactating women.

References

1. Wills S. Cannabis use and abuse by man: an historical perspective. In: Brown D T, ed. *Cannabis: The Genus* Cannabis. Amsterdam: Harwood Academic Publishers, 1998, 1–28.
2. Flach A J. Delta-9-tetrahydrocannabinol (THC) in the treatment of end-stage open-angle glaucoma. *Trans Am Ophthalmol Soc* 2002; 100: 215–222; discussion 222–224.
3. Campbell F A, Tramer M R, Carroll D, *et al*. Are cannabinoids an effective and safe treatment option in the management of pain? A qualitative systematic review. *BMJ* 2001; 323: 13–16.
4. Buggy D J, Toogood L, Maric S. Lack of analgesic efficacy of oral delta-9-tetrahydrocannabinol in postoperative pain. *Pain* 2003; 106: 169–172.
5. Zajicek J, Fox P, Sanders H, *et al*. Cannabinoids for treatment of spasticity and other symptoms related to multiple sclerosis (CAMS study): multicentre randomised placebo-controlled trial. *Lancet* 2003; 362: 1517–1526.
6. Killestein J, Uitdehaag B M, Polman C H. Cannabinoids in multiple sclerosis: do they have a therapeutic role? *Drugs* 2004; 64: 1–11.
7. Page S A, Verhoef M J, Stebbins R A, *et al*. Cannabis use as described by people with multiple sclerosis. *Can J Neurol Sci* 2003; 30: 201–205.
8. Carlini E A, Cunha J M. Hypnotic and antiepileptic effects of cannabidiol. *J Clin Pharmacol* 1981; 21(suppl): S417–427.

9. Nakano S, Gillespie H K, Hollister L E. A model for evaluation of anti-anxiety drugs with the use of experimentally induced stress: Comparison of nabilone and diazepam. *Clin Pharmacol Ther* 1978; 23: 54–62.

10. United Nations Office on Drugs and Crime. *Global Illicit Drug Trends 2003.* Vienna: UNODC, 2004 (available from http://www.unodc.org/pdf/trends2003_www_E.pdf; accessed 17 November 2004).

11. *Statistics on Drug Use in Australia 2002. Drug Statistics Series No. 12.* Cat no. PHE 43. Canberra: Australian Institute of Health and Welfare, February 2003.

12. Aust R, Sharp C, Goulden C. *Prevalence of Drug Use: Key Findings from the 2001/02 British Crime Survey.* Home Office Research Study 182. London: Home Office, 2002.

13. Boreham R, Shaw T, eds. *Drug Use, Smoking and Drinking Among Young People in England 2001.* London: The Stationery Office, 2002.

14. *National Survey on Drug Use and Health,* Substance Abuse and Mental Health Services Administration (SAMHSA), Report ref. 30415. Rockville, MD: Office of Applied Studies, 2002.

15. Johnston L D, O'Malley P M, Bachman J G, *et al. Ecstasy Use Falls for Second Year in a Row, Overall Teen Drug Use Drops.* National press release, University of Michigan News and Information Services, Ann Arbor, 19 December 2003.

16. ElSohly M A, Ross S A, Mehmedic Z, *et al.* Potency trends of delta 9-THC and other cannabinoids in confiscated marijuana from 1980–1997. *J Forens Sci* 2000; 45: 24–30.

17. Ashton C H. Adverse effects of cannabis and cannabinoids. *Br J Anaesth* 1999; 83: 637–649.

18. Division of Mental Health and Prevention of Substance Abuse. *Cannabis: A Health Perspective and Research Agenda.* Geneva: WHO, 1997.

19. Ellis G M Jr, Mann M A, Judson B A, *et al.* Excretion patterns of cannabinoid metabolites after last use in a group of chronic users. *Clin Pharmacol Ther* 1985; 38: 572–578.

20. Kielland K B. Urinary excretion of cannabis metabolites. *Tidsskr Nor Laegeforen* 1992; 10: 1585–1586 [in Norwegian; English abstract].

21. Schwartz R H, Hayden G F, Riddile M. Laboratory detection of marijuana use: experience with a photometric immunoassay to measure urinary cannabinoids. *Am J Dis Child* 1985; 139: 1093–1096.

22. Huestis M A, Mitchell J M, Cone E J. Detection times of marijuana metabolites in urine by immunoassay and GC-MS. *J Anal Toxicol* 1995; 19: 443–449.

23. Mechoulam R, Fride E, DiMarzo V. Endocannabinoids. *Eur J Pharmacol* 1998; 359: 1–18.

24. Schwartz R H, Gruenewald P J, Klitzner M, *et al.* Short-term memory impairment in cannabis-dependent adolescents. *Am J Dis Child* 1989; 143: 1214–1219.

25. Pope H G, Yurgelun-Todd D. The residual cognitive effects of heavy marijuana use in college students. *JAMA* 1996; 275: 521–527.

26. Pope H G Jr, Gruber A J, Hudson J I, *et al.* Neuropsychological performance in long-term cannabis users. *Arch Gen Psychiatry* 2001; 58: 909–915.

27. Chan G C, Hinds T R, Impey S, *et al*. Hippocampal neurotoxicity of delta-9-tetrahydrocannabinol. *J Neurosci* 1998; 18: 5322–5332.

28. Rottanburg D, Ben-Arie O, Robins A H, *et al*. Cannabis-associated psychosis with hypomanic features. *Lancet* 1982; ii: 1364–1366.

29. Andreasson S, Allebeck P, Engstrom A, *et al*. Cannabis and schizophrenia – a longitudinal study of Swedish conscripts. *Lancet* 1987; ii: 1483–1485.

30. Ernst E. Does regular cannabis use cause schizophrenia? *Focus Alt Complement Ther* 2002; 7: 334–336.

31. Johns A. Psychiatric effects of cannabis. *Br J Psychiatry* 2001; 178: 116–122.

32. Campbell A M G, Evans M, Thomson J L G, *et al*. Cerebral atrophy in young cannabis smokers. *Lancet* 1971; ii: 1219–1225.

33. Co B, Goodwin D W, Gado M, *et al*. Absence of cerebral atrophy in chronic cannabis users by computerized transaxial tomography. *JAMA* 1977; 237: 1229–1230.

34. Kuehnle J, Mendelson J H, Davis K R, *et al*. Computed tomographic examination of heavy marihuana smokers. JAMA 1977; 237: 1231–1232.

35. Bovasso G B. Cannabis abuse as a risk factor for depressive symptoms. *Am J Psychiatry* 2001; 158: 2033–2037.

36. Troisi A, Pasini A, Saracco M, *et al*. Psychiatric symptoms in male cannabis users not using other illicit drugs. *Addiction* 1998; 93: 487–492.

37. Degenhardt L, Hall W, Lysnkey M. The relationship between cannabis use, depression and anxiety among Australian adults: findings from the National Survey of Mental Health and Well-Being. *Soc Psychiatry Psychiatr Epidemiol* 2001; 36: 219–227.

38. Green B E, Ritter C. Marijuana use and depression. *J Health Soc Behav* 2000; 41: 40–49.

39. Merritt J C. Orthostatic hypotension after delta-9-tetrahydrocannabinol marihuana inhalation. *Ophthal Res* 1982; 14: 124–128.

40. Mathew R J, Wilson W H, Humphreys D, *et al*. Middle cerebral artery velocity during upright posture after marijuana smoking. *Acta Psychiatr Scand* 1992; 86: 173–178.

41. Collins J S A, Higginson J D S, Boyle D M C, *et al*. Myocardial infarction during marijuana smoking in a young female. *Eur Heart J* 1985; 6: 637–638.

42. Macinnes D C, Miller K M. Fatal coronary artery thrombosis associated with cannabis smoking. *J R Coll Gen Pract* 1984; 34: 575–576.

43. Coutselinis A, Michalodimitrakis M. Myocardial infarction and marijuana. *Clin Toxicol* 1981; 18: 389–390.

44. Pearl W, Choi Y S. Marijuana as a cause of myocardial infarction. *Int J Cardiol* 1992; 34: 353.

45. Tashkin D P, Coulson A H, Clark V A, *et al*. Respiratory symptoms and lung function in habitual heavy smokers of marijuana alone, smokers of marijuana and tobacco, smokers of tobacco alone, and non-smokers. *Am Rev Respir Dis* 1987; 135: 209–216.

46. Wu T-Z, Tashkin D P, Djahed B, *et al*. Pulmonary hazards of smoking marijuana compared with tobacco. *N Engl J Med* 1988; 318: 347–351.

47. Tashkin D P, Gliederer F, Rose J, *et al*. Tar, CO, and delta-9-THC delivery from the 1st and 2nd halves of a marijuana cigarette. *Pharmacol Biochem Behav* 1991; 40: 657–661.

48. Gong H, Fligiel S, Tashkin DP, *et al.* Tracheobronchial changes in habitual, heavy smokers of marijuana with and without tobacco. *Am Rev Respir Dis* 1987; 136: 142–149.

49. Hall W. The respiratory risks of cannabis smoking. *Addiction* 1998; 93: 1461–1463.

50. Chusid M J, Gelford J A, Nutter C, *et al.* Pulmonary aspergillosis, inhalation of contaminated marijuana smoke, chronic granulomatous disease. *Ann Intern Med* 1975; 82: 682–683.

51. Hamadeh R, Ardelai A, Locksley R M, *et al.* Fatal aspergillosis associated with smoking contaminated marijuana in a marrow transplant recipient. *Chest* 1988; 94: 432–433.

52. Llamas R, Hart D R, Schneider N S. Allergic bronchopulmonary aspergillosis associated with smoking moldy marihuana. *Chest* 1978; 73: 871–872.

53. Stokes J R, Hartel R, Ford L B, *et al.* Cannabis (hemp) positive skin tests and respiratory symptoms. *Ann Allergy Asthma Immunol* 2000; 85: 238–240.

54. Kolodny R C, Masters W H, Kolodner R, *et al.* Depression of plasma testosterone levels after chronic intensive marihuana use. *N Engl J Med* 1974; 290: 872–874.

55. Wills S. Side effects of cannabis use and abuse. In: Brown D T, ed. *Cannabis: The Genus* Cannabis. Amsterdam: Harwood Academic Publishers, 1998, 253–277.

56. Abel E L. Marihuana and sex: a critical survey. *Drug Alcohol Depend* 1981; 8: 1–22.

57. Harmon J, Aliapoulios M A. Gynecomastia in marihuana users. *N Engl J Med* 1972; 287: 936.

58. Fergusson D M, Horwood L J, Swain-Campbell N. Cannabis use and psychosocial adjustment in adolescence and young adulthood. *Addiction* 2002; 97: 1123–1135.

59. Fergusson D M, Horwood L J. Does cannabis use encourage other forms of illicit drug use? *Addiction* 2000; 95: 505–520.

60. Degenhardt L, Hall W, Lysnkey M. The relationship between cannabis use and other substance use in the general population. *Drug Alcohol Depend* 2001; 64: 319–327.

61. Lysnkey M T, Heath A C, Bucholz K K, *et al.* Escalation of drug use in early-onset cannabis users vs co-twin controls. *JAMA* 2003; 289: 427–433.

62. News. Teens cite illicit drugs as major worry, see marijuana as gateway. *Am J Health Syst Pharm* 1995; 52: 2170, 2174.

63. Miller N S, Gold M S. The diagnosis of marijuana (cannabis) dependence. *J Subst Abuse Treat* 1989; 6: 183–192.

64. McRae A L, Budney A J, Brady K T. Treatment of marijuana dependence: a review of the literature. *J Subst Abuse Treat* 2003; 24: 369–376.

65. Smith N T. A review of the published literature into cannabis withdrawal symptoms in human users. *Addiction* 2002; 97: 621–632.

66. Beaconsfield P, Ginsburg J, Rainsbury R. Marijuana smoking: cardiovascular effects in man and possible mechanisms. *N Engl J Med* 1972; 287: 209–212.

67. Benowitz N, Jones R T. Effects of delta-9-tetrahydrocannabinol on drug distribution and metabolism: antipyrine, pentobarbital and ethanol. *Clin Pharmacol Ther* 1977; 22: 259–268.

68. Johnstone R E, Lief P L, Kulp R A, *et al*. Combination of delta-9-tetrahydro-cannabinol with oxymorphone or pentobarbital: effects on ventilatory control and cardiovascular dynamics. *Anesthesiology* 1975; 42: 674–684.

69. Lemberger L, Dalton B, Martz R, *et al*. Clinical studies of the interaction of psychopharmacologic agents with marihuana. *Ann N Y Acad Sci* 1976; 281: 219–228.

70. Lukas S E, Sholar M, Kouri E, *et al*. Marihuana smoking increases plasma cocaine levels and subjective reports of euphoria in male volunteers. *Pharmacol Biochem Behav* 1994; 48: 715–721.

71. Lacoursiere R B, Swatek R. Adverse interaction between disulfiram and marijuana: a case report. *Am J Psychiatry* 1983; 140: 243.

72. Rosenberg C M, Gerrein J R, Schnell C. Cannabis in the treatment of alcoholism. *J Stud Alcohol* 1978; 39: 1955.

73. Stoll A L, Cole J O, Lukas S E. A case of mania as a result of fluoxetine-marijuana interaction. *J Clin Psychiatry* 1991; 52: 280–281.

74. Cornelius J R, Salloum I M, Haskett R F, *et al*. Fluoxetine versus placebo for the marijuana use of depressed alcoholics. *Addict Behav* 1999; 24: 111–114.

75. Kosel B W, Aweeka F T, Benowitz N L, *et al*. The effects of cannabinoids on the pharmacokinetics of indinavir and nelfinavir. *AIDS* 2002; 16: 543–550.

76. Ratey J J, Ciraulo D A, Shader R I. Lithium and marijuana. *J Clin Psychopharmacol* 1981; 1: 32–33.

77. Chetty M, Miller R, Moodley S V. Smoking and body weight influence the clearance of chlorpromazine. *Eur J Clin Pharmacol* 1994; 46: 523–526.

78. Knudsen P, Vilmar T. Cannabis and neuroleptic agents in schizophrenia. *Acta Psychiatr Scand* 1984; 69: 162–174.

79. Zullino D F, Delessert D, Eap C B, *et al*. Tobacco and cannabis smoking cessation can lead to intoxication with clozapine or olanzapine. *Int Clin Psychopharmacol* 2002; 17: 141–143.

80. McLeod A L, McKenna C J, Northridge D B. Myocardial infarction following the combined recreational use of Viagra and cannabis. *Clin Cardiol* 2002; 25: 133–134.

81. Jusko W J, Schentag J J, Clark J H, *et al*. Enhanced biotransformation of theophylline in marijuana and tobacco smokers. *Clin Pharmacol Ther* 1978; 24: 406–410.

82. Jusko W J, Gardner M J, Mangione A, *et al*. Factors affecting theophylline clearances: age, tobacco, marijuana, cirrhosis, congestive heart failure, obesity, oral contraceptives, benzodiazepines, barbiturates, and ethanol. *J Pharm Sci* 1979; 68: 1358–1366.

83. Wilens T, Biederman J, Spencer T J. Case study: adverse effects of smoking marijuana while receiving tricyclic antidepressants. *J Am Acad Child Adolesc Psychiatry* 1997; 36: 45–48.

84. Kizer K W. Possible interaction of TCA and marijuana. *Ann Emerg Med* 1980; 19: 444.

85. Hillard J R, Vieweg W V R. Marked sinus tachycardia resulting from the synergistic effects of marijuana and nortriptyline. *Am J Psychiatry* 1983; 140: 626–627.

86. Mannion V. Case report: adverse effects of taking tricyclic antidepressants and smoking marijuana. *Can Fam Physician* 1999; 45: 2683–2684.

87. Tashkin D P, Shapiro B J, Frank I M. Acute effects of smoked marijuana and oral delta-9-tetrahydrocannabinol on specific airway conductance in asthmatic subjects. *Am Rev Respir Dis* 1974; 109: 420–428.

88. Hollister L E, Reaven G M. Delta-9-tetrahydrocannabinol and glucose tolerance. *Clin Pharmacol Ther* 1974; 16: 297–302.

89. Podolsky S, Pattavina C G, Amaral M A. Effect of marijuana on the glucose-tolerance test. *Ann N Y Acad Sci* 1971; 191: 54–60.

90. Hollister L E, Richards R K, Gillespie H K. Comparison of tetrahydrocannabinol and synhexyl in man. *Clin Pharmacol Ther* 1968; 9: 783–791.

91. Keeler M H, Reifler C F. Grand mal convulsions subsequent to marijuana use. *Dis Nerve Syst* 1967; 18: 474–475.

92. Consroe P F, Wood G C, Buchsbaum H. Anticonvulsant nature of marihuana smoking. *JAMA* 1975; 234: 306–307.

93. Feeney D M. Marihuana use among epileptics. *JAMA* 1976; 235: 1105.

94. Brust J C M, Ng S K C, Hauser A W, *et al.* Marijuana use and the risk of new onset seizures. *Trans Am Clin Climatol Assoc* 1992; 103: 176–181.

95. Carlini E A, Cunha J M. Hypnotic and antiepileptic effects of cannabidiol. *J Clin Pharmacol* 1981; 21(suppl): S417–427.

96. Hollister L E. Marijuana and immunity. *J Psychoactive Drugs* 1992; 24: 159–164.

97. DiFranco M J, Sheppard H W, Hunter D J, *et al.* The lack of association of marijuana and other recreational drugs with progression to AIDS in the San Francisco men's health study. *Ann Epidemiol* 1996; 6: 283–289.

98. Ronald P J M, Robertson J R, Elton R A. Continued drug use and other co-factors for progression to AIDS among injecting drug users. *AIDS* 1994; 8: 339–343.

99. Robison L L, Buckley J D, Daigle A E, *et al.* Maternal drug use and risk of childhood nonlymphoblastic leukaemia among offspring: an epidemiologic investigation implicating marijuana. *Cancer* 1989; 63: 1904–1911.

100. Perez-Reyes M, Wall M E. Presence of tetrahydrocannabinol in human milk. *N Engl J Med* 1982; 307: 819–820.

101. Tennes K, Avitable N, Blackard C, *et al.* Marijuana: prenatal and postnatal exposure in the human. *NIDA Res Monogr* 1985; 59: 48–60.

102. Astley S J, Little R E. Maternal marijuana use during lactation and infant development at one year. *Neurotoxicol Teratol* 1990; 12: 161–168.

103. Haclerode J. The effect of marijuana on reproduction and development. *NIDA Res Monogr* 1980; 31: 137–166.

104. Mendelson J H, Mello N K, Elingboe J. Acute effects of marijuana smoking on prolactin levels in human females. *J Pharmacol Exp Ther* 1985; 123: 220–222.

5

Cocaine

Save for the occasional use of Cocaine he had no vices, and he only turned to the drug as a protest against the monotony of existence ...
Dr Watson describing Sherlock Holmes in 'The Adventure of the Yellow Face', Sir Arthur Conan Doyle, 1893

History

Cocaine occurs naturally in the leaves of the coca plant, *Erythroxylum coca*, and certain related species originating from South America, especially Peru, Bolivia and Colombia (Figure 5.1). The Incas considered the plant a divine gift and only the higher echelons of society were allowed to use it. Conversely, all levels of Andean Indian society have used the leaves as a masticatory for thousands of years. The leaves are combined with slaked lime or plant ash to produce an alkaline medium, which enables the cocaine base to form a solution in saliva and thus enter the circulation. Chewing the leaves helps the Indians tolerate hunger, exposure and fatigue at high altitudes, where the working environment can be hostile. Cocaine provides a stimulus to manual labour, therefore, as well as inducing feelings of pleasure. The leaves contain around 1% cocaine.

In about 1860, the alkaloid cocaine was isolated and identified as the active constituent of the coca plant. It was subsequently employed medicinally as a local anaesthetic. Karl Koller was probably the first to use it in humans, when he performed eye surgery in 1884. Not surprisingly, the psychoactive properties of the drug were soon discovered and taken advantage of by healthcare professionals – Sigmund Freud famously abused it. As with opium, the advent of cocaine abuse in the general population was initially facilitated by its inclusion in a variety of over-the-counter (OTC) medicines and tonics, including the first form of the beverage Coca Cola. Eventually the availability of cocaine was restricted by legislation. There was a resurgence in cocaine abuse in the 1960s and usage has progressively increased since then.

When the recreational use of cocaine developed outside South America, the form initially involved was a water-soluble salt: crystalline

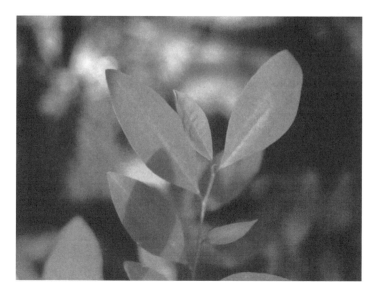

Figure 5.1 A small coca bush (*Erythroxylum coca*). The leaves contain about 1% cocaine.

cocaine hydrochloride (Figure 5.2). This is still the commonest form of the drug used; it is often mixed with various diluents and adulterants on the street to form a white or off-white powder and is usually known as coke, snow, or C. 'Crack' is a highly pure form of the freebase of cocaine (i.e. it is not a salt of cocaine like cocaine hydrochloride). The name is thought to originate from the cracking noises that lumps of freebase make when heated up. This noise is probably caused by impurities in the cocaine remaining from the extraction process (e.g. sodium bicarbonate, sodium chloride). 'Crack' began to be available on a large scale in the USA in the mid-1980s (Figure 5.3).

Until the 1980s cocaine was viewed as an expensive drug, used more by the wealthier sections of the population. However, the number of users at all levels of society has increased. This is probably because cocaine has a reputation as a 'clean' drug and the street price has decreased considerably. Other factors influencing the greater demand for the drug may include the increased availability of very pure forms of cocaine such as 'crack', and the fact that various forms of the drug can produce rapid-onset, short-lived, but intense effects without the need for injection.

The annual quantity of cocaine produced worldwide was judged to be approximately 800 tonnes in 2002,[1] and all of it originated from South America – 72% from Colombia, 20% from Peru and 8% from

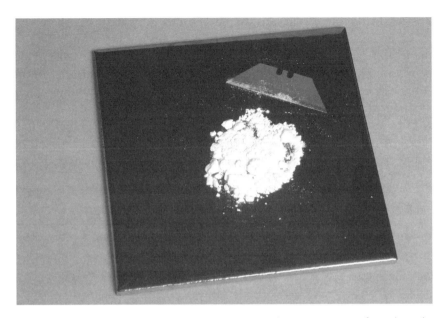

Figure 5.2 Cocaine hydrochloride powder (Photo courtesy of Multimedia Research Partners Ltd).

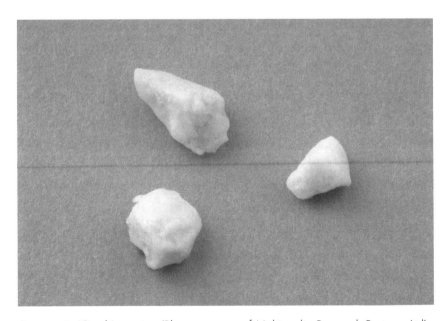

Figure 5.3 'Crack' cocaine (Photo courtesy of Multimedia Research Partners Ltd).

Bolivia. In the same year, the United Nations estimated that there was 173,000 hectares of land devoted to coca bush cultivation.[1] This is the lowest estimate since 1988. Cocaine is abused by about 14 million people across the globe but these users are mainly concentrated in the American continents. In 2003, about 4% of patients demanding treatment for an illicit substance abuse problem in Europe had a problem with cocaine; in Asia and Australasia this was 1% or less. However, in North America the figure was 40% and in South America nearly 60%. Table 5.1 gives data on population prevalence of cocaine use in Australia, England/Wales and the USA.

Table 5.1 Cocaine use amongst the population in national surveys

Country (year)	Used at least once in lifetime by adults	Used in last year by adults	Ref.
Australia (2001)	4.4%	1.3%	2
England + Wales (2002)	–	2.0% for cocaine 0.2% for crack cocaine	3
USA (2002/3)	14.4% for cocaine 3.6% for crack cocaine	2.5% for cocaine 0.7% for crack cocaine	4

Effects sought

When cocaine hydrochloride is injected or crack cocaine is smoked, users experience a sudden 'rush' of exhilaration as the drug enters the brain. This occurs because the drug reaches the central nervous system (CNS) very quickly. The sudden intense 'rush' is not a feature of nasal insufflation of the hydrochloride salt because absorption across the nasal mucous membranes is slow and a feeling of euphoria takes longer to develop (it is probably partly retarded by the vasoconstrictor actions of cocaine, which restrict blood flow to the site).

The desired effects of cocaine are heralded by a series of adrenaline-like reactions caused by stimulation of the sympathetic nervous system and release of adrenaline. Generally, the mental effects produced by cocaine are feelings of euphoria, alertness, excitement and rapid flow of thought. This may manifest as hyperactivity, increased confidence, talkativeness and, sometimes, emotional lability. When intoxicated, users may feel indifferent to matters that normally cause them great concern.

Cocaine is a stimulant; it helps to combat fatigue and subjectively there may be feelings of increased capacity to do work, great physical strength and mental supremacy. It is commonly taken with opioids because they seem to enhance the effects of cocaine. A 'speedball' is a mixed injection of heroin and cocaine favoured by some users.

Administration

The usual method of using cocaine hydrochloride is to arrange the powder in a line on a flat surface and inhale it nasally via a small tube (e.g. a drinking straw or rolled paper). This method of nasal insufflation is called 'snorting'. Sometimes the small amount remaining on the surface after inhaling is rubbed onto the gums.

The hydrochloride salt of cocaine has a high melting point (197°C) and is not very stable when heated to high temperature. It is therefore costly and wasteful to smoke because large amounts need to be used. The freebase form of cocaine has greater thermal stability and a lower melting point (98°C), making it a more suitable preparation to smoke. Individuals can produce base cocaine by treating ('washing back') cocaine hydrochloride with an alkali (ammonia), followed by heating. When base cocaine is produced in this way, it is called 'freebase', and the technique is called 'freebasing'. 'Crack' cocaine is ready prepared base cocaine that has been manufactured on a large scale and sold on the street. In large-scale manufacture, the alkali used tends to be sodium bicarbonate.

'Crack' and 'freebase' may be smoked in a pipe, heated on foil and the vapour inhaled, or smoked with tobacco in a cigarette.

Injection of cocaine is a less popular method of abuse than smoking or insufflation. The hydrochloride is generally used because it is much more water-soluble than 'crack'. However, in one study, over 20% of crack users were found to have attempted to inject the freebase.[5] After injection the time to onset of action and peak effects are similar to those seen with crack smoking.

Cocaine is active when taken orally but is not commonly taken by this route because the onset of action is too slow and the effects are much less intense.

When a user 'freebases', smokes 'crack' or injects cocaine hydrochloride, the psychoactive effects begin within seconds but peak after a few minutes. To maintain the desired euphoria the technique must be repeated frequently. Repeated use of drug in this way is described as a 'run' or a 'binge'. It may continue until the individual is exhausted or until the supply of drug runs out. The peak effects from nasal insufflation or oral administration take longer to develop: 15–30 minutes for nasal insufflation, up to an hour when taken orally. Hence abuse via these routes is less likely to be associated with a 'run'. After a 'run' or a single dose, an individual may 'crash', i.e. experience post-cocaine dysphoria.

Pharmacokinetics and pharmacology

The half-life of cocaine *in vivo* varies from 30 to 90 minutes in humans.[6-8] The average is probably about 60 minutes. There may be a moderate increase in half-life as the dose increases.[7] The psychotropic effects of the drug last for varying lengths of time, depending on the method of administration, as shown in Table 5.2.

The majority of a cocaine dose (about 90%) undergoes hydrolysis. This occurs via both spontaneous hydrolysis in plasma and enzyme action.[8] Plasma and liver esterases catalyse the breakdown of cocaine to metabolites that may have some action on the sympathetic nervous system but which are not thought to be psychoactive. The major hydrolytic metabolites are benzoylecgonine, ecgonine methyl ester, and ecgonine.[8,9] These are excreted in urine. The remaining proportion, which is not hydrolysed, is metabolised in the liver by N-demethylation. The ultimate product of this minor metabolic pathway, norcocaine nitroxide, has been proposed as the cause of cocaine-induced hepatotoxicity (see below).[10]

Cocaine inhibits reuptake of dopamine, noradrenaline and serotonin in central and peripheral nerve synapses and so effectively prolongs and augments their effects. It seems particularly to increase the concentration of neurotransmitters in dopaminergic areas of the brain. The inhibition of dopamine reuptake is believed to cause euphoria and this is the main reason why users continue to take the drug. Mice that have been genetically manipulated so that they lack a central dopamine reuptake mechanism at synapses do not respond to cocaine at all.[11] Cocaine may also increase the release of noradrenaline into sympathetic

Table 5.2 Time course of psychoactive effects of cocaine

Form of cocaine	Administration method	Time to peak effects	Duration of effects
Hydrochloride	Intravenous	< 5 min	30–45 min
Hydrochloride	'Snorted'	10–15 min	60–90 min
'Crack'	Smoked	< 3 min	15–20 min

nervous system synapses and stimulate the release of adrenaline from the adrenals.

In the laboratory setting, many experienced users, given unidentified drugs to inject, cannot distinguish between the effects of cocaine and those of amfetamine. This is not surprising as they produce similar net effects at the synapse level, although by different mechanisms. Both drugs increase the activity of similar CNS neurotransmitters, have stimulant properties and enhance the peripheral sympathetic nervous system. Their similarity is further supported by study of side-effect profiles, which are remarkably alike. The main obvious difference between them is that cocaine has a much shorter duration of action.

Adverse effects

The importance and prevalence of serious side-effects to cocaine is underscored by an analysis of emergency department attendances due to illicit drugs in the USA, where cocaine use is common: for many years it has been the illicit drug responsible for the greatest number of emergency department attendances.[12]

As with many drugs of abuse, the most serious side-effects are often a consequence of acute overdosage or chronic use of high doses. Potential acute adverse reactions, occurring within a few hours of taking cocaine, are summarised in Table 5.3. There is no specific antidote for cocaine intoxication or overdose *per se*, at least not in the same way that naloxone can be given to counteract heroin overdose.

Note that some of the painful adverse effects of cocaine, particularly injuries local to the upper airway if smoked or to the site of injection, may be masked initially by the local anaesthetic effect of the drug.

The **cardiac toxicity** of cocaine has been studied in some detail because many deaths have been attributed to this adverse effect. The effects upon the heart in any one person are unpredictable but cocaine has been reported to cause a variety of cardiac adverse effects (see Table 5.3), of which myocardial infarction (MI) is the most commonly reported in the medical literature. MI has been documented in numerous case reports and the likelihood of infarction does not seem to be related to duration of use, frequency of use, or method of administration. The risk of MI is greatest during the hour after administration.

Analysis of published cases reveals a comparatively young age at diagnosis, with an average of 34 years.[17] Victims are typically healthy, without significant risk factors for cardiovascular disease other than tobacco smoking, and most are male; a thrombus and atherosclerosis is

Table 5.3 Adverse reactions to cocaine

Acute reactions
- Initial adrenaline-like effects such as tachycardia, mydriasis, sweating, tremor, flushing, reduced appetite, headaches
- Nausea, vomiting, abdominal pain, gastrointestinal ischaemia and haemorrhage
- Chest pain, black sputum, wheeziness, shortness of breath, respiratory arrest
- Hypertension, palpitations, tachyarrhythmias, myocarditis, ventricular fibrillation, cardiac arrest, sudden death
- Stroke, convulsions
- Muscle twitches, dystonic or choreoathetoid movements, rhabdomyolysis (with or without hyperpyrexia and sequelae)[13]
- Anxiety, agitation, paranoia, insomnia; hallucinations (visual, auditory, tactile) after large doses; acute psychotic reactions, panic reactions, violence[14]
- Liver damage
- Cocaine may induce heightened sexual interest, which may result in acquisition of sexually transmitted diseases or unwanted pregnancies; it can also cause priapism[15]
- Intoxication may facilitate accidents or participation in risk-taking behaviour[16]
- After a 'run' there is frequently a 'crash', characterised by dysphoria, depression, irritability and craving for the drug; this is often followed by fatigue and sleep

Long-term use
- Gastrointestinal ulcers, dental erosions
- Anorexia, weight loss, malnutrition
- Hypertension, cardiomyopathy
- Perforation of nasal septum, rhinitis, anosmia, nosebleeds
- 'Crack lung' and other forms of respiratory damage
- Chronic anxiety, depression, psychotic-like reactions, anhedonia
- Thrombocytopenia
- Dependence

---

often absent at post-mortem. Four main mechanisms for cocaine causing MI have been proposed:[18]

1. Cocaine stimulates platelet aggregation by various mechanisms, which could result in thrombosis. Platelet-rich thrombi may be found in the coronary vessels of some victims.
2. Increased blood pressure and heart rate caused by cocaine, via peripheral and/or central mechanisms, could trigger myocardial ischaemia. In patients with pre-existing ischaemic heart disease, cocaine can have an apparently sympathomimetic effect on the heart, increasing myocardial oxygen demands to the extent that angina pains occur and sometimes MI. However, the majority of patients who have suffered an MI as a result of

taking cocaine do not have pre-existing symptomatic heart disease but asymptomatic coronary artery disease could be enough to tip the balance.

3. Research has shown that cocaine can cause coronary vasospasm. The exact mechanism of this is uncertain, but it could be a direct vaso-constriction caused by cocaine itself, the catecholamines that it can re-lease, or increased release of a potent vasoconstrictor called endothelin-1. Cocaine abuse can cause endothelial damage and vasospasm could consequently be at least partly due to a reduction in the synthesis of endothelium-derived vasodilators such as nitric oxide or prostacyclin. In one study, coronary vasospasm closely mirrored the time course of cocaine plasma levels. However, spasm also occurred when there was a later peak in cocaine metabolites, so these may also be important in the aetiology of cocaine cardiotoxicity with delayed onset.[19]

4. Prolonged cocaine use is associated with an increased risk of premature atherosclerosis and narrowing of the lumen of coronary vessels.

Arrhythmias produced by cocaine may simply be secondary to the sym-pathomimetic effects of the drug. However, arrhythmias could arise as a result of other adverse cardiovascular effects of cocaine (MI or reper-fusion after coronary artery spasm). Cocaine, as a local anaesthetic, also has direct membrane-stabilising effects on the myocardium itself and can be demonstrated to prolong the QT interval on an electrocardio-gram (ECG). Chronic use of cocaine has been linked to left ventricular hypertrophy and dilated cardiomyopathy.[17]

Chest pain is quite a common complaint. A study of 217 chronic 'crack' smokers showed that 39% suffered pains in the chest within an hour of smoking cocaine; 64% reported a pain that was made worse by taking a deep breath.[20] The cause of the pain is unclear; there may be more than one kind of pain and therefore a variety of causes. The pain is generally short-lived. It could be due to cocaine-induced MI or car-diac ischaemia, but when a series of 100 chest-pain patients were given an ECG, only 8% had a trace typical of an MI.[21] Researchers have sug-gested inflammation of pleural membranes as a cause because of the pain on inspiration.[20] Thoracic muscle rhabdomyolysis has also been suggested,[21,22] and this is consistent with the high creatinine kinase levels observed in such patients. Involvement of pectoral or intercostal muscles would explain why the pain can be more intense on inspiration. In those taking amfetamine derivatives, similar pains have been attributed to spasm of the intercostal muscles.[23] It is not known how cocaine could be toxic to skeletal muscle. If it is capable of causing pro-longed spasm this could give rise to rhabdomyolysis, although why tho-racic muscles should be specifically involved is not understood. The pain might also be caused by various acute respiratory effects (e.g. broncho-constriction, thermal damage, pulmonary infarction). Three cases identified in the UK all had cough, dyspnoea and fever as well as chest pain, and the authors diagnosed pneumonitis.[24] These symptoms were attributed to an 'impurity', although the authors failed to explain why they believed this was the cause.

The **respiratory** effects of cocaine are diverse. The adverse effects of smoking are probably caused by a combination of factors such as inhaling the products of cocaine and adulterant pyrolysis, the hot nature of the smoke, the vasoconstricting action of cocaine, and the caustic action of ammonia in 'freebase' cocaine. Chronic smoking or inhalation of hot cocaine vapour can cause sore throats and a hoarse voice. However, cocaine can produce more extensive effects on the rest of the respiratory tract. Wheezing has been described in up to a third of 'freebase' smokers.[25] A US study of 217 chronic smokers of freebase revealed that 44% of subjects had reported coughing up black sputum within 12 hours of use and that 6% had experienced haemoptysis.[20] Chronic users often have a cough and may suffer from bouts of wheeziness or a hoarse voice. Haemoptysis occurs particularly with crack cocaine and in some of these patients, measurements of lung function can reveal alveolar damage with deterioration in gaseous exchange capacity, alveolar infiltration by eosinophils and a fever. The cause of the condition is not clear, although it may respond to treatment with corticosteroids. Other pulmonary complications appear to be rare but include pulmonary oedema, pneumo-mediastinum, pneumothorax and bronchiolitis.[26]

Regular snorting of cocaine commonly results in perforation of the nasal septum, rhinitis, naso-mucosal ulceration and rhinorrhoea. This may cause discomfort, impaired breathing via the nose and small nosebleeds. It can also cause anosmia.

Neurological reactions include stroke. This is normally rare in patients under 45 years of age, but taking cocaine is associated with an increased risk.[27–30] Haemorrhagic and ischaemic types can both occur – the former may be linked to a cocaine-induced hypertension, the latter perhaps to thrombosis or blood vessel spasm. Convulsions are probably more common when high doses or long 'runs' of cocaine are used. Fitting can occur with any mode of administration and seems to resolve without leaving a permanent propensity to seizures, whether treated with anticonvulsants or not.[30–33] Headache is common shortly after administration, during intoxication and afterwards as a symptom of withdrawal.[30]

Panic attacks are a common acute **psychiatric** problem. However, chronic cocaine abuse may cause a range of psychiatric problems, which may be acute or chronic. Anxiety, nervousness, depression, exhaustion, mania and paranoid psychosis have all been attributed to frequent cocaine use.[29,34,35] Persistent anhedonia or dysphoria can also develop. Subjects may find it difficult to concentrate, suffer from memory loss, experience disturbed sleep patterns, feel exhausted, and become antisocial.

Gastrointestinal effects include gastric and duodenal ulcers.[36] These are believed to arise as a result of cocaine-induced vasoconstriction and can be large. Other related events include gastrointestinal bleeding, perforation and ischaemia. The anorexic properties of the drug frequently give rise to weight loss and malnutrition. Dental erosions have been reported in those who draw snorted cocaine through the nose and then into the mouth, thus partly relying on buccal absorption. This is more likely to occur in those with a perforated nasal septum. The high salivary pH caused by cocaine is thought to be responsible for the resulting damage to teeth.[37]

Cocaine causes dose-dependent **liver** toxicity in mice,[38] and it is believed to have similar effects in humans.[39] Hepatic necrosis is exacerbated by alcohol, and fatty infiltration is usually seen as well. Cocaine-associated liver damage is often associated with other significant adverse reactions such as rhabdomyolysis.

Six cases of thrombocytopenia occurring up to 4 weeks after use of cocaine have been reported.[40] The mechanism is obscure but may be immune-based; the use of cocaine may simply have been coincidental.

Cocaine–ethanol interaction

Interactions between abused substances are often poorly characterised and even when investigated, studies can reveal conflicting or highly subjective interpretations of their importance. However, the interaction between cocaine and alcohol has been the subject of research because of its potential clinical importance. When cocaine is taken with alcohol, greater intoxication and a more pleasurable effect is reported.[41,42] This is because the combination seems to result in higher cocaine levels, a decreased inebriating effect of alcohol, and about 17% of a cocaine dose reacts with alcohol to form cocaethylene. Cocaethylene might potentiate the cardiotoxicity of cocaine and alcohol, but this has not been proved; the administration of the combination may also increase violent behaviour.[42]

Dependence

The dependence potential of cocaine may vary according to the method of administration. 'Snorting' cocaine hydrochloride probably has a lower dependence potential than smoking the freebase ('crack') or injecting the hydrochloride because these latter two methods cause such an intense and short-lived exhilaration. In animal studies, cocaine possesses very potent 'reinforcing properties', i.e. animals will more quickly adopt a certain pattern of behaviour if cocaine is offered as a reward. In humans this is manifested as a 'craving' for the drug. The individual has a strong desire to experience again the euphoric effects of the drug (positive reinforcement) and may also be driven by the desire to reverse the dysphoric aftermath (negative reinforcement). 'Crack' cocaine has been associated with a particularly strong craving; heavy users may go without food or sleep for long periods in order to continue to use the drug.

Craving may persist for weeks after cessation of chronic administration and is a prominent feature of withdrawal. Other symptoms include depression (which may be profound), fatigue, malaise, irritability, anxiety, insomnia and dysphoria.

Research has aimed to identify a drug that will facilitate cocaine abstinence, maintain abstinence, prevent craving or treat withdrawal, but for cocaine users and dependents there are no widely accepted pharmacological interventions that have successfully demonstrated a consistent beneficial effect in rigorous large-scale clinical trials. A variety of medicines has been used to assist the cocaine-dependent patient. On the whole, the studies of these medicines are too small to give much confidence in these interventions; where there is a series of small studies these may show conflicting effects and most of them have high patient drop-out rates. Even when a beneficial effect is claimed from a small study there is typically a lack of follow-up with larger studies that might provide better quality data. Table 5.4 lists some of these. Most users of cocaine who seek abstinence simply stop taking the drug abruptly, with or without counselling or other non-pharmacological support. Antidepressants during this withdrawal period may ease withdrawal symptomatically for some patients, especially if depression is marked or if it has been an important factor in encouraging abuse, but they do not prevent craving.[43] Many cocaine users have a psychiatric illness and it is important to control this effectively during the withdrawal period if possible. Patients with schizophrenia who abuse cocaine may need bigger doses of existing neuroleptics or a reappraisal of therapy if cocaine has exacerbated psychosis.[44] Alternatively, treatment for neuroleptic

Table 5.4 Examples of pharmacological interventions for cocaine dependence that have been investigated in small-scale clinical trials

Antidepressants	Drugs used have included fluoxetine, desipramine, imipramine and venlafaxine. A systematic review of published studies has shown there is no evidence that antidepressants prevent those dependent upon cocaine from resuming their intake.[43]
Carbamazepine	There is no clinical evidence that this drug is effective in cocaine dependence.[45]
Disulfiram	Systematic review shows no evidence of benefit.[46]
Dopamine agonists	Drugs used have included bromocriptine, amantadine and pergolide. Dopamine is known to have a key role in the positive reinforcement produced by cocaine but a systematic review of published trials has shown no evidence to support their use.[47]
Neuroleptics	A study of 20 patients suggested that the dopamine antagonist haloperidol could reduce craving.[48] However a randomised placebo-controlled trial of risperidone in 193 cocaine dependents failed to show a beneficial effect.[49]
Vaccination	In 1995, a team of researchers showed that it was possible to vaccinate against the action of cocaine in rats such that CNS concentrations and response to the drug were markedly reduced.[50] If a human version could be developed it might find a role in preventing relapse in those who have passed through the most acute phase of cocaine withdrawal.

adverse reactions may be needed if cocaine has been taken to counteract them; for example, this may require a change in neuroleptic.

Non-pharmacological approaches are important and include counselling, behavioural therapy, psychotherapy and psychosocial interventions. These are beyond the scope of this book, but are reviewed elsewhere.[51,52] It has been suggested that although pharmacological agents seem ineffective in the treatment of cocaine dependence, psychotherapeutic support may encourage more patients to stay in treatment.[46]

Interactions with medicines

A full medication and substance-abuse history is necessary before investigating drug interactions in an individual patient. The main factors that may predispose cocaine to interact are its pronounced cardiovascular and psychotropic effects. However, few interactions between cocaine and medicines have been reliably or consistently reported.

Beta-blockers

Propranolol was found to significantly enhance the coronary vaso-constriction caused by cocaine in one study of 30 volunteers.[53] The explanation proposed for this is that vasoconstriction imposed by cocaine is mediated by alpha adrenoceptors but is normally partly off-set by vasodilatation via beta-2 adrenoceptors; beta-blockers prevent the attenuating beta-2 effects. The authors suggested that beta-blockers 'probably should be avoided in patients with cocaine-associated myocardial ischaemia or infarction'. Propranolol was reported to cause hypertension in one patient with hyperadrenergic cocaine toxicity and the same mechanism was proposed.[54] However, in a study of 108 dependent patients using cocaine but without overt cardiovascular adverse effects, oral propranolol was used safely for 8 weeks.[55]

Carbamazepine

One study of six cocaine users showed that smoking cocaine after 5 days of oral carbamazepine 400 mg daily caused a significant elevation in blood pressure and heart rate.[56] The authors advocated caution with the combination, but other much bigger studies have not shown this interaction.[57]

Fluoxetine

Some medicines may subjectively decrease the psychoactive effects of cocaine, and fluoxetine is perhaps the most notable example of this.[58,59]

Neuroleptics

A small prospective study of 29 selected psychiatric patients noted that cocaine users developed significantly more neuroleptic-induced acute dystonias than non-users.[60] Case reports have also suggested a similar link.[61]

A study of eight patients reported that clozapine increased cocaine levels in a dose-dependent manner, but paradoxically also attenuated the usual psychoactive and pressor effects of cocaine.[62] One patient on the combination nearly fainted and had to leave the study.

Opioids

Opioids are generally believed by cocaine users to enhance the drug's psychoactive effects. Prescribed methadone has been reported to enhance the psychotropic effects of cocaine and some of its physiological effects (e.g. heart rate).[63] At street level a mixture of cocaine with heroin ('speedball' or 'snowball') is commonly used.

Stimulants

If taken with other stimulants, cocaine would be expected to have additive side-effects, and so stimulant medicines should be avoided in patients taking cocaine (e.g. methylphenidate, dexamfetamine, pseudoephedrine).

Use and concurrent illness

Asthma

Drugs that are inhaled or smoked are likely to cause at least some respiratory symptoms. Cocaine 'snorting' or smoking has been associated with serious bronchospasm and acute exacerbations of existing asthma.[64–66] The inhalation routes for cocaine can cause cough[20] and wheezing.[25]

Diabetes

Stimulant drugs such as cocaine can cause loss of appetite, which could lead to hypoglycaemia in diabetics who do not reduce doses of insulin or sulphonylurea once food intake declines. Drug-induced vomiting could exacerbate this. Furthermore, cocaine increases stamina, which could result in hypoglycaemia due to overactivity. Intoxication may prevent a diabetic recognising and/or dealing with a hypoglycaemic episode. The hypoglycaemic episode can also resemble intoxication, so bystanders may not seek medical attention.

Cocaine use is linked to an increased risk of cardiovascular disease, and patients with diabetes are already at greater risk of this problem compared to the general population. Chronic cocaine use is likely to magnify the risk.

The apathy and poor motivation engendered in some individuals by chronic drug dependence may mitigate against adequate control of blood glucose. Non-compliance with diet, failure to administer medication correctly or inadequate monitoring could result from this. For example, a case control study of 720 hospital admissions for diabetic ketoacidosis identified that 102 of these occurred in cocaine users, and that a significant predictor for presentation was the failure to administer insulin during the previous 24 hours.[67] The increased circulating levels of catecholamines caused by cocaine may also be important in increasing the risk of diabetic ketoacidosis.

Epilepsy

Of all the illicit drugs, cocaine has the strongest association with drug-induced convulsions. Various studies have estimated the incidence in cocaine users to be up to 8%.[30] Although the mechanism for cocaine causing convulsions is unknown, presumably this risk would be even greater in patients who already suffer from epilepsy. Most episodes are single tonic-clonic fits. One study described 23 cases in San Francisco, where cocaine was the sole drug taken;[68] seizures were reported following administration of cocaine by any route. Other reviews have similarly established a link between cocaine abuse and convulsions.[69,70] The reaction is also a well-known symptom of cocaine overdose.[71]

Hepatic disease

Cocaine can be hepatotoxic in humans[39] – an effect that may be potentiated by alcohol. Cocaine is largely metabolised by esterase enzymes that are concentrated in the liver but also found elsewhere throughout the body, so liver disease may not necessarily impair cocaine clearance significantly.

Hypertension

Cocaine is known to increase blood pressure and should be avoided by those with hypertension. One theory has suggested that those with hypertension have impaired reflex baroreceptor responses to hypertensive stimuli and so are at much greater risk of hypertensive crisis and its cardiovascular complications after cocaine administration compared to those without pre-existing hypertension.[72]

Immunity impairment

Compared to non-users, those who abuse cocaine are more prone to infections, but this effect is probably mostly a result of the user's lifestyle. However, one study suggests that cocaine might have some ability to compromise the human immune system because it seems to impair the release of a key immune cascade trigger called interleukin-6.[73]

Renal disease

Cocaine can occasionally cause acute myoglobinuric renal failure, secondary to rhabdomyolysis. This can occur because of convulsions, by stimulation of over-exercise, muscular ischaemia due to intra-arterial injection, or secondary to pressure-related muscle damage caused by unconsciousness. Cocaine tends to raise blood pressure and it can cause renal damage secondary to uncontrolled hypertension, usually in the form of nephrosclerosis or glomerulosclerosis. Renal infarction can also occur.

Given the mode of cocaine metabolism and excretion it would be anticipated that it would not accumulate in patients with renal impairment. However, patients with renal failure typically become more sensitive to the CNS actions of many drugs, probably because of the accumulation of urea. Consequently, cocaine could exert more powerful psychotropic effects in this situation. The effect of renal dysfunction on the clearance of cocaine metabolites is unknown.

Pregnancy and breastfeeding

Pregnancy

Cocaine has potent vasoconstricting and hypertensive properties, and can restrict blood flow to the uterus or cause fetal hypoxia. These may be important actions in the aetiology of many of the adverse effects suggested to occur in pregnancy. Cocaine has been associated with a range of adverse effects during human pregnancy, including increased incidence of prematurity, intra-uterine growth retardation, placental abruption and premature rupture of the membranes. These adverse effects may not be directly the result of cocaine itself, because cocaine users are particularly likely to be polydrug users. Lifestyle factors may also be important and several studies suggest that providing prenatal care to cocaine-using women during pregnancy reduces or eliminates many of the risks. A meta-analysis of 33 published studies showed that a link with most effects could not be established when cocaine-exposed children were compared to children exposed to polydrug use but no cocaine – only placental abruption and premature rupture of the membranes were specifically associated with cocaine.[74]

It has been suggested that cocaine can cause a wide variety of congenital defects, but it is very difficult to ascertain which of these are true drug-related effects. Gut, genitourinary and heart defects are most commonly described and many are attributed to cocaine's effects upon fetal circulation. Fetal CNS infarction and other brain anomalies have also been reported, and may be related to cocaine-induced brain haemorrhage or ischaemia.[75] Cocaine may have teratogenic effects but the magnitude of any risk is not clear. The meta-analysis already referred to could not confirm a link between cocaine and major congenital defects when cocaine-exposed infants were compared to infants exposed to polydrug use with no cocaine.[74]

Babies exposed to cocaine may be irritable at birth and exhibit symptoms such as tremor, fever, abnormal reflexes, tachypnoea, autonomic instability, vomiting, diarrhoea, seizures and poor feeding. Cocaine has often been linked to developmental delay and mental retardation in infants born to cocaine-abusing women, but a review of 36 studies concluded that: 'Among children aged 6 years or younger, there is no convincing evidence that prenatal cocaine exposure is associated with developmental toxic effects that are different in severity, scope, or kind from the sequelae of multiple other risk factors. Many findings once thought to be specific effects of *in utero* cocaine exposure are correlated with other factors, including prenatal exposure to tobacco, marijuana, or alcohol, and the quality of the child's environment'.[76]

Breastfeeding

Cocaine is a weak base, which would be expected to accumulate in milk, and analysis of milk from drug users shows that it can be present in significant concentrations.[77] Prolonged cocaine intoxication lasting 60 hours has been reported in one infant receiving breast milk from a woman who had taken cocaine.[78] The baby experienced tachycardia, tachypnoea, hypertension, irritability and tremor. The infant's urine contained cocaine and metabolites. Another published account describes agitation in a baby who was probably breastfed by a cocaine-using woman, and her milk was shown to contain cocaine.[79] A third publication gives details of cocaine in the urine of a baby who was breastfed by a woman who used cocaine, although no adverse effects in the baby are documented.[80]

Young babies are relatively deficient in some of the esterase enzymes needed to metabolise cocaine. Cocaine should not be used during breastfeeding.

References

1. United Nations Office on Drugs and Crime. *Global Illicit Drug Trends 2003.* Vienna: UNODC, 2004 (available from http://www.unodc.org/pdf/trends2003_ www_E.pdf; accessed 17 November 2004).
2. *Statistics on Drug Use in Australia 2002. Drug Statistics Series No. 12.* Cat no. PHE 43. Canberra: Australian Institute of Health and Welfare, February 2003.
3. Aust R, Sharp C, Goulden C. *Prevalence of Drug Use: Key Findings from the 2001/02 British Crime Survey.* Home Office Research Study 182. London: Home Office, 2002.
4. *National Survey on Drug Use and Health,* Substance Abuse and Mental Health Services Administration (SAMHSA), Report ref. 30415. Rockville, MD: Office of Applied Studies, 2002.
5. Pickering H, Donoghoe M, Green A, *et al.* Crack injection. *Druglink* 1993; 8: 12.
6. Resnick R B, Kestenbaum R S, Schwartz L K. Acute systemic effects of cocaine in man – a controlled study by intranasal and intravenous routes. *Science* 1977; 195: 696–698.
7. Jones R T. The pharmacology of cocaine. *NIDA Res Monogr* 1984; 50: 27–34.
8. Warner A, Norman A B. Mechanisms of cocaine hydrolysis and metabolism *in vitro* and *in vivo*: a clarification. *Ther Drug Monit* 2000; 22: 266–270.
9. Stewart D J, Inaba T, Lucassen M, *et al.* Cocaine and norcocaine hydrolysis by liver and serum esterases. *Clin Pharmacol Ther* 1979; 25: 464–468.
10. Kloss M W, Rosen G M, Rauckman E J. Cocaine mediated hepatotoxicity. A critical review. *Biochem Pharmacol* 1984; 33: 169–173.
11. Leshner A I. Molecular mechanisms of cocaine addiction. *N Engl J Med* 1996; 335: 128–129.
12. The Drug Abuse Warning Network. Emergency department mentions for selected drug categories by year (available at http://www.dawninfo. samhsa.gov).
13. Roth D, Alarcon F J, Fernandez J A, *et al.* Acute rhabdomyolysis associated with cocaine intoxication. *N Engl J Med* 1988; 319: 673–677.
14. Giannini A J, Miller N S, Loiselle R H, *et al.* Cocaine-associated violence and relationship to route of administration. *J Subst Abuse Treat* 1993; 10: 67–69.
15. Altman A L, Seftel A D, Brown S L, *et al.* Cocaine associated priapism. *J Urol* 1999; 161: 1817–1818.
16. Marzuk P M, Tardiff K, Smyth D, *et al.* Cocaine use, risk taking and fatal Russian roulette. JAMA 1992; 267: 2635–2637.
17. Lange R A, Hillis L D. Cardiovascular complications of cocaine use. *N Engl J Med* 2001; 345: 351–359.
18. Vasica G, Tennant C C. Cocaine use and cardiovascular complications. *Med J Aust* 2002; 177: 260–262.
19. Brogan W C, Lange R A, Glamann D B, *et al.* Recurrent coronary vasoconstriction caused by intranasal cocaine: possible role for metabolites. *Ann Intern Med* 1992; 116: 556–561.
20. Khalsa M E, Tashkin D P, Perrochet B. Smoked cocaine: patterns of use and pulmonary consequences. *J Psychoactive Drugs* 1992; 24: 265–272.

21. Gitter M J, Goldsmith S R, Dunbar D N, *et al*. Cocaine and chest pain: clinical features and outcome of patients hospitalized to rule out myocardial infarction. *Ann Intern Med* 1991; 115: 277–282.

22. Rubin R B, Neugarten J. Cocaine-induced rhabdomyolysis masquerading as myocardial ischaemia. *Am J Med* 1989; 86: 551–553.

23. Rittoo D, Rittoo D B, Rittoo D. Misuse of ecstasy. *BMJ* 1992; 305: 309–310.

24. Kon O M, Redhead J B G, Gillen D, *et al*. 'Crack lung' caused by an impure preparation. *Thorax* 1996; 51: 959–960.

25. Suhl J, Gorelick D A. Pulmonary function in male free base cocaine smokers. *Am J Respir Dis* 1988; 137: 488 [abstract].

26. Ettinger N A, Albin R J. A review of the respiratory effects of smoking cocaine. *Am J Med* 1989; 87: 664–668.

27. Klonoff D C. Stroke associated with cocaine use. *Arch Neurol* 1989; 46: 989–993.

28. Kaku D A, Lowenstein D H. Emergence of recreational drug abuse as a major risk factor for stroke in young adults. *Ann Intern Med* 1990; 113: 821–827.

29. Miller B L, Mena I, Giombetti R, *et al*. Neuropsychiatric effects of cocaine: SPECT measurements. *J Addict Dis* 1992; 11: 47–58.

30. Daras M. Neurologic complications of cocaine. In: *Neurotoxicity and Neuropathology Associated with Cocaine Abuse*. NIDA Research Monograph No. 163. Rockville, MD: National Institute on Drug Abuse, 1996, 43–65.

31. Shallash A J, Shih R D, Hoffman R S, *et al*. Grand mal seizures and cocaine use. *Ann Emerg Med* 1993; 22: 758.

32. Harden C L, Daras M, Tuchman A J. Cocaine causing convulsions in a large municipal hospital population. *J Epilepsy* 1992; 5: 175–177.

33. Holland R W, Marx J A, Earnest M P, *et al*. Grand mal seizures temporally related to cocaine use: clinical and diagnostic features. *Ann Emerg Med* 1992; 21: 772–776.

34. Lacayo A. Neurologic and psychiatric complications of cocaine abuse. *Neuropsychiatry Neuropsychol Behav Neurol* 1995; 8: 53–60.

35. Brady K T, Lydiard R B, Malcolm R, *et al*. Cocaine-induced psychosis. *J Clin Psychiatr* 1991; 52: 509–512.

36. Pecha R E, Prindiville T, Pecha B S, *et al*. Association of cocaine and methamphetamine use with giant gastroduodenal ulcers. *Am J Gastroenterol* 1996; 91: 2523–2527.

37. Krutchkoff D J, Eisenberg E, O'Brien J E, *et al*. Cocaine-induced dental erosions. *N Engl J Med* 1990; 322: 408.

38. Evans M A, Harbison R D. Cocaine-induced hepatotoxicity in mice. *Toxicol Appl Pharmacol* 1978; 45: 739–754.

39. Riordan S M, Williams R. Liver disease due to illicit substance use. *Addict Biol* 1998; 3: 47–53.

40. Leissinger C A. Severe thrombocytopenia associated with cocaine use. *Ann Intern Med* 1990; 112: 708–710.

41. Harris D S, Everhart E T, Mendelson J, *et al*. The pharmacology of cocaethylene in humans following cocaine and ethanol administration. *Drug Alcohol Depend* 2003; 72: 169–182.

42. Pennings E J M, Leccese A P, de Wolff F A. Effects of concurrent use of alcohol and cocaine. *Addiction* 2002; 97: 773–783.

43. Lima M S, Reisser A A P, Soares B G O, *et al*. Antidepressants for cocaine dependence (Cochrane review). In: *The Cochrane Library*, Issue 1, 2004. Chichester, UK: John Wiley & Sons Ltd.

44. Schottenfeld R, Carroll K, Rounsaville B. Comorbid psychiatric disorders and cocaine abuse. *NIDA Res Monogr* 1993; 135: 31–47.

45. Lima A R, Lima M S, Soares B G O, *et al*. Carbamazepine for cocaine dependence (Cochrane review). In: *The Cochrane Library*, Issue 1, 2004. Chichester, UK: John Wiley & Sons Ltd.

46. Lima M S, Soares B G O, Reisser A A P, *et al*. Pharmacological treatment of cocaine dependence: a systematic review. *Addiction* 2002; 97: 931–949.

47. Soares B G O, Lima M S, Reisser A A P, *et al*. Dopamine agonists for cocaine dependence (Cochrane review). In: *The Cochrane Library*, Issue 1, 2004. Chichester, UK: John Wiley & Sons Ltd.

48. Berger S P, Mickalian J D, Reid M S, *et al*. Haloperidol antagonism of cue-elicited cocaine craving. *Lancet* 1996; 347: 504–508.

49. Grabowski J, Rhoades H, Silverman P, *et al*. Risperidone for the treatment of cocaine dependence: randomized, double-blind trial. *J Clin Psychopharmacol* 2000; 20: 305–310.

50. Carrera M R, Ashley J A, Parsons L H, *et al*. Suppression of psychoactive effects of cocaine by active immunization. *Nature* 1995; 378: 727–730.

51. Hennessy G O, de Menil V, Weiss R D. Psychosocial treatments for cocaine dependence. *Curr Psychiatry Rep* 2003; 5: 362–364.

52. Higgins S T, Budney A J, Bickel W K. Applying behavioral concepts and principles to the treatment of cocaine dependence. *Drug Alcohol Depend* 1994; 34: 87–97.

53. Lange R A, Cigarroa R G, Flores E D, *et al*. Potentiation of cocaine-induced coronary vasoconstriction by beta-adrenergic blockade. *Ann Intern Med* 1990; 112: 897–903.

54. Ramoska E, Sacchetti A D. Propranolol-induced hypertension in treatment of cocaine intoxication. *Ann Emerg Med* 1985; 14: 1112–1113.

55. Kampman K M, Volpicelli J R, Mulvaney F, *et al*. Effectiveness of propranolol for cocaine dependence treatment may depend on cocaine withdrawal symptom severity. *Drug Alcohol Depend* 2001; 63: 69–78.

56. Hatsukami D, Keenan R, Halikas J, *et al*. Effects of carbamazepine on acute responses to smoked cocaine-base in human cocaine users. *Psychopharmacologia* 1991; 104: 120–124.

57. Halikas J A, Crosby R D, Pearson V L, *et al*. A randomized double-blind study of carbamazepine in the treatment of cocaine abuse. *Clin Pharmacol Ther* 1997; 62: 89–105.

58. Batki S L, Manfredi L B, Jacob P, *et al*. Fluoxetine for cocaine dependence in methadone maintenance: quantitative plasma and urine cocaine/benzoyl-ecgonine concentrations. *J Clin Psychopharmacol* 1993; 13: 243–250.

59. Walsh S L, Preston K L, Sullivan J T, *et al*. Fluoxetine alters the effects of intravenous cocaine in humans. *J Clin Psychopharmacol* 1994; 14: 396–407.

60. van Harten P N, van Trier J C A M, Horwitz E H, *et al*. Cocaine as a risk factor for neuroleptic-induced acute dystonia. *J Clin Psychiatry* 1998; 59: 128–130.

61. Horwitz E H, van Harten P N. Acute dystonia after combined use of cocaine and neuroleptics. *Nederlands Tijdschrift voor Geneeskunde* 1994; 138: 2405–2407.

62. Farren C K, Hameedi F A, Rosen M A, *et al.* Significant interaction between clozapine and cocaine in cocaine addicts. *Drug Alcohol Depend* 2000; 59: 153–163.

63. Preston K L, Sullivan J T, Strain E C, *et al.* Enhancement of cocaine's abuse liability in methadone maintenance patients. *Psychopharmacologia* 123: 15–25.

64. Rubin R B, Neugarten J. Cocaine-associated asthma. *Am J Med* 1990; 88: 438–439.

65. Gaeta T J, Hammock R, Spevack T A, *et al.* Association between substance abuse and acute exacerbation of bronchial asthma. *Acad Emerg Med* 1996; 3: 1170–1172.

66. Averbach M, Casey K K, Frank E. Near-fatal status asthmaticus induced by nasal insufflation of cocaine. *South Med J* 1996; 89: 340–341.

67. Warner E A, Greene G S, Buchsbaum M S, *et al.* Diabetic ketoacidosis associated with cocaine use. *Arch Intern Med* 1998; 158: 1799–1802.

68. Alldredge B K, Lowenstein D H, Simon R P. Seizures associated with recreational drug abuse. *Neurology* 1989; 39: 1037–1039.

69. Myers J A, Earnest M P. Generalized seizures and cocaine abuse. *Neurology* 1984; 34: 675–676.

70. Choy-Kwong M, Lipton R B. Seizures in hospitalized cocaine users. *Neurology* 1989; 39: 425–427.

71. Jonsson S, O'Meara M, Young J B. Acute cocaine poisoning: importance of treating seizures and acidosis. *Am J Med* 1983; 75: 1061–1064.

72. Tuncel M, Wang Z, Arbique D, *et al.* Mechanism of blood pressure-raising effect of cocaine in humans. *Circulation* 2002; 105: 1054–1059.

73. Halpern J H, Sholar M B, Glowacki J, *et al.* Diminished interleukin-6 response to proinflammatory challenge in men and women after intravenous cocaine administration. *J Clin Endocrinol Metab* 2003; 88: 1188–1093.

74. Addis A, Moretti M E, Ahmed Syed F, *et al.* Fetal effects of cocaine: an updated meta-analysis. *Reprod Toxicol* 2001; 15: 341–369.

75. Dixon S D, Bejar R. Echoencephalographic findings in neonates associated with maternal cocaine and methamphetamine use: incidence and clinical correlates. *J Pediatr* 1989; 115: 770–778.

76. Frank D A, Augustyn M, Knight W G, *et al.* Growth, development, and behavior in early childhood following prenatal cocaine exposure: a systematic review. *JAMA* 2001; 285: 1613–1625.

77. Winecker R E, Goldberger B A, Tebbett I R, *et al.* Detection of cocaine and its metabolites in breast milk. *J Forensic Sci* 2001; 46: 1221–1223.

78. Chasnoff I J, Lewis D E, Squires L. Cocaine intoxication in a breast-fed infant. *Pediatrics* 1987; 80: 836–838.

79. Dickson P H, Lind A, Studts P, *et al.* The routine analysis of breast milk for drugs of abuse in a clinical toxicology laboratory. *J Forensic Sci* 1994; 39: 207–214.

80. Shannon M, Lacouture P G, Roa J, *et al.* Cocaine exposure among children seen at a pediatric hospital. *Pediatrics* 1989; 83: 337–342.

6

Amfetamine, metamfetamine, ecstasy and related drugs

> *Bond cursed himself for an impulse that earlier in the day would have seemed unthinkable. Champagne and Benzedrine [amphetamine] – never again.*
>
> Ian Fleming, 'Moonraker', 1955

Amfetamine has been the subject of more intensive chemical manipulation than any other abused drug. As a result, there are a very large number of amfetamine derivatives available. Figure 6.1 illustrates the chemical structure of amfetamine and some of its derivatives that have been, and still are, abused. Quite small changes in chemical structure can result in derivatives with significantly different properties. Amfetamine itself has been abused since the 1930s, but the first derivative to gain acceptance on the street was 3,4-methylenedioxyamfetamine (MDA, tenamfetamine), known at the time as the 'love drug' because it purportedly dispelled feelings of hate or anger and encouraged emotional closeness between users. MDA abuse began in the USA in the mid-1960s. The drug was declared illegal in 1970, but many other amfetamine derivatives were introduced during this period and the banning of MDA merely opened the door to related drugs such as MDMA (3,4-methylenedioxymetamfetamine or ecstasy). DOM is an example of an especially hallucinogenic derivative, while metamfetamine is highly stimulatory. MDMA itself seems to have particularly prominent effects on central serotonergic neurones. This may explain why MDMA intoxication seems to involve an overly emotional element. The drug also has a low hallucinogenic potential with less stimulatory effect than amfetamine.

Other related drugs with less potent sympathomimetic effects and less abuse potential, such as phentermine, are still used as appetite suppressants in the treatment of obesity. Another derivative, methylphenidate, is used to treat attention deficit hyperactivity disorder in children.

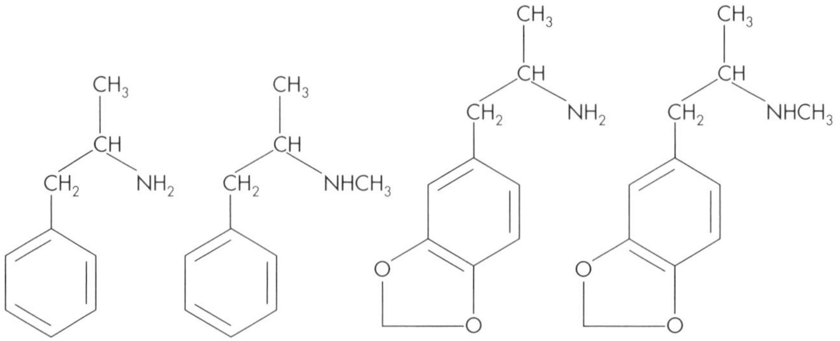

Amfetamine | Metamfetamine (ice) | 3,4-Methylenedioxyamfetamine (MDA) | 3,4-Methylenedioxymethamfetamine (MDMA, ecstasy)

Figure 6.1 Amfetamine and some of its chemical derivatives. Amfetamine is a racemic mixture of dextro- and laevo-rotatory amfetamine. D-amfetamine (dexamfetamine) is the most active and is the form used therapeutically. Many other amfetamine derivatives are abused: 3,4-dimethoxymethylamfetamine (DOM or STP); 3,4-methylenedioxyethamfetamine (MDEA or 'Eve'); methoxymethylenedioxyamfetamine (MMDA); L-acetyl-3,4-methylenedioxyphenylisoprenaline hydrochloride; DMA; MDE; MEDA; POM; TMA.

In this chapter, the main emphasis is placed on amfetamine, metamfetamine and ecstasy. They are all stimulants with broadly similar pharmacological effects, but some of the differences between them are highlighted in Table 6.1.

History

Amfetamine was first synthesised in the 1880s and has since been used to treat a range of medical conditions; some of these are listed in Table 6.2. Amfetamine use proliferated in the 1930s when it was found to have similar, although more potent, effects to the widely used drug ephedrine. At the time, ephedrine was extracted from plants and so supplies were limited and expensive.

Vast quantities of amfetamine were synthesised and issued to troops and workers during World War II for use as a stimulant during periods of strenuous activity. Amfetamine was also widely used to treat comparatively trivial conditions such as rhinitis. Together, these two factors played a large part in facilitating the early rise of amfetamine abuse; the population could obtain amfetamine easily and experiment

Table 6.1 Some differences between amfetamine, metamfetamine and ecstasy

	Amfetamine	Metamfetamine	Ecstasy
Administration routes	Injection, nasal inhalation of powder and oral most common	Injection, nasal inhalation of powder, vaporisation, oral	Oral most common
Usual form	Powder	Powder, crystals, tablets	Tablets
Half-life	12–13 hours	10–12 hours	8–9 hours
Effects sought	All-purpose stimulant	The most pronounced central nervous system (CNS) stimulant effects	Has stimulant actions, but tends to be taken more for its emotional and mystical effects
Pharmacology	Has greatest peripheral actions	Has the most powerful CNS stimulatory effects	Has the most pronounced CNS serotonergic effects
Dependence potential	High	High	Lower – tends to be taken intermittently for specific events (e.g. attending nightclubs)

Table 6.2 Therapeutic uses of amfetamine

Historical uses
- Depression
- Asthma
- Anxiety, lethargy and other 'personality' disorders
- Analeptic in barbiturate poisoning
- Appetite suppressant
- Parkinsonism
- Nasal decongestant
- Stimulant for troops and factory workers in wartime
- Nocturnal enuresis

Modern uses of dexamfetamine
- Narcolepsy and other hypersomnic states
- Attention deficit hyperactivity disorder in children
- 'Space sickness', usually in association with hyoscine or an antihistamine

freely with its psychoactive effects. In the 1960s, amfetamine abuse began to escalate more rapidly towards modern levels. The drug is known on the street under various names such as 'speed', 'whizz' or 'uppers'.

Just as 'crack' represents a highly purified form of alkaloidal cocaine, metamfetamine 'ice' is a very pure form of metamfetamine, which was probably first produced in eastern Asia in the mid-1980s. The synthesis procedure allows crystallisation of the drug into tiny colourless spindle shapes or lumps that resemble small ice crystals, hence the street name. However, the most common form of metamfetamine is a powder. Other street names include 'crystal', 'burn', 'pure', 'p', 'crank' and 'meth'. The main centres for production appear to be in South-East Asia, and Central and North America, where there are a very large number of clandestine laboratories of various sizes. It can be synthesised relatively easily from OTC (over-the-counter) medicines such as pseudoephedrine. Metamfetamine has been particularly popular in Japan.

3,4-methylenedioxymethamfetamine or MDMA has a variety of street names including 'Adam', 'XTC', 'M' and 'AKA'. However, it is usually known as 'ecstasy' or 'E'. Some tablets are known by particular names according to the motif embossed upon them (e.g. 'doves'), or their colour (e.g. 'strawberries'). MDMA was first synthesised by E. Merck Pharmaceuticals just before World War I and investigated as an appetite suppressant. However, it was not until MDA was declared an illegal drug in the USA in 1970 that MDMA became widely available. In the 1970s, MDMA was used legally by US psychotherapists to aid counselling,[1] particularly in the field of disturbed interpersonal relationships, such as marriage guidance. MDMA was claimed to promote emotional harmony and to reduce enmity. By 1985, street abuse had reached such heights in the USA that ecstasy was declared an illegal substance. In the UK, the legislature was one step ahead of the illicit manufacturers; all amfetamine-related compounds (including MDMA) were classified as illegal substances under an amendment to the Misuse of Drugs Act as early as 1977.

The United Nations estimated that 42 million people used amfetamine-type stimulant (ATS) in 2001.[2] This figure is 0.7% of the global population and makes amfetamines the second most popular illicit drugs in the world after cannabis. Of the drugs involved, approximately 7.7 million people were ecstasy users, the remainder using mainly amfetamine and metamfetamine. Analysis of those seeking treatment for substance abuse in 2003 revealed that in Europe, Asia and Australia, 11–18% had an ATS problem.[2] Figures for the Americas and Africa were lower.

Figures for the usage of amfetamine derivatives in Australia, the USA and England/Wales are shown in Table 6.3.

Table 6.3 Use of amfetamine-type stimulants amongst the population in national household surveys

Country (year)	% ever used	% used in past year	Ref.
Australia (2001)	Amfetamines 8.9% Ecstasy, etc. 6.1%	Amfetamines 3.4% Ecstasy, etc. 2.9%	3
England + Wales (2002)	–	Amfetamines 1.6% Ecstasy 2.2%	4
USA (2002)	Stimulants 9.0% Metamfetamine 5.3% Ecstasy 4.3%	Stimulants 1.4% Metamfetamine 0.7% Ecstasy 1.3%	5

Effects sought

Amfetamine and metamfetamine produce mental and physical stimulation. If injected, smoked or vaporised they cause an initial rush of euphoria, within a few seconds, that is not seen after administration by other routes. Nasal inhalation of powder (snorting) produces a less intense euphoria, which takes some minutes to develop. The effects of oral administration may take 20 minutes to begin. The individual typically becomes alert, full of self-confidence, happy and talkative. He or she may also feel energetic, strong, and impulsive and have increased stamina (enabling the user to dance for longer in nightclubs, for example).

Some users seek the stimulating properties of amfetamine for other purposes. Students may use the drug to stop them feeling tired, so that they can study for longer periods; those in monotonous occupations may abuse amfetamine in the workplace; sportsmen or bodybuilders may use amfetamine to enable them to train for longer.

For amfetamine itself, the psychoactive effects usually last for up to 4 hours. Metamfetamine has particularly powerful CNS stimulant actions that can last as long as 12 hours after snorting or oral administration. Unlike the other amfetamines, it is specifically taken by some to extend and intensify the sexual experience, particularly by gay men.

Ecstasy users seek a state of tranquil euphoria in which there is a high degree of emotional empathy between associates, greater insight into personal problems and an expanded mental perspective. Users feel 'at peace with the world' and aggressive and violent feelings are suppressed. Those under the influence of the drug feel benevolent, less defensive and more interested in interacting with others. The hallucinogenic potential is relatively low, but perceptions may be enhanced. There is often a subjectively altered sense of time. These notably different effects of ecstasy compared to other common stimulants such as cocaine and amfetamine have led to suggestions that ecstasy and related drugs ought to be classified differently, for example as 'empathogens' or 'entactogens'. Ecstasy does have more conventional amfetamine-like stimulant properties, which give users increased endurance and so forth, but these effects are less potent than those of amfetamine itself. The effects of ecstasy last approximately 4–6 hours.

Although initially associated with the growth of the 'acid house' music scene, and then an intimate part of 'rave' culture, ecstasy is now more generically referred to as a 'club drug', because of its links with young people who regularly attend nightclubs. Users, largely between the ages of 16 and 25, gather in nightclubs or private parties and dance through the night. The association between ecstasy and music is important: users favour a wide range of repetitive musical styles, often with minimal lyrics, which encourage long periods of dancing. Ecstasy can provide the stamina to dance for lengthy periods, but this prolonged exercise also forms the basis for some of the more serious side-effects (see below).

For all the amfetamines, the stimulant effects gradually dissipate, and as they begin to wear off, they may be succeeded by a period of restlessness, anxiety, fatigue, disinterest or tiredness. Although larger doses can provoke a more exhilarating stimulant feeling, they may also be associated with more intense negative feelings afterwards, such as depression, lethargy, irritability and anxiety (a 'crash'). Regular users develop tolerance to the positive psychoactive effects such that progressively greater doses are needed with time.

Administration

Amfetamine may be taken orally, via nasal inhalation or by injection. It is occasionally smoked. Amfetamine is usually supplied as a white or off-white powder in small card or paper 'wraps' (Figure 6.2). Oral administration is commonly by rubbing the powder around the buccal mucosa with a finger. Amfetamine and metamfetamine may be repeatedly administered at intervals to maintain their effects. This is similar to the 'run' that cocaine users may employ. However, the intervals between doses are greater with the two amfetamines because of their longer duration of action.

Metamfetamine can be administered by nasal inhalation, smoking, orally or by injection. 'Ice' crystals are the purest form of the drug and are more commonly vaporised for inhalation or smoked. The same

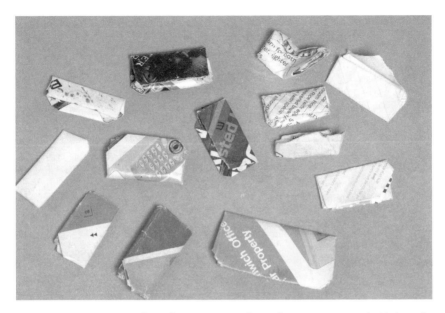

Figure 6.2 'Wraps' of amfetamine powder (Photo courtesy of Multimedia Research Partners Ltd).

sample of drug can be reheated several times and still produce the desired effect because it has a high melting point and is stable to thermal decomposition. Smoking the drug with tobacco greatly reduces the availability of metamfetamine.[6] The more common powder form of metamfetamine is less pure and may have an oily or waxy appearance, with a brownish-yellow colour caused by impurities. Tablets are less common, but oral administration may make them popular as a club drug. Metamfetamine produces a long-lasting 'high' of some 10–12 hours.

Ecstasy is almost invariably taken orally, although occasionally injection is reported. The drug is usually supplied in the form of white or off-white tablets, which may be embossed and/or scored. Some examples are illustrated in Figures 6.3 and 6.4. Capsules are occasionally seen. A typical dose for a first-time user would be 75–100 mg but because of the development of tolerance, the dose needs to be gradually increased to achieve the same effect if taken regularly. A regular user might take up to 200 mg as a single dose followed by a smaller booster dose several hours later in order to maintain the intoxication. Some users may 'binge' on ecstasy, taking the drug repeatedly every few hours and going without sleep for 1–2 days.

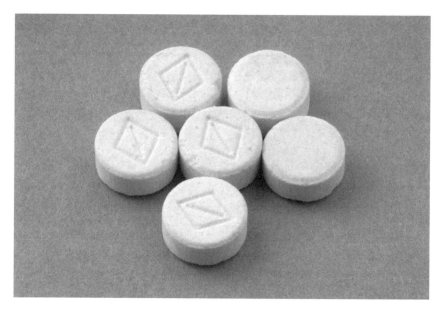

Figure 6.3 Ecstasy tablets. These tablets are well made (Photo courtesy of Multimedia Research Partners Ltd).

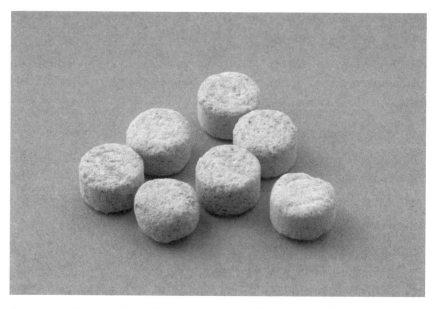

Figure 6.4 Ecstasy tablets. This is a more typical appearance for ecstasy than the tablets in Figure 6.3. The tablets have been pressed inexpertly, such that some have split or crumbled. The surface texture is rough and similar to 'extra strong mints' (Photo courtesy of Multimedia Research Partners Ltd).

Users frequently take ecstasy in association with other drugs, for example alkyl nitrites, LSD (lysergide), gamma hydroxybutyrate (GHB), ketamine and amfetamine. Users may also employ a variety of preparations to make the aftermath of an ecstasy experience tolerable. This is called 'coming down'. Preparations used include proprietary aromatic medicines (e.g. Vicks 'VapoRub'), the caffeine-rich herbal product guarana, and fluoxetine. Some users, aware of the potential serotonin-depleting properties of ecstasy (see below), may take fluoxetine or 'smart drug' drinks containing serotonin precursors in an attempt to prevent CNS damage. Smart drugs are discussed in Chapter 19.

It is clear that many ecstasy tablets do not contain pure ecstasy. A variety of patterns has emerged:[7–9]

- A small proportion of tablets contain no psychoactive drugs at all.
- Most tablets contain ecstasy together with a variety of adulterants including caffeine, paracetamol, amfetamine, metamfetamine, MDEA, ephedrine, selegiline and ketamine.
- Some tablets contain ecstasy alone.
- Other tablets contain a psychoactive substitute for ecstasy, e.g. ketamine, MDEA, MDA or any one of the bewildering array of amfetamine derivatives that exist.

This lack of purity makes it difficult to identify the substance abused and to anticipate adverse effects.

Pharmacokinetics and pharmacology

The amfetamines are sympathomimetic agents that cause the release of monoamines from central and peripheral neurones. The main neurotransmitters involved are noradrenaline, dopamine and serotonin. The detailed pharmacology of many of the amfetamine-related drugs remains to be investigated but many of them have fewer peripheral actions than amfetamine itself and users report subjective differences between them. The stimulant effects of amfetamines are probably mediated by noradrenaline. The distinctive mental effects of ecstasy are thought to occur because of its more powerful action on central serotonin – it seems to be able to inhibit the reuptake of serotonin from nerve synapses after its release.

All amfetamines sold at street level are racemic mixtures. It is not always clear what differences there are between stereoisomers, but usually one is more potent than the other. In amfetamine, for example, dexamfetamine is the most psychoactive isomer.

The half-lives of amfetamine derivatives are strongly affected by the pH of urine. They are basic compounds, so an acidic urine tends to 'trap' them in urine in an ionised water-soluble form that hinders their reabsorption into blood and facilitates clearance from the body. Conversely, an alkaline urine tends to delay clearance and prolong the half-life. Some users employ this knowledge to prolong the effects of amfetamines by taking sodium bicarbonate (baking soda) or any other substance that alkalinises the urine to prolong drug effects. Similarly, users may employ vitamin C, cranberry juice or ammonium chloride to terminate the effects of amfetamines more quickly if required.

The half-lives of both laevo- and dextrorotatory amfetamine are approximately 12–13 hours. The metabolic fate of amfetamine is partly determined by urinary pH, but deamination, N-hydroxylation, and aromatic p-hydroxylation all occur to varying extents and CYP2D6 is involved in metabolism. When urinary pH is unregulated, about 15% of a dose is excreted as unchanged drug.[10]

Although subject to liver metabolism, a substantial proportion of metamfetamine is excreted in the urine unchanged. In normal urine, 37–54% is excreted as metamfetamine and 4–7% as dexamfetamine, but the pH of urine significantly affects the proportion cleared as parent compound.[11] The half-life of metamfetamine has been estimated at 10–12 hours in normal urine.[6,12] Aromatic hydroxylation, N-dealkylation and deamination occur in the liver and cytochrome P450 isoenzyme CYP2D6 is involved in metabolism; metabolites are excreted renally.

The average half-life of ecstasy is 8–9 hours.[13,14] The enzyme CYP2D6 is thought to be a key enzyme involved in ecstasy metabolism. However, a small study of healthy volunteers given a range of ecstasy doses revealed that at high doses, non-renal clearance mechanisms seem to become saturated, such that a small increase in dose can cause a very marked increase in plasma levels.[15] The CYP2D6 status of all volunteers was characterised as 'extensive metaboliser', suggesting that some other saturatable enzyme may be involved or that ecstasy can significantly inhibit its own metabolism at high dose. These non-linear elimination kinetics may be important in patients who take large doses and suffer side-effects.

A significant proportion of an ecstasy dose is eliminated unchanged in the urine and this proportion seems to increase as the dose of ecstasy increases.[15] A small amount of ecstasy is converted to a psychoactive metabolite, MDA, by the enzyme CYP3A4.

Adverse effects

Ecstasy, amfetamine and metamfetamine are closely related chemically, and pharmacologically they exert many similar effects. They therefore have similar side-effects. However, there are differences between the three drugs, some of which are outlined in Table 6.1. These are important for determining the type of side-effects that occur and their frequency. Some of these differences are highlighted in the text below.

The onset of amfetamine-type stimulant effects is typically heralded by a range of adrenergic 'fight-or-flight' actions, such as sweating and tachycardia; initial side-effects can also include nausea, headache and abdominal cramps. Bruxism (grinding of the teeth) or trismus (uncomfortable rigidity of the jaw muscles) are more common with ecstasy than with amfetamine. All these 'introductory' effects may be short-lived or more persistent. A detailed list of adverse reactions is given in Table 6.4.

The adverse **cardiovascular** effects of amfetamines and cocaine are similar, although the effects of amfetamines have been investigated and described in much less detail. Amfetamines do not have local anaesthetic actions on the heart like cocaine but are considerably longer-acting and commonly cause hypertension and tachycardia. One study of ecstasy showed it to produce these effects without inotropism.[16] The increased strain imposed on the myocardium by this could increase the risk of heart damage. Despite this, amfetamines have only rarely been linked to specific cardiac effects. Examples include myocardial infarction (MI),[17–19] cardiac arrhythmias,[20,21] and acute and chronic cardiomyopathy.[19,22] Analysis of post-mortem findings in metamfetamine users suggests that, like cocaine, amfetamines may predispose users to coronary artery disease.[23] Haemorrhagic stroke has also been described.[23–25] In one case series, this was related to an underlying cerebral aneurysm or arteriovenous malformation in 10 out of 11 patients.[24]

Severe central chest pain has been reported in those taking amfetamines.[26] A similar effect has been described in patients who abuse cocaine and the cause of the pain is not understood, although intercostal muscle spasm has been proposed (see also Chapter 5).[26]

Most psychoactive drugs will occasionally produce unpleasant short-lived effects reminiscent of **psychiatric** illness and many of these are probably at least partly determined by the mental state of the user, and their surroundings. Amfetamines are no exception: extreme anxiety, frightening hallucinations or panic reactions may occur. Interestingly, paranoid delusions seem particularly common and some regular users

Table 6.4 Potential side-effects of amfetamine, metamfetamine, ecstasy and related drugs

Minor adverse effects
Relatively common and generally short-lived reactions, which occur shortly after taking a dose:
- Mydriasis, photophobia, blurred vision, headache, numbness
- Anorexia, nausea, dry mouth, abdominal cramps, diarrhoea
- Sweating
- Tachycardia, palpitations
- Tremor, bruxism, trismus, gait disturbance, ataxia
- Confusion, anxiety

Serious acute adverse effects
- Unpleasant hallucinations, severe anxiety, agitation, panic attacks, paranoia
- Risk-taking, accidents, violent behaviour (especially with metamfetamine)
- Hypertension, cardiac arrhythmias, cardiomyopathy, MI
- Strokes, convulsions, CNS neurotoxicity (ecstasy and metamfetamine)
- Severe central chest pain
- Severe abdominal cramps, gastrointestinal ulcers, aspiration of vomit
- Urinary retention (one case reported after a large dose of ecstasy[34])
- Jaundice, hepatotoxicity
- Over-exertion leading to dehydration, collapse, or spontaneous pneumomediastinum[35]
- Hyperpyrexia and sequelae (see Figure 6.5)
- Rhabdomyolysis and sequelae (see Figure 6.5)
- Polydipsia, hyponatraemia and stupor
- Lead poisoning due to lead acetate contamination of metamfetamine from the production process

Reactions associated with chronic exposure
- Chronic exhaustion, fatigue, muscular aches (may persist for several days even after a single dose)
- Insomnia (may be persistent)
- Anxiety and/or depression (associated with withdrawal and with continued regular use; may become chronic)
- Psychosis (may be an acute short-lived reaction or a more persistent problem), 'flashbacks' (with ecstasy and metamfetamine)
- Cardiomyopathy
- Weight loss (associated with repeated use; due to increased exercise while intoxicated and anorexic effects of amfetamines)

find that a certain sense of paranoia can persist beyond the acute phase of intoxication. Other common ongoing problems in chronic amfetamine users include mood swings, depression and anxiety. Psychosis may develop after single or repeated use of any of the amfetamine derivatives but is more common after chronic high-dose use. It can be reproduced in healthy volunteers without a history of mental illness if they are given high doses of dexamfetamine for several days running.[27] It can also be rapidly reproduced in those who have suffered from clinical amfetamine-induced psychosis if a high enough dose is given.[28] The psychosis is characterised by paranoia and delusions; hallucinations are common and violence is sometimes seen. It can become a long-term problem in up to 15% of sufferers who fail to recover completely.[29] Patients with mental health symptoms before using amfetamines are at greater risk of developing psychosis. Some metamfetamine users presenting for treatment report flashbacks or delusions, hallucinations and other psychotic symptoms when no longer intoxicated,[30] while ecstasy users may describe a similar although milder phenomenon.[31]

Metamfetamine has more pronounced stimulatory effects on the CNS than amfetamine and users may become particularly restless and agitated. Metamfetamine is also more closely linked to impaired judgement than other amfetamines. Studies have tended to associate it with **risk-taking** behaviour. A high level of interpersonal violence is frequently reported amongst metamfetamine users[32] and an increased sexual activity linked to greater numbers of sexual partners, higher-risk sex, and decreased likelihood of condom use.[33]

The **neurological** toxicity of amfetamines gives cause for much concern. Animal studies have shown that ecstasy is neurotoxic.[36,37] In various mammals, destruction of central serotonergic neurones and decreased synthesis of serotonin has been demonstrated. Primates appear to be even more sensitive to this effect than rats, because the effects may be permanent. When damaged nerve tissue regrows after exposure to ecstasy in animals, it does so slowly and is also incomplete. The axons generated do not make the same connections to adjacent nerves as their predecessors.[38] The implications of this drug-induced 'rewiring' are unclear.

It is not known to what extent these changes will occur in humans, whether they are reversible, and what the implications are for affected individuals. However, several studies suggest that neurological damage does occur in humans exposed to the drug.[39] For example:

1. Regular users of ecstasy have lower concentrations of the serotonin metabolite 5-hydroxyindole acetic acid in their cerebrospinal fluid, suggesting a lower serotonergic activity in the brain.[40]
2. Positron emission topography targeted at serotonin transporters in the brains of chronic ecstasy users show significantly depleted numbers.[41,42] The transporters are an intimate part of serotonergic neurones and reduced numbers of transporters suggests significant neuronal loss.

3. Serotonin agonists have less effect on neuroendocrine responses (e.g. pro-
    lactin release) in ecstasy users.[39]
4. Ecstasy is toxic to human serotonergic neurones grown *in vitro*, but not
    dopaminergic neurones.[43]

If ecstasy causes long-lasting damage to central serotonergic pathways
in humans, drug abuse might result in a range of chronic disorders. For
example, serotonergic neurones are prevalent in areas of the brain connected with emotions and CNS turnover of this neurotransmitter is
reduced in those suffering from depression. Many antidepressants exert
their beneficial effects by boosting serotonin activity in the brain. The
long-term legacy of ecstasy abuse might be a tendency towards affective
disorders. Short-term lethargy and depression after the effects of ecstasy
have worn off are quite common reactions. This might be a psychological response in individuals who feel so content and cheerful during
an ecstasy trip that 'real life' seems very unsatisfactory by comparison.
On the other hand, it might equally be due to an ecstasy-induced
destruction of central serotonin neurones. If this is the case then affected
individuals might be predisposed to endogenous depression in later life.
Although not always consistent, a range of studies have also suggested
that ecstasy may cause impulsivity and have adverse effects on mood
and cognitive function (particularly memory).[44–46] At least one study
suggests that the frequency of these problems is related to the frequency
of ecstasy use.[44] It is very difficult to design such studies to take account
of all potential confounders, and more research is needed to clarify
the impact that ecstasy and its probable neurotoxicity might have for
individuals.

Metamfetamine is also known to have neurotoxic effects but it
seems to destroy both serotonergic and dopaminergic neurones. Initial
studies in animals showed this effect, and positron emission tomography
in human users has shown a reduced number of dopamine neuronal
transporters.[47,48] Magnetic resonance spectroscopy of the brains of
abstinent metamfetamine users also suggests neuronal loss compared to
non-using controls.[49] As with ecstasy, the time course of any reversibility, and its extent, is unknown, but it has been suggested that this
damage may predispose affected individuals to persistent psychosis,
personality change and violence.[49] Reduced motor skills and memory
impairment has been demonstrated in former metamfetamine
users with dopamine neuronal transporter deficits.[48] This may predispose some former metamfetamine users to Parkinson's disease in later
life.

Convulsions can occur as a result of amfetamine abuse.[50,51] They can also occur as a consequence of the hyperprexia or hyponatraemia that has been associated most commonly with ecstasy (see below).

Hepatotoxicity has been a particular feature of ecstasy abuse. The spectrum of disease varies from a mild hepatitis with jaundice that resolves within a few weeks, to fatal liver failure, and does not seem to be dependent on dose or duration of abuse.[52,53] Some cases are associated with hyperpyrexia (see below).

Rhabdomyolysis, hyperpyrexia and hyponatraemia

Many of the more severe adverse effects of ecstasy are linked in aetiology (see Figure 6.5). The stimulant properties of the drug can lead individuals to over-exercise on the hot dance floor. This may lead simply to dehydration or later exhaustion and muscle aches but, depending on the level of activity, it can progress to rhabdomyolysis and/or hyperpyrexia.[54,55] Once established, hyperpyrexia may trigger further major complications such as convulsions, collapse, disseminated intravascular coagulation, and renal failure. It also fuels the process of rhabdomyolysis. Rhabdomyolysis, in turn, may result in acute renal failure via muscle breakdown products (myoglobin) accumulating in the kidney tubules. Increased body temperature may also accelerate other forms of ecstasy toxicity (e.g. hepatotoxicity, CNS neurotoxicity). Rhabdomyolysis is not always easy to diagnose initially because, although it often produces muscle pain, swelling and tenderness, many patients are asymptomatic.

Hyperpyrexia may simply be the result of over-exercise in a hot environment, but it might also be caused or exacerbated by ecstasy disrupting serotonin transmission in the hypothalamus, so incapacitating central thermoregulatory control in some way.

The distinctive pattern of hyperpyrexia/rhabdomyolysis adverse effects can occur with other amfetamine-related drugs, but has been described most consistently with ecstasy, perhaps because of the close association between ecstasy and dance music (i.e. high levels of physical activity) and the drug's pronounced serotonergic effects. The chain of events is not necessarily linked to the dose, although higher doses probably increase the risk. First-time users are just as vulnerable as those who abuse the drug regularly. Many fatalities have been reported. Rhabdomyolysis and hyperpyrexia associated with amfetamine and metamfetamine seem less common than that associated with ecstasy, is

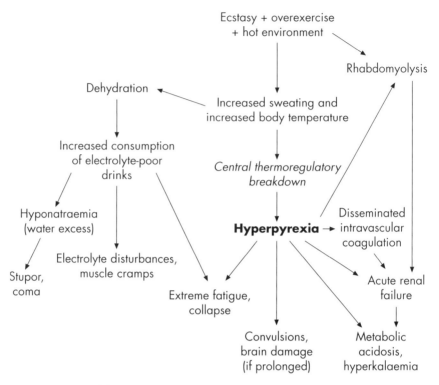

Figure 6.5 Simplified aetiological relationship between some of the more serious adverse effects of ecstasy. Many of these effects have also been described with other amfetamine derivatives.

not linked to over-exercise in a hot environment, and typically results from overdose.[56–60]

Hyponatraemia is another problem that occurs in ecstasy users and is linked to a similar set of circumstances to those producing rhabdomyolysis and hyperpyrexia.[21,61–65] It occurs when, as a result of prolonged exercise in a hot environment, the subject loses large amounts of salt and water through sweating and becomes very thirsty. If the fluid loss is corrected by taking excessive quantities of salt-poor drinks, it can result in hyponatraemia and water intoxication. The thirst could simply be a result of becoming hot while dancing, but it is conceivable that ecstasy may in some way stimulate drinking behaviour via a central action. It has also been suggested that ecstasy can cause the syndrome of inappropriate secretion of antidiuretic hormone,[61–63] but this has been disputed.[66,67] Serotonin may have a role in the aetiology of this condition because the selective serotonin reuptake inhibitor (SSRI) antidepressants, which have a predominant serotonergic action, are also associated with a (less dramatic) hyponatraemia. Whatever the precise mechanism of hyponatraemia, the effects of it can be severe in ecstasy users. Agitation, variable consciousness, stupor, dystonias, cerebral oedema, convulsions and coma are notable sequelae. Deaths have occurred.

The risks of death or serious injury due to hyperpyrexia, rhabdomyolysis or hyponatraemia can be reduced by encouraging ecstasy users to follow some straightforward advice, including:

- Avoid dancing for prolonged periods of time. Do not get too hot. Take regular rests and relax in a cool place for a while. Many club owners and hosts of events provide 'chill out' areas for this purpose.
- Drink plenty of fluid to reduce dehydration, but avoid overhydration. Taking electrolyte replacement solutions is preferable.
- Wear light, loose clothing.
- Keep an eye on your friends.

Dependence

Both amfetamine and metamfetamine commonly cause dependence, but there are no pharmacological agents shown to effectively encourage abstinence.[68] Cessation of chronic use of amfetamine and metamfetamine can produce a withdrawal reaction similar to that seen with cocaine and which occurs in about 90% of users.[70] It is characterised by depression, craving for the drug, anxiety, insomnia or tiredness, paranoia, and irritability, which are most intense during the first week but may persist for months. There are no objective physical signs. This reaction can be managed symptomatically. For example, even though a systematic review failed to recover published evidence to support the practice,[69] it is common to prescribe an antidepressant to counteract the depression that frequently arises and which may be intense and persistent. Sometimes withdrawal may provoke suicidal ideation, especially in metamfetamine users.

There has been limited experience with prescribing dexamfetamine to those who are dependent on amfetamine, but it may encourage retention in treatment and cessation of illicit and intravenous amfetamine use.[70] UK guidelines advocate that only experienced practitioners should consider prescribing substitute dexamfetamine,[71] and that it should be limited to the following cases:

- Primary amfetamine users.
- Injecting users.

- Heavy dependent use for over 3 months (more than 1 g daily at least 3 days each week).
- Evidence of escalating use, increased tolerance and craving.

Substitute dexamfetamine prescribing must be avoided in some groups (e.g. polydrug users and those with a history of mental illness). The aim is not to give an equivalent dose to that used illicitly but to minimise withdrawal symptoms and craving,[71] and a maximum daily dose of 60 mg as a liquid formulation has been advocated.[70] A time limit to achieve abstinence is essential, but this may require a stabilisation period first.

Ecstasy has been reported to cause dependence. In one study, 22 out of 52 ecstasy users met diagnostic criteria for dependence.[72] However, ecstasy should be less likely to be associated with dependence than amfetamine and metamfetamine. This is not particularly because of pharmacological differences between ecstasy and the other amfetamines, it is primarily because of the way that ecstasy is used. Firstly, ecstasy is normally taken by mouth, and oral administration produces less intense effects, which reduces the dependence potential compared to, say, intravenous use of amfetamines. Secondly, and more importantly, ecstasy is not usually taken on a daily basis because the culture surrounding its use typically promotes administration associated with specific events, e.g. attendance at nightclubs. This encourages intermittent use, which may be concentrated at selected weekends, and a daily habit is thus less likely to arise. Finally, many users report that frequent use seems not to produce the desired pleasurable effects – this could be because ecstasy provokes such drastic depletion of CNS stores of serotonin that a considerable period may be required for replenishment.

Other amfetamine derivatives

Methcathinone

This is sometimes called 'cat' and should not be confused with khat, a plant with psychoactive effects (see Chapter 17). Its abuse was prevalent in Russia and the Baltic countries in the 1970s, but has gradually expanded into the USA in particular.[73] It can be synthesised easily from over-the-counter (OTC) sympathomimetics such as ephedrine, and is supplied as a slightly sticky, white or off-white powder. It is normally taken orally or by inhalation, where it may produce a characteristic burning sensation in the nose, but intravenous use is also possible.

Methcathinone has similar pharmacological effects to amfetamine and causes similar adverse reactions, but it has a particularly long duration of action, reported to be even longer than that of metamfetamine.[73] Methcathinone, like metamfetamine, seems to be toxic to central dopaminergic neurones.[47]

Other illicit amfetamines and related compounds

There are a very large number of these, some of which are named in Figure 6.1. A chemist named Alexander Shulgin has experimented with the production of a wide range of these compounds. This resulted in him writing a text known as *Phenethylamines I Have Known And Loved*, or PIHKAL for short. Parts of the text describing the compounds can be found at several locations on the Internet by simply typing PIHKAL into a search engine. It gives an insight into the wide range of derivatives that can be and are manufactured. Often they are sold as other amfetamines such as ecstasy, either by themselves or as mixtures with similar drugs. For example, the 2C series of phenethyl-amines has begun to attract the attention of users in Europe.[74]

Amfetamine-related medicines

Diethylpropion, phentermine, methylphenidate and pemoline have only mild amfetamine-like properties and so large doses are needed for the purpose of abuse. Because black market availability of these drugs is limited, street abuse is a comparatively minor problem.

Methylphenidate is probably the most widely abused of the pre-scription amfetamine derivatives. A survey of 2250 college students in the USA in 2003 revealed that 3% had abused methylphenidate from an illicit source.[75] The drug has only weak amfetamine effects when taken orally because of poor bioavailability. However, these drawbacks are overcome when it is abused by the intravenous route. The injection is prepared by crushing tablets and dissolving the drug in water. When injected, methylphenidate has a range of side-effects similar to those seen with other amfetamines. Intranasal abuse has also been reported.[76]

An 'eosinophilic syndrome' has been described in 16 intravenous methylphenidate users.[77] This was characterised by eosinophilia, fever, musculoskeletal complaints (e.g. arthralgia) and pulmonary symptoms (e.g. pleuritic chest pain, dyspnoea, wheezing). The exact presentation varied quite widely between patients. The reaction may have been at least partly due to tablet excipients. Similarly, retinopathy was described in another series of 12 patients abusing methylphenidate.[78] Emboli of insoluble tablet excipients were probably responsible (see Chapter 2). Sufficient emboli can wedge in the blood vessels of the lungs to cause pulmonary hypertension and a death has been reported.[78] In a group of 22 intravenous methylphenidate users, the average daily dose was 200 mg (range 40–700 mg).[79] Users, who all had a history of drug abuse, often obtained the drug initially after their children were prescribed it for hyperactivity. Later, supplies were maintained by duping a variety of physicians into prescribing it or by altering legitimate prescriptions in their favour.

Several OTC sympathomimetic drugs have amfetamine-like properties and are sometimes abused. Examples include pseudoephedrine, ephedrine and phenylpropanolamine (see Chapter 13).

Plants with amfetamine-like properties

Plants such as *Ephedra*, khat and nutmeg have amfetamine-like chemical constituents and may be abused for this reason (see Chapter 17).

Piperazine derivatives

Benzylpiperazine, trifluoromethylphenylpiperazine and related chemicals are becoming more widely abused orally as stimulants.[80] They are not amfetamines, but seem to have similar actions, and are not illicit substances in many parts of the world. They have been variously known as 'BZP', 'legal E' and 'legal X'.

Interactions with medicines

Interactions between illicit amfetamines and conventional medicines have not been systematically studied in humans. Most data are derived from case reports and so should be interpreted cautiously. A full medication and substance-abuse history is necessary before investigating drug interactions in an individual patient. In terms of the potential to interact, amfetamines have a range of properties that may render interactions more likely:

- Amfetamines have significant side-effects that may be augmented by concurrent use with medicines that have the same effects (e.g. hypertension).

More specifically, ecstasy has especially pronounced serotonergic effects, which may be additive with medicines that have similar properties.

- Ecstasy, amfetamine and metamfetamine can all competitively inhibit the enzyme CYP2D6, but ecstasy has the most potent effects.[81]
- Metamfetamine, amfetamine and ecstasy are themselves metabolised by CYP2D6.

Some documented interactions involving amfetamines and medicines are discussed below.

Beta-blockers

As with cocaine (Chapter 5), concern has been raised about unopposed alpha-adrenoceptor stimulation in patients with ecstasy-induced hypertension and tachycardia requiring emergency treatment.[17] Where indicated, the combination of a beta-blocker plus a vasodilator has been suggested.

Lithium

Two small studies suggest that lithium can prevent the euphoriant effects of amfetamines.[82]

Monoamine oxidase inhibitor (MAOI) antidepressants and moclobemide

The combination of dexamfetamine, metamfetamine or ecstasy with MAOIs has resulted in severe hypertension and some fatalities.[82] Two cases involving ecstasy and phenelzine involved heightened muscle tension as well as hypertension, and other effects reminiscent of the serotonin syndrome.[83,84] Four deaths in ecstasy users who took non-prescribed moclobemide at the same time were similarly attributed to the serotonin syndrome.[85] Patients taking MAOI antidepressants or moclobemide should avoid amfetamines.

Neuroleptics

Amfetamines can cause psychotic reactions (see above), and would be expected to antagonise the effects of neuroleptics in controlling the symptoms of schizophrenia and related conditions. In one study, the introduction of dexamfetamine antagonised the schizophrenia control wrought by chlorpromazine.[86]

Interestingly, neuroleptics may also attenuate the effects of amfet-amines. In an investigation involving 14 volunteers, pre-treatment with haloperidol changed the subjective effects of ecstasy from pleasurable and euphoric, to dysphoric with some anxiety.[87]

Ritonavir

Two cases suggest that ritonavir may increase plasma levels of ecstasy by inhibiting its metabolism. Ritonavir inhibits the activity of CYP2D6, the major isoenzyme involved in ecstasy metabolism, as well as CYP3A4, which is responsible for a minor metabolic route. In the first case, a young man recently started on ritonavir took a dose of ecstasy that he had taken previously without ill effects (180 mg).[88] He developed convulsions and tachycardia, then vomited before dying of cardiac arrest. His ecstasy plasma levels at post-mortem were very high, an effect possibly at least partly due to his reduced liver function. In the second case a man recently started on ritonavir took two ecstasy tablets and developed agitation that lasted for over 29 hours.[89] He had taken similar doses of ecstasy before without this effect, suggesting that ritonavir may have delayed the excretion of ecstasy. (He later took a familiar dose of GHB and its metabolism may also have been inhibited by ritonavir because he became unconscious).

One case report also describes the death of a patient taking ritonavir who was known to have injected metamfetamine.[90] At post-mortem a precise cause of death could not be ascertained, but his metamfetamine levels were high and it was proposed that ritonavir inhibited its metabolism via CYP2D6 and contributed to his death.

SSRI antidepressants and venlafaxine

The potential interactions between SSRIs and amfetamines are complex. It seems that SSRIs may block the psychoactive effects of ecstasy, but can also cause symptoms similar to serotonin excess in some patients using amfetamines. Fluoxetine can inhibit the metabolism of amfetamines.

One case report and a small study in 16 volunteers showed that the psychotropic effects of ecstasy can be blocked by citalopram;[91,92] a similar effect was also described in one patient who took paroxetine.[91] However, a case report suggested that the use of ecstasy in a long-term citalopram recipient caused agitation, aggression, psychotic-like symptoms, poor movement control and compulsive movements that may have been caused by serotonin excess.[93] Another report described symptoms of serotonin excess in a patient prescribed venlafaxine plus dexamfetamine (sweating, movement disorders, tachycardia, tremor), which abated when venlafaxine was stopped and cyproheptadine given, but which returned when citalopram was substituted for venlafaxine.[94] Finally, the self-administration of amfetamine by two patients who had used amfetamine before but had recently taken fluoxetine, resulted in symptoms of overdose including psychotic symptoms.[95] This may have happened because fluoxetine is such a potent inhibitor of CYP2D6 (citalopram is not).

It should also be noted that SSRI antidepressants can cause hyponatraemia and so may be best avoided by patients who are known to take ecstasy and attend venues for prolonged dance activity, because of the risk of an additive effect.

Despite all these potential risks, fluoxetine and other SSRIs are known to be taken by ecstasy users in an attempt to minimise neurotoxicity; SSRIs also may have amfetamine-like effects if abused (see Chapter 12).

Stimulants

If taken with other stimulants, amfetamines would be expected to have additive side-effects, and so stimulant medicines should be avoided in these patients (e.g. methylphenidate, pseudoephedrine).

Use and concurrent illness

Asthma

If smoked, amfetamines might exacerbate existing asthma.

Diabetes

The amfetamine-related drugs are all stimulants and so commonly cause loss of appetite, which could lead to hypoglycaemia in patients with diabetes who do not reduce doses of insulin or sulphonylurea when food intake declines. Stimulants also increase stamina, which could then result in hypoglycaemia caused by overactivity. The balance of food intake and dose of hypoglycaemic drug can also be disrupted by vomiting, which is a recognised side-effect of most drugs of abuse, including occasionally amfetamines.

As with cocaine, the adverse cardiovascular effects of amfetamines may effectively be magnified in patients with diabetes because of their increased propensity to these conditions.

The apathy and poor motivation engendered in some individuals by chronic drug dependence may mitigate against adequate control of blood glucose. Non-compliance with diet, failure to administer medication correctly or inadequate monitoring could result. Intoxication may prevent a diabetic recognising and/or dealing with a hypoglycaemic episode. The hypoglycaemic episode can also resemble intoxication, so bystanders may not seek medical attention.

Epilepsy

Amfetamines, especially ecstasy, can cause fits as part of the hyper-pyrexia or hyponatraemia chain of events described above. Outside these situations, amfetamines have been occasionally associated with drug-induced convulsions, but the link is less well established than for cocaine. Eight suspected cases linked to amfetamine in non-epileptics were reported in one US study,[50] and two cases associated with ecstasy.[51]

Hepatic disease

The number of reported cases of liver disease linked to amfetamine and metamfetamine is relatively small compared to those described with ecstasy users.[52,53,96,97] Ecstasy can cause a range of liver problems, ranging from acute hepatitis to fatal liver failure. Drug-induced hyper-pyrexia may be present at the same time.

Amfetamine, metamfetamine and ecstasy are partly metabolised by the liver, so moderate to severe hepatic disease would be expected to result in some accumulation to a greater or lesser extent. However, a proportion of these drugs is excreted unchanged by the kidney, so the effect of hepatic impairment on plasma levels may be limited.

Hypertension

Amfetamine derivatives are known to increase blood pressure and should be avoided by those with hypertension.

Immunity impairment

Ecstasy seems to have adverse effects on the human immune system, which might predispose individuals to infection or immune-based diseases.[98] Anecdotally, immunosuppressant properties have been attributed to ecstasy because users seem more likely to contract colds and other minor infections. However, these effects could be more related to the user's lifestyle than to the drug itself. Dancing in a hot, crowded environment is very conducive to the spread of minor infectious diseases and to the development of 'chills' after leaving the gathering.

Renal disease

Stimulants can cause myoglobinuric renal failure, secondary to rhabdomyolysis, often linked to over-exercise or hyperpyrexia. The reaction is particularly associated with ecstasy but has been reported with other amfetamine derivatives. Rhabdomyolysis can also arise after intra-arterial injection due to skeletal muscle ischaemia, and unconsciousness secondary to intoxication can lead to pressure-related muscle damage. There are very rare reports of amfetamines causing renal dysfunction by other means.[99,100]

Amfetamine, metamfetamine and ecstasy could accumulate in patients with renal impairment, because although subject to liver metabolism, a significant proportion of the parent drug and its metabolites (some of which are active) are cleared renally. In renal failure, patients typically become more sensitive to the CNS effects of many drugs, probably because of the accumulation of urea. Consequently, the amfetamine derivatives might exert more powerful effects in this situation.

Pregnancy and breastfeeding

Pregnancy

When studies of amfetamine use during human pregnancy are analysed collectively there is insufficient evidence to prove them teratogenic.[101] Fetal abnormalities do occur in association with amfetamine exposure,[102,103] but separating out a definite pattern of deformations linked to amfetamines alone, rather than other factors, has never been satisfactorily achieved. Amfetamines have vasoconstrictive properties and are known to cause hypertension and reduced blood flow to the fetus;

they also cause maternal anorexia (which can result in relative malnutrition). These actions may help to explain associations between amfetamines abuse and growth retardation, low birth weight, prematurity and cranial scan abnormalities in some newborns, but the effects have been inadequately studied.[104] Some studies suggest that maternal amfetamines abuse near term is associated with neonatal drowsiness, and even various withdrawal symptoms, but information on this is also limited. More study of abuse of amfetamines during human pregnancy is needed to reach definite conclusions about the extent and nature of the risks for mother and fetus.

Breastfeeding

There is only one detailed case report in the literature of amfetamine administration to a breastfeeding mother. Milk from a woman receiving 20 mg of dexamfetamine daily for therapeutic reasons was analysed.[105] The drug was found to be much more concentrated in milk than in plasma. This would be expected because amfetamines are weak bases and breast milk is slightly more acidic than blood. Despite this, no adverse effects were reported in the baby, who was periodically assessed for 2 years. Similarly, an investigation of 103 infants receiving milk from mothers who took amfetamines (various forms and doses) revealed no acute side-effects in the recipients – but this study has never been published in full.[106] Theoretically, amfetamines could cause stimulation (irritability, poor sleep pattern) or sedation (poor feeding) in infants. On the whole, children tend to be sedated by amfetamines rather than stimulated.

Although the effects upon lactation have not been studied specifically, high doses of amfetamine do suppress prolactin secretion in patients with hyperprolactinaemia.[107] If this effect were to happen in lactating women the drug might reduce milk production.

There is no specific information on any of the amfetamine derivatives such as ecstasy and metamfetamine in human lactation.

References

1.   Saunders N. *Ecstasy and the Dance Culture*. Exeter: Nicholas Saunders Publishers, 1995, 14–15, 124–137.
2.   United Nations Office on Drugs and Crime. *Global Illicit Drug Trends 2003*. Vienna: UNODC, 2004 (available from http://www.unodc.org/pdf/trends 2003_www_E.pdf; accessed 17 November 2004).

3. *Statistics on Drug Use in Australia 2002. Drug Statistics Series No. 12.* Cat no. PHE 43. Canberra: Australian Institute of Health and Welfare, February 2003.

4. Aust R, Sharp C, Goulden C. *Prevalence of Drug Use: Key Findings from the 2001/02 British Crime Survey.* Home Office Research Study 182. London: Home Office, 2002.

5. *National Survey on Drug Use and Health*, Substance Abuse and Mental Health Services Administration (SAMHSA), Report ref. 30415. Rockville, MD: Office of Applied Studies, 2002.

6. Cook C E. Pyrolytic characteristics, pharmacokinetics, and bioavailability of smoked heroin, cocaine, phencyclidine and methamphetamine. *NIDA Res Monogr* 1991; 115: 6–24.

7. Wolff K, Hay A W M, Sherlock K, *et al.* Contents of ecstasy. *Lancet* 1995; 346: 1100–1101.

8. Saunders N. *Ecstasy and the Dance Culture.* Exeter: Nicholas Saunders Publishers, 1995, 149–50, 161–163.

9. Milroy C M, Clark J C, Forrest A R W. Pathology of deaths associated with 'ecstasy' and 'eve' misuse. *J Clin Pathol* 1996; 49: 149–153.

10. Dollery C, ed. *Therapeutic Drugs*, 2nd edn. Edinburgh: Churchill Livingstone, 1999, D59–62.

11. Oyler J M, Cone E J, Joseph R E, *et al.* Duration of detectable methamphetamine and amphetamine excretion in urine after controlled oral administration of methamphetamine to humans. *Clin Chem* 2002; 48: 1703–1714.

12. Harris D S, Boxenbaum H, Everhart E T, *et al.* The bioavailability of intranasal and smoked methamphetamine. *Clin Pharmacol Ther* 2003; 74: 475–486.

13. Mas M, Farre M, de la Torre R, *et al.* Cardiovascular and neuroendocrine effects and pharmacokinetics of 3,4-methylendioxy-methamphetamine in humans. *J Pharmacol Exp Ther* 1999; 290: 136–145.

14. de la Torre R, Farre M, Roset PN, *et al.* Pharmacology of MDMA in humans. *Ann N Y Acad Sci* 2000; 914: 225–237.

15. de la Torre R, Farre M, Ortuno J, *et al.* Non-linear pharmacokinetics of MDMA ('ecstasy') in humans. *Br J Clin Pharmacol* 2000; 49: 104–109.

16. Lester S J, Baggott M, Welm S, *et al.* Cardiovascular effects of 3,4-methylene-dioxymethamphetamine: a double-blind, placebo-controlled trial. *Ann Intern Med* 2000; 133: 969–973.

17. Farnsworth T L, Brugger C H, Malters P. Myocardial infarction after intranasal methamphetamine. *Am J Health Syst Pharm* 1997; 54: 586–587.

18. Hung M J, Kuo L T, Chering W J. Amphetamine-related acute myocardial infarction due to coronary artery spasm. *Int J Clin Pract* 2003; 57: 62–64.

19. Hong R, Matsuyama E, Nur K. Cardiomyopathy associated with the smoking of crystal methamphetamine. *JAMA* 1991; 265: 1152–1154.

20. Dowling G P, McDonough E T, Bost R O. Eve and Ecstasy: a report of five deaths associated with the use of MDEA and MDMA. *JAMA* 1987; 257: 1615–1617.

21. Milroy C M, Clark J C, Forrest A R W. Pathology of deaths associated with 'ecstasy' and 'eve' misuse. *J Clin Pathol* 1996; 49: 149–153.

22. Call T D, Hartneck J, Dickinson W A, *et al.* Acute cardiomyopathy secondary to intravenous amphetamine abuse. *Ann Intern Med* 1982; 97: 559–560.

23. Karch S B, Stephens B G, Ho C-H. Methamphetamine-related deaths in San Francisco: demographic, pathologic, and toxicologic profiles. *J Forensic Sci* 1999; 44: 359–368.

24. McEvoy A W, Kitchen N D, Thomas D G T. Intracerebral haemorrhage caused by drug abuse. *Lancet* 1998; 351: 1029.

25. Harries D P, de Silva R N. Ecstasy and intracerebral haemorrhage. *Scott Med J* 1992; 370: 150–152.

26. Rittoo D, Rittoo D B, Rittoo D. Misuse of ecstasy. *BMJ* 1992; 305: 309–310.

27. Griffith J D, Cavanaugh J, Held J, *et al.* Dextroamphetamine: evaluation of psychotomimetic properties in man. *Arch Gen Psychiatry* 1972; 26: 97–100.

28. Bell D S. The experimental reproduction of amphetamine psychosis. *Arch Gen Psychiatry* 1973; 29: 35–40.

29. Srisurapanont M, Kittiratanapaiboon P, Jarusuraisin N. Treatment for amphetamine psychosis (Cochrane review). In: *The Cochrane Library*, Issue 1, 2004. Chichester, UK: John Wiley & Sons Ltd.

30. Yui K, Ikemoto S, Goto K, *et al.* Spontaneous recurrence of methamphetamine-induced paranoid-hallucinatory states in female subjects: susceptibility to psychotic states and implications for relapse of schizophrenia. *Pharmacopsychiatry* 2002; 35: 62–71.

31. Creighton F J, Black D L, Hyde C E. 'Ecstasy' psychosis and flashbacks. *Br J Psychiatry* 1991; 159: 713–715.

32. Cohen J B, Dickow A, Horner K, *et al.* Abuse and violence history of men and women in treatment for methamphetamine dependence. *Am J Addict* 2003; 12: 377–385.

33. Freese T E, Obert J, Dickow A, *et al.* Methamphetamine abuse: issues for special populations. *J Psychoactive Drugs* 2000; 32: 177–182.

34. Bryden A A, Rothwell P J N, O'Reilly P H. Urinary retention with misuse of ecstasy. *BMJ* 1995; 310: 504.

35. Rezvani K, Kurbaan A S, Brenton D. Ecstasy induced pneumomediastinum. *Thorax* 1996; 51: 960–961.

36. Ricaurte G, Bryan G, Strauss L, *et al.* Hallucinogenic amphetamine selectively destroys brain serotonin nerve terminals. *Science* 1985; 229: 986–968.

37. Steele T D, McCann U D, Ricaurte G A. 3,4-methylenedioxymethamphetamine (MDMA, ecstasy): pharmacology and toxicology in animals and humans. *Addiction* 1994; 89: 539–551.

38. Fischer C, Hatzidimitriou G, Wlos J, *et al.* Reorganisation of ascending 5-HT axon projections in animals previously exposed to the recreational drug (±)3,4-methylenedioxymethamphetamine (MDMA, 'Ecstasy'). *J Neurosci* 1995; 15: 5476–5485.

39. Boot B P, McGregor I S, Hall W. MDMA (ecstasy) neurotoxicity: assessing and communicating the risks. *Lancet* 2000; 355: 1818-1821.

40. McCann U D, Ridenour A, Shaham Y, *et al.* Seronergic neurotoxicity after (±)3,4-methylenedioxymethamphetamine (MDMA; "ecstasy"): a controlled study in humans. *Neuropsychopharmacology* 1994; 10: 129–138.

41. McCann U D, Szabo Z, Scheffel U, *et al.* Positron emission tomographic evidence of toxic effect of MDMA ("ecstasy") on brain serotonin neurons in human beings. *Lancet* 1998; 352: 1433–1437.

42. Semple D M, Ebmeier K P, Glabus M F, *et al*. Reduced *in vivo* binding to the serotonin transporter in the cerebral cortex of MDMA ('ecstasy') users. *Br J Psychiatry* 1999; 175: 63–69.

43. Simantov R, Tauber M. The abused drug MDMA (ecstasy) induces programmed death of serotonergic cells. *FASEB J* 1997; 11: 141–146.

44. Parrott A C, Buchanan T, Scholey A B, *et al*. Ecstasy/MDMA attributed problems reported by novice, moderate and heavy recreational users. *Hum Psychopharmacol* 2002; 17: 309–312.

45. Morgan M J. Recreational use of "ecstasy" (MDMA) is associated with elevated impulsivity. *Neuropsychopharmacology* 1998; 19: 252–264.

46. *Ecstasy: What We Know and Don't Know About MDMA. A Scientific Review*. Rockville, MD: National Institute on Drug Abuse, 2003, 36–43.

47. McCann U D, Wong D F, Yokoi F, *et al*. Reduced striatal dopamine transporter density in abstinent methamphetamine and methcathinone users: evidence from positron emission tomography studies with [11C]WIN-35,428. *J Neurosci* 1998; 18: 8417–8422.

48. Volkow N D, Chang L, Wang G-J, *et al*. Association of dopamine transporter reduction with psychomotor impairment in methamphetamine abusers. *Am J Psychiatry* 2001; 158: 377–382.

49. Ernst T, Chang L, Leonido-Yee M, *et al*. Evidence for long-term neurotoxicity associated with methamphetamine abuse: a ^{1}H MRS study. *Neurology* 2000; 54: 1344–1349.

50. Alldredge B K, Lowenstein D H, Simon R P. Seizures associated with recreational drug abuse. *Neurology* 1989; 39: 1037–1039.

51. Sawyer J, Stephens W P. Misuse of ecstasy. *BMJ* 1992; 305: 310.

52. Riordan S M, Williams R. Liver disease due to illicit substance use. *Addict Biol* 1998; 3: 47–53.

53. Kalant H. The pharmacology and toxicology of "ecstasy" (MDMA) and related drugs. *Can Med Assoc J* 2001; 165: 917–928.

54. Henry J A, Jeffreys K J, Dawling S. Toxicity and deaths from 3,4-methylenedioxymethamphetamine ('ecstasy'). *Lancet* 1992; 340: 384–387.

55. Henry J A. Ecstasy and the dance of death. *BMJ* 1992; 305: 5–6.

56. Ginsberg M D, Hertzman M, Schmidt-Nowara W W. Amphetamine intoxication with coagulopathy, hyperthermia, and reversible renal failure. *Ann Intern Med* 1970; 73: 81–85.

57. Kojima T, Une I, Yashiki M, *et al*. A fatal methamphetamine poisoning associated with hyperpyrexia. *Forensic Sci Int* 1984; 24: 87–93.

58. Scandling J, Spital A. Amphetamine-associated myoglobinuric renal failure. *South Med J* 1982; 75: 237–240.

59. Callaway C W, Clark R F. Hyperthermia in psychostimulant overdose. *Ann Emerg Med* 1994; 24: 68–76.

60. Richards J R, Johnson E B, Stark R W, *et al*. Methamphetamine abuse and rhabdomyolysis in the ED: a 5-year study. *Am J Emerg Med* 1999; 17: 681–685.

61. Holden R, Jackson M A. Near-fatal hyponatraemic coma due to vasopressin oversecretion after 'ecstasy' (3,4-MDMA). *Lancet* 1996; 347: 1052.

62. Satchell S C, Connaughton M. Inappropriate antidiuretic hormone secretion and extreme rises in serum creatinine kinase following MDMA ingestion. *Br J Hosp Med* 1994; 51: 495.

63. Matthai S M, Davidson D C, Sills J A, *et al*. Cerebral oedema after ingestion of MDMA ('ecstasy') and unrestricted intake of water. *BMJ* 1996; 312: 1359.

64. Maxwell D L, Pikey M I, Henry J A. Hyponatraemia and catatonic stupor after taking 'ecstasy'. *BMJ* 1993; 307: 1399.

65. Kessel B. Hyponatraemia after ingestion of 'ecstasy'. *BMJ* 1994; 308: 414.

66. Cook T M. Cerebral oedema after MDMA ('ecstasy') and unrestricted water intake. *BMJ* 1996; 313: 689.

67. Wilkins B. Hyponatraemia must be treated with low water input. *BMJ* 1996; 313: 689–670.

68. Srisurapanont M, Jarusuraisin N, Kittiratanapaiboon P. Treatment for amphetamine dependence and abuse (Cochrane review). In: *The Cochrane Library*, Issue 1, 2004. Chichester, UK: John Wiley & Sons Ltd.

69. Srisurapanont M, Jarusuraisin N, Kittiratanapaiboon P. Treatment for amphetamine withdrawal (Cochrane review). In: *The Cochrane Library*, Issue 1, 2004. Chichester, UK: John Wiley & Sons Ltd.

70. Walters C. *Amphetamine Use: Literature Review and Recommendations for Intervention*. Auckland: Regional Alcohol and Drug Services, 2002.

71. Department of Health UK, Scottish Office Department of Health, Welsh Office, Department of Health and Social Services Northern Ireland. *Drug Misuse and Dependence – Guidelines on Clinical Management*. London: The Stationery Office, 1999.

72. Cottler L B, Womack S B, Compton W M, *et al*. Ecstasy abuse and dependence among adolescents and young adults: applicability and reliability of DSM-IV criteria. *Hum Psychopharmacol* 2001; 16: 599–606.

73. Calkins R F, Aktan G B, Hussain K L. Methcathinone: the next illicit stimulant epidemic? *J Psychoactive Drugs* 1995; 27: 277–285.

74. de Boer D, Bosman I. A new trend in drugs-of-abuse; the 2C-series of phenethylamine designer drugs. *Pharm World Sci* 2004 ; 26: 110–113.

75. Teter C J, McCabe S E, Boyd C J, *et al*. Illicit methylphenidate use in an undergraduate student sample: prevalence and risk factors. *Pharmacotherapy* 2003; 23: 609–617.

76. Coetzee M, Kaminer Y, Morales A. Megadose intranasal methylphenidate (Ritalin) abuse in adult attention deficit hyperactivity disorder. *Subst Abus* 2002; 23: 165–169.

77. Gunby P. Methylphenidate abuse produces retinopathy. *JAMA* 1979; 241: 546.

78. Parran T V, Jasinski D R. Intravenous methylphenidate abuse – prototype for prescription drug abuse. *Arch Intern Med* 1991; 151: 781–783.

79. Wolf J, Fein A, Fehrenbacher L. Eosinophilic syndrome with methylphenidate abuse. *Ann Intern Med* 1978; 89: 224–225.

80. *Drugs and Chemicals of Concern: Benzylpiperazine, Trifluromethylphenyl-piperazine (BZP, TFMPP)*. US Department of Justice, Drug Enforcement Administration, August 2001 (available at http://www.deadiversion. usdoj.gov/drugs_concern/bzp_tmp/bzp_tmp.htm (accessed 30 November 2004).

81. Wu D, Otton S V, Inaba T, *et al*. Interactions of amphetamine analogs with human liver CYP2D6. *Biochem Pharmacol* 1997; 53: 1605–1612.

82. Stockley I H (ed). *Stockley's Drug Interactions*, 6th edn. London: Pharmaceutical Press, 2002, 680–682.
83. Kaskey G B. Possible interaction between an MAOI and "ecstasy". *Am J Psychiatry* 1992; 149: 411–412.
84. Smilkstein M J, Smolinske S C, Rumack B H. A case of MAO inhibitor? MDMA interaction: agony after ecstasy. *Clin Toxicol* 1987; 25: 149–159.
85. Vuori E, Henry J A, Ojanpera I, *et al.* Death following ingestion of MDMA (ecstasy) and moclobemide. *Addiction* 2003; 98: 365–368.
86. Casey J F, Hollister L E, Klett C J, *et al.* Combined drug therapy of chronic schizophrenics: controlled evaluation of placebo, dextro-amphetamine, imipramine, isocarboxacid and trifluoperazine added to maintenance dose of chlorpromazine. *Am J Psychiatry* 1961; 117: 997–1003.
87. Liechti M E, Vollenweider F X. Acute psychological and physiological effects of MDMA ("ecstasy") after haloperidol pretreatment in healthy humans. *Eur Neuropsychopharmacol* 2000; 10: 289–295.
88. Henry J A, Hill I R. Fatal interaction between ritonavir and MDMA. *Lancet* 1998; 352: 1751–1752.
89. Harrington R D, Woodward J A, Hooton T M, *et al.* Life-threatening interactions between HIV-1 protease inhibitors and the illicit drugs MDMA and gamma-hydroxybutyrate. *Arch Intern Med* 1999; 159: 2221–2224.
90. Hales G, Roth N, Smith D. Possible fatal interaction between protease inhibitors and methamphetamine. *Antivir Ther* 2000; 5: 19.
91. Stein D J, Rink J. Effects of "ecstasy" blocked by serotonin reuptake inhibitors. *J Clin Psychiatry* 1999; 60: 485.
92. Liechti M E, Baumann C, Gamma A, *et al.* Acute psychological effects of 3,4-methylenedioxymethamphetamine (MDMA, "ecstasy") are attenuated by the serotonin uptake inhibitor citalopram. *Neuropsychopharmacology* 2000; 22: 513–521.
93. Lauerma H, Wuorela M, Halme M. Interaction of serotonin reuptake inhibitor and 3,4-methylenedioxymethamphetamine? *Biol Psychiatry* 1998; 43: 929.
94. Prior F H, Isbister G K, Dawson A H, *et al.* Serotonin toxicity with therapeutic doses of dexamphetamine and venlafaxine. *Med J Aust* 2002; 176: 240–241.
95. Barrett J, Meehan O, Fahy T. SSRI and sympathomimetic interaction. *Br J Psychiatry* 1996; 168: 253.
96. Jones A L, Simpson K J. Review article: Mechanisms and management of hepatotoxicity in ecstasy (MDMA) and amphetamine intoxications. *Aliment Pharmacol Ther* 1999; 13: 129–133.
97. Kamiio Y, Soma K, Nishida M, *et al.* Acute liver failure following intravenous methamphetamine. *Vet Hum Toxicol* 2002; 44: 216–217.
98. Pacifici R, Zuccaro P, Farre M, *et al.* Cell-mediated immune response in MDMA users after repeated dose administration: studies in controlled versus noncontrolled settings. *Ann N Y Acad Sci* 2002; 965: 421–423.
99. Foley R J, Kapatkin K, Verani R, *et al.* Amphetamine-induced acute renal failure. *South Med J* 1984; 77: 258–260.
100. Bingham C, Beaman M, Nicholls A J, *et al.* Necrotizing renal vasculopathy resulting in chronic renal failure after ingestion of methamphetamine and

3,4-methylenedioxymethamphetamine ('ecstasy'). *Nephrol Dial Transplant* 1998; 13: 2654–2655.

101. Briggs G G, Freeman R K, Yaffe S J. *Drugs in Pregnancy and Lactation*, 6th edn. Baltimore, MD: Williams & Wilkins, 2002, 66a–72a.

102. McElhatton P R, Bateman D N, Evans C, *et al*. Congenital anomalies after prenatal ecstasy exposure. *Lancet* 1999; 354: 1441–1442.

103. Schaefer C, ed. *Drugs During Pregnancy and Lactation. Handbook of Prescription Drugs and Comparative Risk Assessment*. Amsterdam: Elsevier, 2001, 221.

104. Dixon S D, Bejar R. Echoencephalographic findings in neonates associated with maternal cocaine and methamphetamine use: incidence and clinical correlates. *J Pediatr* 1989; 115: 770–778.

105. Steiner E, Villen T, Hallberg M, *et al*. Amphetamine secretion in breast milk. *Eur J Clin Pharmacol* 1984; 27: 123–124.

106. Ayd F J. Excretion of psychotropic drugs in human breast milk. *Int Drug Ther News Bull* 1973; 8: 33–40.

107. DeLeo V, Cella S G, Camanni F. Prolactin lowering effect of amphetamine in normoprolactinemic subjects and in physiological and pathological hyperprolactinaemia. *Horm Metab Res* 1983; 15: 439–443.

7

LSD

When I closed my eyes, an unending series of colourful, very realistic and fantastic images surged in upon me. A remarkable feature was the manner in which all acoustic perceptions (e.g. the noise of a passing car) were transformed into optical effects, every sound evoking a corresponding coloured hallucination constantly changing in shape and colour like pictures in a kaleidoscope.
Albert Hofmann, from notes made following self-administration of LSD, 1943

History

LSD has many street names but is most commonly referred to as 'acid' or 'trips'. It is also known as lysergic acid diethylamide or lysergide, and was first synthesised by Hofmann and Stoll of Sandoz in 1938. It was derived from lysergic acid, a non-psychoactive compound found in ergot (*Claviceps purpurea*), a common fungal contaminant of rye and other cereal crops. The initials LSD are derived from the German name for the drug: 'Lyserg Säure Diäthylamid-25', it being the 25th compound synthesised from the ergot derivative. Following investigation as a 'psycho-therapeutic' aid in Europe and the USA during the 1950s and 1960s,[1] recreational use began to spread rapidly, resulting in the drug becoming an illicit substance.

In the USA, a national household survey in 2002 revealed that 10.4% of the population over 12 years of age had used LSD at least once during their lifetime, but only 0.4% had used the drug in the past year.[2] A similar survey in Australia in 2001 showed that 7.6% of the adult population had used hallucinogens at least once in their lives.[3] This was presumably mainly LSD, because ecstasy, amfetamines and designer drugs were excluded from the definition of 'hallucinogen'. In the UK, 0.4% of the adult population under 60 years of age had used LSD in the past year, according to a survey in 2001/2.[4] However, in a survey of 16 to 24-year-olds in England and Wales in 2003, a total of 6% had used LSD at least once in their lifetime, with 1% using it in the past year.[5]

Effects sought

As with amfetamine derivatives, LSD often produces an initial burst of adrenaline-like activity characterised by flushing, hypertension, dry mouth, tachycardia, sweating, tremor, etc. These actions usually begin within 10 minutes of taking an oral dose and may persist through the rest of the experience. Sometimes the user may feel nauseous at the outset. As this initial stage progresses, the individual may begin to experience a range of psychotropic effects (the 'trip'). LSD is the most potent mind-altering substance known. Its precise effects are to some extent conditioned by the user's environment and expectation, but can include:

- Emotional lability – users may swing rapidly from one emotion to another, or appear to experience more than one emotion simultaneously.
- Time distortions, including perceptions of rapid ageing (of self or others), or time slowing down.
- Visual and auditory illusions (colours, smells and sounds may be enhanced or magnified; real images may assume unusual colours or patterns).
- Synaesthesia (a mixing of sensory input, so that the user may 'see' sounds or smells, and 'hear' or 'feel' colours, etc.).
- The events may have mystic, religious or philosophical overtones. The individual may become depersonalised and detached from reality, feel 'at peace with the world' or undergo 'out-of-body' experiences.

During the recovery period, as the effects of an LSD dose begin to wear off, the subject may experience episodes of normality alternating with psychedelic effects.

Most of the mind-altering properties of LSD involve distortion or misinterpretation of real sensory stimuli (i.e. illusions) rather than completely false perceptions without any sensory stimulus (hallucinations), although true hallucinations can occur. LSD also causes delusions (false beliefs), such as believing one to be invincible or able to fly. Consequently, although LSD is typically described as an hallucinogenic drug, this is rather misleading. Alternative descriptions are illusionogenic or illusogenic (illusion-producing) and psychedelic (producing an expansion of the mind and widening of perception).

Administration

LSD is nearly always administered orally, although nasal inhalation, injection, smoking and conjunctival instillation have been reported.[6] The dose required is small, usually between 50 and 200 mcg, but smaller doses may be taken by the inexperienced; sometimes as little as 20 mcg. LSD solution is used to impregnate small pieces of paper that are then dried, and this is the main means by which the drug is taken orally. These paper squares are often adorned with brightly coloured designs or motifs such as animals, geometric shapes, signs of the zodiac or cartoon characters. They are chewed and then swallowed. Tiny tablets or microdots are occasionally available (Figure 7.1). Conventional tablets, gelatin squares, sugar cubes, capsules or liquid preparations are less commonly seen. The drug is odourless, colourless and almost tasteless.

Taking LSD is an occasional activity for the majority of users. The drug may be taken as a club or rave drug, often with other substances such as ecstasy or cannabis, but it may also be taken in a quieter, more personal, environment to provoke contemplation, enjoyment of the senses, spiritual awareness or creativity.

There have been a number of 'scares' in the past that LSD might be given to unsuspecting schoolchildren en masse by drug dealers in the form of skin transfers or stickers 'to get them hooked'. LSD is not administered transdermally at street level, and no published research has demonstrated that it is absorbed through normal, intact human skin in amounts sufficient to cause intoxication. It is also most unlikely that

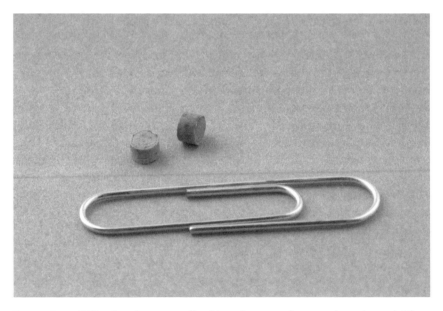

Figure 7.1 LSD microdots – small tablets that may be round or shaped (Photo courtesy of Multimedia Research Partners Ltd).

drug dealers would give away supplies of LSD, and because the drug is known not to cause physical dependence, the idea seems fanciful. Unfortunately, many parents have been unnecessarily alarmed by hoaxes of this kind, which have been reported regularly from the USA, Canada, Germany, France and the UK. All have been without foundation.[7,8]

Pharmacokinetics and pharmacology

The mechanism of action of the drug is becoming clearer. It is thought to interact principally with serotonergic systems in the central nervous system (CNS), particularly via $5HT_2$ receptors, but dopaminergic effects are also seen. LSD appears to be absorbed by mouth very quickly. The psychedelic effects of LSD usually take 30–90 minutes to begin after an oral dose and they last 3–12 hours, depending on the dose and the individual. The average duration is 6–8 hours. The half-life is about 3 hours, but can extend to 5 hours in some people[9,10] and the main route of elimination is via the liver. Although the exact enzyme system involved is not known, hydroxylation and conjugation is followed by excretion into bile.[11]

Adverse effects

Table 7.1 summarises the adverse effects. Apart from the adrenergic-like actions already mentioned, exhaustion, headaches, muscular weakness and inability to concentrate are quite common. However, most adverse effects are related to the mind-altering properties of the drug. Bad 'trips' may involve prolonged panic attacks, fear of insanity or death, general dysphoria, acute depression or frightening illusions. Unpleasant mental events were categorised in one US study of 107 LSD users who described their experiences.[12] Results were as follows: terror, 39%; crawling insects or animals, 18%; Satan's face appearing, 18%; ageing of others' faces, 12%; delusion of insanity, 5%. Distress or panic in the affected individual tends to make bad trips worse. Consequently, it has been advocated that pharmacological intervention should be avoided in patients presenting with distressing experiences of this kind and that those affected should be 'talked down' in a quiet place. In extreme situations, low-dose haloperidol or benzodiazepines have been used.[6,8,13]

LSD users tend to remain conscious and relatively communicative when prompted, even at the height of intoxication. However, temporary unawareness of intoxication is recognised as a significant problem: users may confuse the drugged state with reality.[13]

Table 7.1   Adverse effects of LSD

Common acute reactions
- Adrenergic 'fight or flight' effects (tachycardia, flushing, dry mouth, sweating, etc.)
- Exhaustion, tiredness, weakness
- Headache, inability to concentrate, disorientation, confusion
- Anxiety, dysphoria, panic, frightening illusions, delusions or hallucinations, psychosis
- Self-harm, accidents or violence while intoxicated

Rare acute reactions
- Ataxia, convulsions
- Paraesthesiae
- Hyperpyrexia, neuroleptic malignant syndrome (one case report associated with LSD plus alcohol[14])

Post-exposure reactions
- 'Flashbacks'
- Depression, feelings of isolation, psychotic symptoms extending beyond the period of intoxication
- Impaired concentration, insomnia/tiredness
- Weakness, exhaustion

Psychedelic effects occasionally result in curious injuries or acts of reckless behaviour or violence (against self or others) while in the intoxicated state. For example, delusions of being able to fly or of being invincible can have serious consequences. In the study of LSD users referred to above, 23 from a total of 107 declared that they or a close friend had been involved in a serious accident or had made a suicide attempt while under the influence of LSD.[12] Acute depression and feelings of loneliness after the effects of LSD have worn off may also lead to suicide attempts. Weakness, tiredness or sleeplessness can develop afterwards as well. The psychedelic effects may take some time to completely stop and may recur periodically for a few hours.

Psychosis more commonly occurs after chronic use of LSD, but can develop after a single dose and may become a long-term problem. As with amfetamines, it is not clear whether this represents a true drug-induced condition or the unmasking of a latent mental illness. In Germany, 3200 people contacted psychosocial services for treatment of psychiatric problems after using LSD and related substances in 1997; there were fewer than 50 such cases in 1992, possibly reflecting an increasing popularity of the drug there.[15]

'Flashbacks' can also be a problem.[16–18] These phenomena are psychedelic effects experienced long after the drug has been eliminated from the body and the mechanism underlying their development is obscure. They are more likely to occur in those who have used the drug on several occasions (more than ten times) and are generally not reported by people who have taken LSD on only a few occasions. Where flashbacks become a troublesome, persistent problem, they may be referred to by the more grandiose title of 'hallucinogen persisting perception disorder' (HPPD). In one study, 64% of 107 chronic users reported flashbacks but only 16% found them persistent or worrying.[12] Flashbacks can develop a few days after LSD intoxication or up to 1 year later and involve any aspect of a previous 'trip'. They can be induced at will by some individuals and may continue for years after exposure, but tend to diminish in intensity and frequency with time. Flashbacks most commonly take the form of visual aberrations and frequently reported components include the illusion that stationary objects are moving, haloes, the sudden appearance of bright patterns, time distortions, specific detailed images, and other visual or auditory hallucinations and illusions. They can be accompanied by emotional reactions (e.g. euphoria, anxiety) and illusions of changes to the body. Sometimes flashbacks are brought on by later abuse of other drugs (e.g. alcohol, cannabis), by physical or emotional stress, or particular environmental conditions (e.g. sudden darkness).

Research on HPPD treatments comprises small open studies and case reports. Various pharmacological methods have been used to suppress HPPD including benzodiazepines (especially clonazepam), clonidine, phenothiazines and naltrexone.[18–21] The neuroleptic drug risperidone has been consistently reported to exacerbate both the visual and emotional aspects of HPPD;[22–24] Selective serotonin reuptake inhibitors (SSRI) type antidepressants and phenothiazines may do this as well.[17,25,26] These exacerbations can be transient and may remit despite continued treatment.

LSD overdose is reported infrequently. Features on presentation may include mydriasis, hypertension, tachycardia, respiratory arrest, convulsions, hyperpyrexia or coma.

Dependence

Dependence is not recognised to occur in practice and withdrawal reactions have not been described. Tolerance may occur in the repeat user, but a few days' abstinence will restore full CNS sensitivity to the drug.

Interactions with medicines

Interactions between illicit drugs and conventional medicines have not been systematically studied in humans. Most data are derived from case reports and small-scale laboratory research and so should be interpreted cautiously. A full medication and substance-abuse history is necessary before investigating drug interactions in an individual patient. Investigation or prediction of LSD interactions is hampered by the poor understanding of its mode of action and the lack of details regarding its metabolism. Factors that may predispose LSD to interactions include:

- It is a very potent psychoactive drug with pronounced ability to cause hallucinations/illusions; elements of these effects may recur as 'flashbacks' for years afterwards. As noted above, some medicines may exacerbate LSD flashbacks.
- LSD acts via the serotonergic system.
- It is metabolised and excreted via the liver.

Antidepressants

Small studies of the experiences of LSD users when prescribed anti-depressants suggest that chronic administration of tricyclic antidepressants and lithium may subjectively increase the physical, hallucinatory and psychological responses to LSD while chronic administration of SSRI antidepressants, trazodone or monoamine oxidase inhibitors (MAOIs) subjectively decreases the response to LSD and may even eliminate its effects.[27,28]

A single case report described the advent of convulsions in a young man without a history of fitting who had been taking fluoxetine uneventfully for 1 year. He took LSD regularly while on fluoxetine, but developed convulsions on one occasion shortly after taking twice his normal dose of LSD.[29] If this was an interaction between the two drugs, it must be rare as it has never been described again.

Abuse and concurrent illness

Asthma

There are no reports in the medical literature of LSD exacerbating asthma.

Diabetes

Intoxication may prevent a diabetic recognising and/or dealing with a hypoglycaemic episode. The hypoglycaemic episode can also resemble intoxication, so bystanders may not seek medical attention.

Epilepsy

LSD has rarely been reported to cause convulsions, which may be more common with overdose.

Hepatic disease

There is no evidence that LSD causes liver damage. Hepatic failure could allow LSD to accumulate because the liver is the main route of metabolism and excretion.

Hypertension

LSD is unlikely to exacerbate existing hypertension and has not been reported to do so.

Immunity impairment

LSD is not known to adversely affect immune function.

Renal disease

Accumulation in renal failure is unlikely as long as the liver is functioning normally, but patients with renal failure typically become more sensitive to the CNS effects of many drugs, probably because of the accumulation of urea. LSD might exert more powerful psychotropic effects in this situation.

Pregnancy and breastfeeding

Pregnancy

Of the commonly abused illicit substances, LSD has been studied the least in human pregnancy. There are several case reports in the medical literature ascribing various congenital anomalies to the effects of LSD but there is no consistent pattern to these, rendering an association unproven. All of the human studies are small, relatively old and are poorly conducted and reported, by modern standards. The evidence from these does not support a link between maternal LSD use and fetal malformations or other adverse pregnancy outcome but neither do they provide reassurance about safety. More research is needed to ascertain any risk.

Breastfeeding

The use of LSD during breastfeeding has not been reported in the medical literature. Consequently, use in breastfeeding should be avoided because the effects upon the infant are completely unknown. LSD is a very potent psychoactive compound even in small doses.

References

1.   Dyer C. Patients given LSD may be able to claim compensation (news). *BMJ* 1995; 311: 1185–1186.
2.   *National Survey on Drug Use and Health*, Substance Abuse and Mental Health Services Administration (SAMHSA), Report ref. 30415. Rockville, MD: Office of Applied Studies, 2002.
3.   *Statistics on Drug Use in Australia 2002. Drug Statistics Series No. 12.* Cat no. PHE 43. Canberra: Australian Institute of Health and Welfare, February 2003.
4.   Aust R, Sharp C, Goulden C. *Prevalence of Drug Use: Key Findings from the 2001/02 British Crime Survey.* Home Office Research Study 182. London: Home Office, 2002.
5.   *Statistics on young people and drug misuse: England, 2003.* Statistical Bulletin 2004/13. London: National Statistics Office and Department of Health, 2004.
6.   Kulig K. LSD. *Emerg Med Clin North Am* 1990; 8: 551–558.
7.   Babin L. Blue star LSD: a psychedelic hoax. *Roy Can Mounted Police Bull* October 1988; 23–25.
8.   Schwartz R H. LSD: its rise, fall, and renewed popularity among high school students. *Pediatr Clin North Am* 1995; 42: 403–413.
9.   Aghajanian G K, Bing O H C. Persistence of lysergic acid diethylamide in the plasma of human subjects. *Clin Pharmacol Ther* 1964; 5: 611–614.
10. Papac D I, Foltz R L. Measurement of lysergic acid diethylamide (LSD) in human plasma by gas chromatography/negative ion chemical ionization mass spectrometry. *J Anal Toxicol* 1990; 14: 189–190.
11. Renkel M. Pharmacodynamics of LSD and mescaline. *J Nerv Ment Dis* 1957; 125: 424–427.
12. Schwartz R H. LSD: patterns of use by chemically dependent adolescents. *J Pediatr* 1987; 111: 936–938.

13. Miller P L, Gay G R, Ferris K C, Anderson S. Treatment of acute, adverse psychedelic reactions: 'I've tripped and I can't get down'. *J Psychoactive Drugs* 1992; 24: 277–279.

14. Bakheit A M O, Behan P O, Prach A T, *et al*. A syndrome identical to the neuroleptic malignant syndrome induced by LSD and alcohol. *Br J Addict* 1990; 85: 150–151.

15. Prepeliczay S. Socio-cultural and psychological aspects of contemporary LSD use in Germany. *J Drug Issues* Spring 2002; 431–458.

16. Horowitz M J. Flashbacks: recurrent images after the use of LSD. *Am J Psychiatry* 1969; 126: 565–569.

17. Abraham H D. Visual phenomenology of the LSD flashback. *Ann Gen Psychiatry* 1983; 40: 884–889.

18. Lerner A G, Gelkopf M, Skladman I, *et al*. Flashback and hallucinogen persisting perception disorder: clinical aspects and pharmacological treatment approach. *Isr J Psychiatry Relat Sci* 2002; 39: 92–99.

19. Lerner A G, Gelkopf M, Skladman I, *et al*. Clonazepam treatment of lysergic acid diethylamide-induced hallucinogen persisting perception disorder with anxiety features. *Int Clin Psychopharmacol* 2003; 18: 101–105.

20. Lerner A G, Oyffe I, Isaacs G, *et al*. Naltrexone treatment of hallucinogen persisting perception disorder. *Am J Psychiatry* 1997; 154: 437.

21. Lerner A G, Gelkopf M, Oyffe I, *et al*. LSD-induced hallucinogen persisting perception disorder treatment with clonidine: an open pilot study. *Int Clin Psychopharmacol* 2000; 15: 35–37.

22. Abraham H D, Mamen A. LSD-like panic from risperidone in post-LSD visual disorder. *J Clin Psychiatry* 1996; 16: 238–241.

23. Morehead D B. Exacerbation of hallucinogen-persisting perception disorder with risperidone. *J Clin Psychiatry* 1997; 17: 327–328.

24. Lerner A G, Shufman E, Kodesh A, *et al*. Risperidone-associated, benign transient visual disturbances in schizophrenic patients with a past history of LSD abuse. *Isr J Psychiatry Relat Sci* 2002; 39: 57–60.

25. Markel H, Lee A, Holmes R D, *et al*. LSD flashback syndrome exacerbated by selective serotonin reuptake inhibitor antidepressants in adolescents. *J Pediatr* 1994; 125: 817–819.

26. Young C R. Sertraline treatment of hallucinogen persisting perception disorder. *J Clin Psychiatry* 1997; 52: 85.

27. Bonson K R, Buckholz J W, Murphy D L. Chronic administration of serotonergic antidepressants attenuates the subjective effects of LSD in humans. *Neuropsychopharmacology* 1996; 14: 425–436.

28. Bonson K R, Murphy D L. Alterations in responses to LSD in humans associated with chronic administration of tricyclic antidepressants, monoamine oxidase inhibitors or lithium. *Behav Brain Res* 1996; 73: 1–2.

29. Picker W, Lerman A, Hajal F. Potential interaction of LSD and fluoxetine. *Am J Psychiatry* 1992; 149: 843–844.

8

Gamma hydroxybutyrate

Poisons and medicine are oftentimes the same substance given with
different intents.
Peter Mere Latham (1789–1875), *General Remarks*
on the Practice of Medicine

History

Gamma hydroxybutyrate (GHB) is known by various alternative chemical names including 4-hydroxybutyrate, 4-hydroxybutanoic acid, hydroxybutyric acid and sodium oxybate. The related compounds gamma butyrolactone (known as GBL) and 1,4-butanediol are converted into GHB by human metabolism after ingestion. GHB itself is known to occur naturally in the human body in the brain, but also in other tissues such as the kidneys, muscles and the heart.

GHB has attracted great interest from medical researchers and has been used therapeutically as a sedative pre-medicant before surgery, an intravenous anaesthetic, to alleviate the symptoms of narcolepsy, to treat acute alcohol withdrawal, to reduce cravings for alcohol in alcoholics, to maintain abstinence from heroin in those dependent upon it and to ameliorate the effects of cerebral ischaemia in patients with head injuries. In addition, it has been sold as a non-prescription dietary supplement for bodybuilding, to promote weight loss, or to treat insomnia. However, it is perhaps most well known as a psychoactive drug, and is one of a number of substances collectively referred to as 'club drugs' because of its association with young people attending nightclubs and raves. It has also been implicated in cases of drug-facilitated sexual assault ('date rape').

GBL and 1,4-butanediol are both marketed as dietary supplements with similar claims to GHB. They are also used as solvents in cleaning products.

Effects sought

Street names for this drug include 'GBH', 'liquid X', 'liquid ecstasy', 'fantasy', and 'G'. GHB is abused because it has relaxant, sedative and euphoric properties. It can produce disinhibition, relaxation, and a prolonged euphoria. The sedative effects, if undesirable, can be counteracted by administration with a stimulant such as amfetamine. Psychoactive effects are generally potentiated when taken with other psychotropic substances, especially alcohol, but begin about 15–60 minutes after ingestion. Some users find that it increases libido.

In addition, GHB is claimed to be an alternative to anabolic steroids because it purportedly increases muscle bulk and reduces body fat by stimulating the secretion of growth hormone. GBL and 1,4-butanediol have been marketed with similar claims.

Administration

GHB is usually supplied as an odourless white powder, sometimes as capsules or occasionally tablets, and is taken orally, usually dissolved in water. Sometimes it is supplied ready dissolved in water. It has a slightly salty taste, but this is easily disguised in any flavoured drink. Occasional reports of injection are described. Doses range from 2 g to over 30 g. GHB is not subject to illicit drug regulations in many countries.

Pharmacokinetics and pharmacology

GHB is actually a product of normal human metabolism. It is a catabolite of the inhibitory central nervous system (CNS) neurotransmitter gamma-aminobutyric ascid (GABA) and is found at 1000-fold lower concentrations than GABA itself. GHB is known to increase dopamine concentrations in the brain and to interact with endogenous CNS opioids. It may also increase CNS levels of other neurotransmitters (e.g. serotonin) and have agonist activity at certain GABA receptors. It is probably a neurotransmitter in its own right, as transport mechanisms and receptor sites have been identified in the brain.[1,2]

In humans, the absorption of GHB solution from the gastro-intestinal tract is significantly impaired by food.[3] In rats the oral bioavailability of GHB is 59–65% because of the effects of first-pass metabolism, and GHB is probably subject to significant first-pass metabolism in humans as well.[2] The average human elimination half-life has been measured as 20–53 minutes,[2] but it has been suggested that the elimination pathway is saturable and that at high doses the half-life would effectively be increased as a result.[4] This may explain the long duration of effects after administration of high doses. Acute effects generally last for up to 6 hours, but some milder psychotropic effects may persist beyond this. GHB is ultimately metabolised to carbon dioxide and water; there are no psychoactive metabolites.

GBL is metabolised to GHB in the body by enzymatic and non-enzymatic hydrolysis but has greater bioavailability than GHB because it is better absorbed from the gastrointestinal tract.[5] It is therefore more potent on an equimolar basis. 1,4-butanediol also requires metabolism for conversion to GHB: firstly by the enzyme alcohol dehydrogenase and then aldehyde dehydrogenase.[6]

Adverse effects

Side-effects are summarised in Table 8.1. As has already been noted, the products GBL and 1,4-butanediol are both converted to GHB and so produce the same adverse effects.[5-7] Note that side-effects seem particularly to be potentiated by alcohol.

The sedative effects of GHB should not be underestimated and its earlier use as an anaesthetic bear witness to its potential potency. One US study of 42 users identified that 66% reported loss of consciousness as a side-effect.[8] Reports of coma requiring ventilation and admission to intensive care were first described from the USA in the early 1990s,[9] and there have been further reports since then.[5,7,10,11] Doses greater than 50 mg/kg body weight are more likely to cause decreased cardiac output, respiratory depression, seizure-like episodes and coma.[11] One death caused by cardiac arrest was reported in 1997.[11] Other deaths caused by circulatory/respiratory failure have been described and attributed to GHB or precursor ingestion; sometimes, but not always, alcohol was also taken.[7,12,13] Aspiration of stomach contents while under the influence of GHB may be particularly troublesome because home-made

Table 8.1 Adverse effects of GHB

- Drowsiness, hypnagogic states, confusion, agitation, combativeness, fluctuating level of consciousness or mood, delirium, amnesia, unconsciousness, respiratory depression, coma
- Headache, tunnel vision, vertigo, dizziness
- Ataxia, hypotonia, myoclonic movements, seizure-like episodes, tremors
- Bradycardia, cardiac arrest, hypotension
- Nausea, vomiting, diarrhoea
- Urinary and faecal incontinence
- Hypothermia

GHB can contain appreciable quantities of the caustic alkali sodium hydroxide.[11]

GHB was first reported to cause a **withdrawal** reaction in 1994.[14] A 30-year-old woman who had taken 25 g daily in five divided doses for 2 years decreased the dose to 10 g per day before stopping completely. Twelve hours after the last dose she experienced tremor, anxiety and insomnia, which persisted for 12 days after cessation, but then resolved. Since this report many other similar cases have been described, and it is now known that GHB can cause dependence and a withdrawal reaction.[15–17] Because of tolerance, long-term users tend to escalate both the dose and the frequency of administration, such that large doses are often taken every few hours around the clock. Daily doses in excess of 100 g/day have been described. Often other substances are abused at the same time. The withdrawal reaction is not apparent in all long-term users, but can begin within 6 hours of the last dose of GHB and may last for up to 2 weeks. It includes symptoms such as:

- anxiety, agitation, dysphoria, confusion, hallucinations, delirium, paranoia
- insomnia
- tremors, muscle cramps
- nausea, vomiting, diarrhoea
- sweating
- tachycardia, hypertension.

The management of withdrawal is symptomatic and supportive, and benzodiazepines, for example, have often been used. One case of death during a particularly severe withdrawal reaction has been described.[16]

Interactions with medicines

Sedative medicines and alcohol

GHB and its precursors can produce a range of adverse reactions that could be additive with other medicines or drugs with similar effects. In particular, GHB has pronounced CNS depressant actions and although individual GHB–medicine combinations have not been studied in humans, all medicines with this property should be avoided by GHB users. For example, GHB is commonly taken with alcohol but this may facilitate a rapidly decreased level of consciousness and other sequelae of CNS depression. GHB has been used therapeutically to reduce cravings for alcohol in alcoholics, suggesting that the two drugs may have similar CNS actions. The effect of alcohol is particularly important for 1,4-butanediol because alcohol also competitively inhibits its metabolism, effectively prolonging its effects. In an affected individual, the full onset of CNS depression due to 1,4-butanediol may be delayed until alcohol has been metabolised, thus freeing alcohol dehydrogenase to initiate the conversion of 1,4-butanediol to active GHB.[6]

HIV (human immunodeficiency virus) medication

One case report describes a patient who developed near-fatal severe CNS depression after taking 10 mg/kg of GHB.[18] He had previously taken much bigger doses without these effects. This potentiation of GHB was attributed to the drugs ritonavir and saquinavir, both of which had been recently initiated. These two protease inhibitors may have inhibited the cytochrome P450-mediated first-pass metabolism of GHB, leading to increased GHB plasma levels.

Use and concurrent illness

Asthma

There are no specific studies on the abuse of GHB by people with asthma. However, because respiratory depression can occur at high dose its use is inadvisable.

Diabetes

There have been no studies of GHB abuse in patients suffering from diabetes. However, the balance of food intake and dose of hypoglycaemic drug in diabetic patients can be disrupted by vomiting, which is a recognised side-effect of GHB and of GHB withdrawal. Intoxication may prevent a diabetic patient recognising and/or dealing with a hypoglycaemic episode, particularly because GHB can cause such profound sedation. The hypoglycaemic episode can also resemble intoxication, so bystanders may not seek medical attention. The apathy and poor motivation engendered in some individuals by chronic drug dependence may mitigate against adequate control of blood glucose. Non-compliance with diet, failure to administer medication correctly or inadequate monitoring could result from this.

Epilepsy

GHB should be avoided by those suffering from epilepsy because it can cause seizure-like episodes. In fact, one of the reasons it was abandoned as an anaesthetic agent in the 1960s was its propensity to cause this problem.[19] GHB also acts via GABA, as do many anticonvulsant medicines, and the effects of co-administration are unknown.

Hepatic disease

In 16 patients with moderate to severe liver damage (cirrhosis), the rate of clearance of GHB was approximately halved compared to healthy subjects and the area under the curve doubled after a single dose.[20] The mean terminal half-life was 22 minutes in controls, 32 minutes in non-ascitic patients and 56 minutes in ascitic patients. Despite these effects, adverse reactions were mild and transient both in liver disease patients and in controls, and GHB plasma concentrations fell to negligible levels within 6–8 hours in all patients. GHB is not known to cause liver damage.

Hypertension

GHB abuse is not known to cause hypertension, although withdrawal may be associated with an elevated blood pressure.

Immunity impairment

The effects of GHB on immunity do not appear to have been studied, but no adverse effects have been described in the medical literature.

Renal disease

The use of GHB in patients with renal disease has not been investigated, but patients with renal failure typically become more sensitive to the CNS effects of many drugs, particularly those with sedative properties, probably because of the accumulation of urea. Consequently, GHB might exert more powerful psychotropic effects in this situation. GHB has not been linked to drug-induced kidney damage.

Pregnancy and breastfeeding

There have been no studies of GHB abuse in pregnant or lactating humans.

References

1. Wong C G T, Bottiglieri T, Snead III O C. GABA, gamma-hydroxybutyric acid, and neurological disease. *Ann Neurol* 2003; 54(Suppl. 6): S3–12.
2. Mason P E, Kerns II W P. Gamma hydroxybutyric acid (GHB) intoxication. *Acad Emerg Med* 2002; 9: 730–739.
3. Borgen L A, Okerholm R, Morrison D, *et al*. The influence of gender and food on the pharmacokinetics of sodium oxybate oral solution in healthy subjects. *J Clin Pharmacol* 2003; 43: 59–65.
4. Ferrara S D, Zotti S, Tedeschi L, *et al*. Pharmacokinetics of gamma-hydroxy-butyric acid in alcohol dependent patients after single and repeated oral doses. *Br J Clin Pharmacol* 1992; 34: 231–235.
5. From the Centers for Disease Control and Prevention. Adverse events associated with ingestion of gamma-butyrolactone – Minnesota, New Mexico, and Texas, 1998–1999. *JAMA* 1999; 281: 979–980.
6. Tancredi D N, Shannon M W. Case 30 – 2003: a 21-year old man with sudden alteration of mental status. *N Engl J Med* 2003; 349: 1267–1271.
7. Zvosec D L, Smith S W, McCutcheon J R, *et al*. Adverse events, including death, associated with the use of 1,4-butanediol. *N Engl J Med* 2001; 344: 87–94.
8. Miotto K, Darakjian J, Basch J, *et al*. Gamma-hydroxybutyric acid: patterns of use, effect and withdrawal. *Am J Addict* 2001; 10: 232–241.
9. From the Food and Drug Administration. Warning about GHB. *JAMA* 1991 265: 1802.
10. Thomas G, Bonner S, Gascoigne A. Coma induced by abuse of gamma-hydroxybutyrate (GBH or liquid ecstasy): a case report. *BMJ* 1997; 314: 35–36.
11. From the Centers for Disease Control and Prevention. Gamma hydroxy butyrate use – New York and Texas, 1995–1996. *JAMA* 1997; 277: 1511.
12. Timby N, Eriksson A, Bostrom K. Gamma-hydroxybutyrate-associated deaths. *Am J Med* 2000; 108: 518–519.
13. Theron L, Jansen K, Skinner A. New Zealand's first fatality linked to use of 1,4-butanediol (1,4-B, fantasy): no evidence of coingestion or comorbidity. *N Z Med J* 2003; 116: U650.
14. Galloway G P, Frederick S L, Staggers F Jr. Physical dependence on sodium oxybate. *Lancet* 1994; 343: 57.
15. Galloway G P, Frederick S L, Staggers FE Jr, *et al*. Gamma-hydroxybutyrate: an emerging drug of abuse that causes physical dependence. *Addiction* 1997; 92: 89–96.
16. Dyer J E, Roth B, Hyma B A. Gamma-hydroxybutyrate withdrawal syndrome. *Ann Emerg Med* 2001; 37: 147–153.
17. McDaniel C H, Miotto K A. Gamma hydroxybutyrate (GHB) and gamma butyrolactone (GBL) withdrawal: five case studies. *J Psychoactive Drugs* 2001; 33: 143–149.
18. Harrington R D, Woodward J A, Hooton T M, *et al*. Life-threatening interactions between HIV-1 protease inhibitors and the illicit drugs MDMA and gamma-hydroxybutyrate. *Arch Intern Med* 1999; 159: 2221–2224.

19. Dyer J E. Gamma-hydroxybutyrate: a health-food product producing coma and seizure like activity. *Am J Emerg Med* 1991; 9: 321–324.
20. Ferrara S D, Tedeschi L, Frison G, *et al*. Effect of moderate or severe liver dysfunction on the pharmacokinetics of gamma-hydroxybutyric acid. *Eur J Clin Pharmacol* 1996; 50: 305–310.

9

Phencyclidine

It produces profound analgesia to a degree that even some major surgical procedures may be done without supplemental drugs. It has the decided disadvantage of producing in some patients severe excitement on emergence and severe hallucinatory disturbances.
Description of the first clinical study of phencyclidine use in humans as an anaesthetic (1958)[1]

History

Phencyclidine (PCP or 'angel dust') was investigated as an intravenous anaesthetic in the 1950s but was withdrawn from the market because it produced unpleasant hallucinations, agitation and delirium in humans. The product was later used as a veterinary anaesthetic but is no longer available. All supplies now encountered at street level therefore derive from illicit manufacture.

Abuse has never been a major problem in the UK, Europe or Australia but in the USA, phencyclidine was a popular drug in the late 1960s and early 1970s, with a resurgence in the early 1980s. Yet by 2001, a US survey reported that only 1.8% of senior pupils at high school had ever used phencyclidine, compared with 7% in 1979.[2,3] To some extent phencyclidine has been supplanted by newer drugs such as ketamine, metamfetamine, methcathinone, crack cocaine and ecstasy. However, despite a relative lull for two decades there is evidence of a renewed interest in the drug amongst the US population. The number of emergency-room (casualty department) visits linked to phencyclidine increased by 78% from 1998 to 2001 (n = 3436 vs 6102), and initial analysis of 2002 data suggested this might increase further.[3] Nonetheless, only 0.1% of adults had used phencyclidine within the previous 12 months in a 2002 nationwide US household survey; 3.2% of the population surveyed had used it at least once during their lifetime.[3] Where there is increased use of the drug it seems to be localised to certain parts of the country, with most of it being manufactured in the Los Angeles area.

A large number of phencyclidine derivatives have been developed illicitly but none of these has gained widespread acceptance on the street. An example is 1-(1-phenylcyclohexyl)pyrrolidine or PHP; others include PCC, PCE and TCP.

Effects sought

Users seek euphoria, which develops within a few minutes of smoking but may take up to half an hour to culminate. When taken by mouth, intoxicating effects begin within an hour and peak at around 2 hours. The acute effects last some 4–8 hours but it may take a few days for the effects to wear off completely. Phencyclidine has a dissociative action – it tends to produce feelings of detachment from oneself and from the environment. This effect is typically accompanied by unusual perceptual distortions, delusions and hallucinations. Some users are attracted by the feelings of power and invulnerability that the drug gives them.

Administration

Phencyclidine is typically supplied as a white or off-white powder, but it is also available in crystalline form or as a liquid. Occasionally tablets or capsules are supplied. The drug is usually smoked, but it must be mixed with leafy material first such as tobacco, cannabis or even dried herbs. It can also be administered by nasal inhalation of dry powder or by mouth, but it has a bitter taste. Intravenous use is unusual. In the USA, phencyclidine has been identified as an adulterant of other illicit drugs because it is cheap and easy to make.

Pharmacokinetics and pharmacology

The mode of action of phencyclidine is not understood, but it is known to affect a range of central neurotransmitters including glutamate, dopamine, serotonin, acetylcholine and endogenous opioids. This probably accounts for the wide variety of side-effects that have been reported (Table 9.1). Of particular note is the fact that it significantly blocks the action of the central nervous system (CNS) neurotransmitter glutamate at NMDA (N-methyl-D-aspartate) receptors and this may explain why phencyclidine can produce symptoms that are so reminiscent of schizophrenia.[4] This observation has led to great interest in using phencyclidine to improve the understanding of this mental illness.

Table 9.1 Adverse effects of phencyclidine

Relatively acute problems
- Hypertension (very common, but hypertensive crises are rare), intracranial haemorrhage
- Tachycardia (very common), cardiac arrest
- Nausea, vomiting
- Hypersalivation, slurred speech
- Flushing, sweating, fever, hyperpyrexia (and sequelae)
- Bronchospasm, aspiration pneumonia, apnoea
- Nystagmus (very common)
- Numbness of the extremities
- Incoordination, rhabdomyolysis (and sequelae), convulsions, catatonia, tremor, dystonias and other movement disorders
- Confusion, amnesia, euphoria, agitation, violence, psychosis, hallucinations, delusions, dysphoria, aggression
- Variable consciousness, stupor, coma
- Bizarre and dangerous behaviour while intoxicated, sometimes with serious or fatal consequences

Problems connected with chronic use
- Dependence
- Chronic anxiety, confusion, depression
- Memory loss, speech difficulties
- Psychosis, various personality changes, 'flashbacks'

The half-life of phencyclidine varies greatly, from 7 hours to 5 days,[5–7] but the average is probably about 20 hours. Excretion is accelerated in the presence of acidified urine.[7] The drug is eliminated primarily by hydroxylation in the liver followed by kidney excretion. About 10% of circulating phencyclidine is excreted as unchanged drug in the urine.

Adverse effects

Several authors have reviewed the adverse effects of procyclidine.[2,5,8,9] As with ketamine, to which phencyclidine is closely related chemically, much concern has centred on the unusual perceptual distortions, mind-altering and behavioural effects of phencyclidine. In the USA particularly, strange dissociative and psychotomimetic effects have resulted in bizarre accidents and acts of self-harm or violence. Actual harm to the user may be disguised by the analgesic properties of phencyclidine. Many people who use phencyclidine for the first time find the experience unpleasant and do not use the drug again.

Phencyclidine-induced psychosis can be peculiarly persistent and may take weeks or even months to dissipate. As with many other drugs of abuse it is unclear whether phencyclidine simply unmasks or exacerbates a tendency to psychosis in an individual, or causes the illness *de novo*.[8,10]

Those intoxicated with phencyclidine typically show frequent changes in behaviour and level of alertness[5,7,9] (see Table 9.1). Phencyclidine is a very lipophilic drug and symptoms of intoxication may sometimes reappear 2 or 3 days after the original exposure, when fatty tissues are metabolised and it is released into the circulation again.

References

1. Greifenstein F E, DeVault M, Yoshitake J, *et al*. A study of 1-aryl cyclohexylamine for anesthesia. *Anesth Analg* 1958; 37: 283–294.
2. Anonymous. PCP (Phencyclidine). *NIDA Capsule (CAP14)*. Bethesda, MD: National Institute on Drug Abuse, 1993, pp. 1–2.
3. *National Survey on Drug Use and Health*, Substance Abuse and Mental Health Services Administration (SAMHSA), Report ref. 30415. Rockville, MD: Office of Applied Studies, 2002.
4. Murray J. Phencyclidine (PCP): a dangerous drug, but useful in schizophrenia research. *J Psychol* 2002; 136: 319–327.
5. Baldridge E B, Bessen H A. Phencyclidine. *Emerg Med Clin North Am* 1990; 8: 541–550.
6. Cook C E, Brine D R, Jeffcoat A R, *et al*. Phencyclidine disposition after intravenous and oral doses. *Clin Pharmacol Ther* 1982; 31: 625–634.
7. Done A K, Aronow R, Miceli J N. Pharmacokinetic bases for the diagnosis and treatment of acute PCP intoxication. In: Smith D E, *et al*., eds. *PCP: Problems and Prevention*. Iowa: Kendall/Hunt Publishing Company, 1982, 64–69.
8. Wright H H, Cole E A, Batey S R, *et al*. Phencyclidine-induced psychosis: eight year follow-up of ten cases. *South Med J* 1988; 81: 565–567.
9. Isaacs S O, Martin P, Washington J A. Phencyclidine (PCP) abuse. *Oral Surg Oral Med Oral Pathol* 1986; 61: 126–129.
10. Erard R, Luisada P V, Peele R. The PCP psychosis: prolonged intoxication or drug-precipitated functional illness? In: Smith D E, *et al*., eds. *PCP: Problems and Prevention*. Iowa: Kendall/Hunt Publishing Company, 1982, 47–63.

10

Volatile substance abuse

Dr Snow gave that blessed chloroform and the effect was soothing,
quieting and delightful beyond measure.
Queen Victoria describing the administration of
anaesthetic chloroform in her Journal

History

Volatile substance abuse (VSA) can be defined as 'deliberate inhalation of a volatile substance to achieve a change in mental state'.[1] The practice is also known as inhalant abuse. It should be noted that alkyl nitrites, which are also volatile substances, will not be discussed here as they are used in a different milieu, have a different mechanism of action and different side-effects: they are considered separately in Chapter 18.

Abuse of volatile compounds is a relatively modern practice, which has arisen in concert with the rise of the chemicals industry. Without the ability to synthesise large quantities of volatile compounds, the problem of abuse cannot exist as these substances do not occur freely in nature. Perhaps the earliest examples of VSA are the compulsive abuse of ether and chloroform, which was known in the 19th century (e.g. in Victorian Britain).

In modern times, the volatile compounds that are abused are mainly solvents, fuels, propellants and gases. They are perhaps unique amongst substances of abuse in that the main users are children and teenagers: most are between 10 and 18 years old. The majority start when aged between 10 and 14. This subject has been particularly well studied in the UK. A population survey of UK adults over the age of 16 in 2001/2 reported that 2% had ever abused volatile substances, but in adults aged 16–24 this was 6%.[2] Similarly, while only 0.1% of the general adult population admitted abusing glues in the past year in 2002,[3] 8% of young people aged 11–15 engaged in VSA during the previous year in 2003.[4] In 1992, the UK Department of Health considered that about 70% of users 'experimented' with volatile substances a small number of times only, but that about 1% of secondary school children became long-term users who abused inhalants regularly for more than 3 months.[5]

A population survey in Australia in 2001 revealed that 2.6% of the general population over 14 years of age had abused inhalants at least once in their lifetime.[6] A similar survey in the USA in 2002 gave a figure of 9.7% in people aged over 12 years.[7] However, in both of these surveys data included alkyl nitrites abuse as well. When specifically asked about VSA in 2002, it was reported that 16% of US schoolchildren aged 12 had used them at least once in their life.[8]

The UK is one of the few countries with a mechanism for collecting data on VSA-related mortality. In fact it was not until mortality data became available in the 1970s that the problem of VSA began to attract higher profile medical and media attention. The annual number of UK deaths attributed to VSA gradually increased until 1990, but there has been a decline since then. In 1990, the number of deaths peaked at 152 for the year. In 1991 this fell to 122 and by 2001 the number of fatalities was 63.[9] This decline is most welcome but the reasons for it are unknown. It may represent a genuine decrease in use as a result of recognition of the potential adverse consequences: in the USA there is also evidence for a gradual decline in the popularity of VSA amongst teenagers since the mid-1990s.[10] Alternatively, and more likely, other abusable substances have become more popular. Tobacco and alcohol are readily available and there is evidence for increased use of tobacco amongst teenage girls in some Western countries; certain alcoholic products are now marketed with teenagers in mind. Ecstasy, which was unknown until the mid-1980s, has become a very important youth drug and cannabis usage has increased since that time. Both of these illicit drugs are relatively cheap and easy to obtain.

Effects sought

The first 'rush' or 'buzz' occurs when a relatively high concentration of inhaled substance reaches the brain quickly and is characterised by the rapid onset of an intense feeling of exhilaration. The subsequent effects can appear similar to drunkenness: feeling merry, playful and uninhibited, and sociability is often increased. The emotions prevalent at the time can be heightened. Unlike alcohol, inhalants commonly cause euphoria, hallucinations and perceptual disturbances. The hallucinations can, to some extent, be controlled and sometimes become a group activity.

All these effects appear very quickly – within minutes – but do not last long. However, the experienced (usually chronic) user can sustain the desirable effects for several hours by repeating inhalations when the effects of previous exposures begin to wear off.

It is not always easy to understand why a particular child or teenager has taken to VSA. Undoubtedly the 'naughtiness' and potential danger associated with a behaviour that would shock or anger parents is an attraction for some. Loneliness, boredom, domestic strife or feelings of inadequacy may sometimes be important causes. For others, solvents are simply an easily obtainable, affordable alternative to the alcohol consumed by older friends and relatives. Inhalants are even more accessible to teenagers than tobacco. The hallucinations and loss of control experienced can be pleasurable or frightening, but either way can represent an appealing escape from reality.

In the UK, there is some evidence that users are more likely to come from families at the lower end of the socioeconomic scale and that the incidence is greater in inner city areas. Inhalant users are also more likely to play truant from school than other children.

Administration

The terms 'glue sniffing' and 'solvent misuse' are misleading as they only cover part of the problem. Numerous products are involved, as volatile substances have a wide variety of uses in the domestic, school and work environment. Some of these preparations are listed in Table 10.1. It is difficult to be certain which ones are used most commonly. The 2001 data for abuse-related deaths in the UK show that gas fuels accounted for the biggest proportion of deaths (72%), followed by aerosols (20%) then glues (6%).[9] In earlier years the mortality statistics showed a greater preponderance of aerosols and glues, which seem to be implicated in progressively fewer deaths. It is not clear whether certain volatile substance-based products, and the methods of using them, are intrinsically more likely to cause harm than others or whether a greater awareness of the problem by suppliers and more controls on the sales of glues, in particular, have limited availability. Some products have also been re-formulated to remove volatile substances. In an attempt to limit the deaths caused by gas fuels, in 1999 the UK introduced legislation to ban sales of cigarette lighter fuel refills to persons aged under 18.

As with many forms of drug abuse, VSA can be either a group or an individual activity. The practice may take place in quiet public areas (such as car parks, recreation grounds and woodland) or in the home.

Table 10.1 Substances that may be abused by inhalation

Substance	Sources
Solvents	
Toluene, xylene, hexane	Many glues with a solvent smell; some paints, paint thinners and paint strippers
1,1,1-trichloroethane, trichloroethylene	Typewriter correction fluids (and thinners for them); solvent-based plaster removers; dry-cleaning fluids, stain removers, degreasers, etc.
Other chlorinated hydrocarbons	Paints, varnishes, paint strippers, dyestuffs, dry-cleaning fluids; chloroform and carbon tetrachloride
Ketones (e.g. acetone)	Nail-varnish remover; polystyrene cements
Esters	Marker pens, adhesives
Propellants, gases and fuels	
Propane, butane	Cigarette-lighter fuel; bottled camping and stove gases; propellant in aerosols
Chlorofluorocarbons	Propellant in aerosols; the active ingredient in some sprays used to relieve the pain of sports injuries; fire extinguishers; gaseous general anaesthetics
Dimethyl ether	Aerosol propellant
Nitrous oxide	Nitrous oxide-based general anaesthetics (e.g. Entonox); propellant in spray canisters of whipped cream (see Chapter 12)
Fuels	Petrol, paraffin
Nitrites	
Amyl nitrite, butyl nitrite	Available in sex shops and other outlets under various brand names (see Chapter 18)

The administration methods adopted depend on the inhalant being abused. The user needs to obtain a high concentration of volatile substance in the lungs quickly in order to experience the sudden 'rush' of intoxication that is the initial desired effect.

A common procedure is to inhale concentrated fumes from a limited space and to re-breathe this air repeatedly until a 'high' is achieved. This can be accomplished by holding a plastic bag containing the inhalant firmly over the mouth and nose and then breathing in and out rapidly several times. This is known as 'bagging'; supermarket carrier bags and crisp packets are commonly used. Other methods have involved placing plastic bags completely over the head or inhaling from underneath bedclothes or similar whole-body covering. Such techniques produce varying degrees of hypoxia, which is known to exacerbate the pro-arrhythmic potential of these agents, but it may also intensify the euphoric effects. Clearly some of these activities also carry the risk of death from suffocation.

The inhalant may also be applied to a rag held over the mouth and nose to allow deep inhalation of the vapour ('huffing'). A similar technique can be used with items of clothing (e.g. cuffs and sleeves of jumpers, scarves, handkerchiefs). Sometimes users breathe fumes directly from the original container ('snorting'); others inhale from hands cupped over the mouth or nose. Chlorofluorocarbons (CFCs) and butane are sometimes sprayed directly down the throat. This is known to be a very hazardous practice and can cause sudden death (see below).

Pharmacokinetics

Following inhalation, vapours are readily absorbed into the bloodstream and access to the brain is rapid because of the high lipophilicity of the substances involved. The lungs are an important route of excretion subsequent to inhalation. Consequently, being volatile, most solvents and related substances do not cause long-lasting central nervous system (CNS) effects following a single 'sniff' because pulmonary excretion is usually rapid. The actions of butane and CFCs disappear after a few minutes but the effect of toluene can last 30–45 minutes following a single 'sniffing' episode.

Adverse effects

The intoxicated individual may appear disorientated, with slurred speech, clumsy movements and unusual behaviour. The irritant properties of certain solvents such as toluene can produce erythema around the mouth and nose, and inflammation of peri-oral abrasions or spots. Coughing, lacrimation and salivation can also occur as a result of this irritancy. Other undesirable effects from the user's point of view include vomiting, confusion, dizziness and drowsiness. Some users become very depressed, aggressive, agitated or frightened.

There may be a subsequent hangover feeling in some users, even after a single exposure. This usually takes the form of drowsiness, headache, loss of appetite and inability to concentrate.

Deaths during the period of intoxication are basically the result of one of three consequences: CNS depression, accidents arising as a result of intoxication or sudden death. CNS depression and sudden death are the principal direct toxic effects of inhalants. Analysis of 30 years of UK mortality data for VSA-related deaths (1971 to 2001; 1986 cases) reveals that direct toxic effects of the inhalant were responsible for 53% of deaths, trauma in 16% of cases, inhalation of vomit in 15%, and suffocation in a plastic bag in 12%.[9]

All of the inhaled products can cause a CNS derangement that appears superficially similar to drunkenness. Historically, trichloroethane, trichloroethylene and chloroform have all been used as general anaesthetics, so the ability of commonly abused inhalants to produce serious CNS depression should not be underestimated. As with all similar drugs, the effects produced in an individual are dose-dependent; greater levels of exposure may result, progressively, in disorientation, ataxia, sedation, unconsciousness and even respiratory depression or coma. In one study of 335 users, 3% had been admitted to hospital in a coma and a further 14% had experienced 'blackouts' without hospital admission.[11] One study suggests that short-term VSA is unlikely to cause neuropsychological problems,[12] but CNS damage may occur with chronic exposure (see below).

Although the direct CNS effects in isolation are rarely fatal, significant repercussions may arise indirectly. Accidental deaths and serious injuries can be sustained by the semiconscious or disorientated user, sometimes as a result of hallucinations or illusions; some believe that they are able to fly or swim[13] and falls from heights and drownings do occur. Aspiration of vomit while sedated, and suffocation in the large plastic bags used by some teenagers, have already been alluded to. In addition, the reduced awareness of danger associated with intoxication increases the risk of fires. Solvents, fuels and butane propellants are highly flammable and many users or their associates smoke.

Apart from the direct or indirect CNS effects, the other major cause of mortality is sudden death. Tragically, some of these deaths are in first-time users and, as has already been stated, many of these are young teenagers who would probably only have abused once or twice as an 'experiment'. There are also many fatal cases documented amongst long-term users. Most of these deaths are thought to be caused by ventricular fibrillation but this has been difficult to confirm because the majority of sufferers are either found dead or die shortly afterwards. Even when the cause and/or diagnosis has been confirmed at an early stage, resuscitation is often unsuccessful.

Many sudden deaths occur shortly after a bout of 'sniffing', when the user is stressed emotionally or physically (particularly by running). This is sometimes called the 'sudden sniffing death syndrome'. It is therefore probable that sympathetic nervous system activity or circulating adrenaline play a role in the aetiology. It seems likely that volatile substances sensitise the myocardium to catecholamines. Animal studies show that both adrenaline[14,15] and asphyxia[14,16] increase the arrhythmogenic actions of solvents and that ethanol may further potentiate some of these effects.[17] Animal work also confirms that myocardial sensitivity may persist for hours after inhalant exposure.[16] This may explain why some documented cases of sudden death seem to occur some time after a sniffing event. The inhalational anaesthetic halothane, itself a CFC, can rarely cause arrhythmias and has even precipitated or exacerbated cardiac problems in those known to have been chronically exposed to solvents,[18] providing further evidence that cardiac sensitisation is not always an acute short-lived effect. Interestingly, trichloroethane was used briefly as a general anaesthetic in the 1960s, but this practice was discontinued because of a high incidence of ventricular arrhythmias. It is structurally related to halothane.

Another form of sudden death with a cardiac origin is believed to result from vagal inhibition as a reflex response to inhalants being sprayed directly against the back of the throat.[19] Very rapid cooling of the larynx can stimulate the vagus nerve to the extent that the pulse rapidly slows and then the heart stops. This is particularly associated with butane and CFC propellants.

Although a range of different arrhythmias has been observed in animals exposed to inhalants, ventricular arrhythmias are reported most consistently in humans. Occasionally those presenting with severe arrhythmia are successfully resuscitated[20–22] but this does depend on help being near at hand. Other rare human cardiac effects have included myocardial infarction (MI).[20]

Given the many serious risks that the user may encounter following inhalation, sniffing alone is potentially more hazardous than a group activity.

Long-term use

Generally, chronic abuse may be associated with a decreased ability to concentrate, insomnia and nightmares. Chronic users are also more likely to have resorted to theft to keep the habit going. Various medical problems may occur as a result of long-term misuse but there is no consistent pattern to these problems and it is not clear why some users suffer and others do not. Adverse effects reported include neurological damage such as structural abnormalities in the brain,[23–25] cognitive impairment,[24] peripheral neuropathy,[23] persistent tremor,[26] dementia,[23] encephalopathy[23] and temporal lobe epilepsy.[27] Other problems that have been linked to chronic VSA are psychosis,[27] renal damage,[28] hepatotoxicity[29] and cardiac myopathy.[30,31] Some inhalants are more toxic than others; chronic exposure to toluene seems to cause a particularly wide array of adverse effects. Benzene toxicity and lead poisoning have been described in persons regularly exposed to petrol.

Tolerance seems to develop in the chronic user such that much larger amounts of inhalant are required to achieve a 'high'. This tolerance quickly reverses if inhalants are withheld for a few days. A possible withdrawal reaction has been described consisting of irritability, headaches, sleep disturbance, tremor, sweating, nausea, tachycardia and delusions.[32,33] This appears to be rare but usually takes 1 or 2 days to develop following abstinence and may last a few days or weeks. A withdrawal reaction has also been described in babies born to women who were chronic users of volatile substances during pregnancy (see below).[34] Animal work suggests that withdrawal may occur only with certain solvents.[1] On the whole, VSA has a low dependence potential and usually is not associated with chronic daily usage or a compulsion to continue administration.

Pregnancy and breastfeeding

Pregnancy

Much information has been published on solvent exposure during pregnancy but most of it does not relate to deliberate abuse. Notably, various studies of occupational exposure to solvents have been performed. These have reported differing results depending upon the solvent involved, the extent of exposure and other factors. For example, some have described an increased risk of miscarriage, others have not.[35] Some studies suggest an increased risk of specific congenital defects but there is no consistent link to a definite anomaly and some studies show no association.

Unfortunately there are no large prospective studies of VSA in pregnancy. The small studies available suggest that VSA during human pregnancy may increase the risk of adverse outcomes. Some have specifically assessed the effects of toluene abuse during human pregnancy.[35] From these, there is evidence that toluene might cause prematurity, low birth weight and a mild facial dysmorphism. Follow-up of a proportion of these cases suggested that growth and developmental retardation might ensue in infancy. However, the total number of published cases is small.

The largest detailed study of VSA on pregnancy outcomes is from Canada.[36] A retrospective analysis of 56 cases where VSA was confirmed in pregnancy showed these adverse outcomes, although it should be noted that half of the women also abused alcohol and other substances:

Maternal
Renal tubular acidosis	5.3%
Grand mal seizure at 23 weeks	3.6%

Neonatal
Premature delivery	21.4%
Delayed metabolic acidosis	17.8%
Intra-uterine growth retardation	16.1%
Major congenital anomaly	16.1%
Dysmorphic facial features	12.5%
Hearing loss	10.7%

Other cases of maternal renal tubular acidosis during pregnancy have been described in known heavy users of toluene, which may also cause hyperchloraemic acidosis in the neonate.[37]

In 1996, a team of researchers in Canada suggested that VSA can be associated with a neonatal withdrawal syndrome that may respond to treatment with phenobarbital.[34] This was identified in 32 babies born over a 4-year period and was characterised by a high-pitched cry, lack of sleep, tremor, hypotonia, poor feeding and a hyperactive Moro reflex. Treatment was typically initiated about 24 hours after birth and lasted for about 6 days. The authors stated that the aroma of solvents in mother or baby may be a marker for this syndrome. In the case series of 56 births described above, 24 babies suffered from a withdrawal reaction (43%).[36]

Breastfeeding

VSA in lactating women has not been studied, but solvents are small lipophilic molecules and there is almost certain to be some passage into breast milk. However, the very short half-lives of most volatile substances suggest that breastfeeding should not cause problems for the infant unless it occurs while the mother is actually intoxicated, or shortly afterwards. Even if breast milk containing solvent is ingested by the infant it is not known what proportion might subsequently enter the infant bloodstream.

Reducing the abuse problem

In most countries it is not illegal to abuse inhalants in public unless the law is broken in other respects (e.g. breach of the peace, criminal damage, trespass). Given the range of potentially abusable substances available, it is virtually impossible to restrict supplies via legislation. For example in England and Wales the Intoxicating Substances Supply Act of 1985 makes it illegal for any shopkeeper to sell volatile substances with the knowledge that they are likely to be abused, but a breach of the law is difficult to prove. As with over-the-counter (OTC) medicine abuse some products (e.g. adhesives) could be kept behind the counter or out of sight, giving shop owners the opportunity to refuse a sale if necessary.

The retailer needs to appreciate which substances on his/her premises are open to abuse and ensure that all staff understand the nature of the problem. Some products are clearly a greater attraction to users than others. For example, aerosol hairsprays and air fresheners contain a proportionately larger amount of available propellant for abuse than, say, shaving foam or spray paint. These latter products are thus much less likely to be abused. Some products contain virtually pure volatile substances and are particularly open to abuse, e.g. camping-stove gas refills, cigarette-lighter fuel refills, dry-cleaning fluid, coolant sprays used to relieve sports injuries, and some 'thinners' for typewriter correction fluid or paint. Many of these are unusual products for a

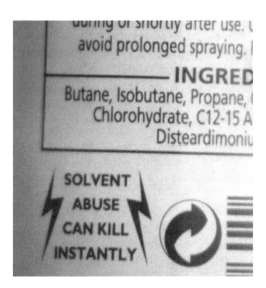

Figure 10.1 Many products manufactured in the UK are now labelled with the warning: 'Solvent abuse can kill instantly'.

Table 10.2 Pointers to inhalant abuse

- The smell of volatile substances persists on the breath for several hours after inhalation; the smell may also arise from clothes or a cloth about the person
- Frequent purchase of potentially abusable substances by the same individual; groups of teenagers buying inhalants together or suspected shop-lifting of these products
- Signs of intoxication (see text)
- Obvious truancy
- Facial erythema and spots, inflammation or abrasions around the mouth and nose
- Runny nose, watery or bloodshot eyes
- Finding empty containers of abusable substances or used plastic bags 'hidden' where the teenager has been; signs of glues, paints, etc. on skin, clothes or bedclothes
- Regular signs of 'hangover' (e.g. headaches, drowsiness) or of repeated sore throats, coughing or colds
- Sudden changes in mood, lifestyle and appetite, or secrecy concerning absences from home; inability to concentrate

young teenager to buy and so arouse suspicion. A national report in the UK in 1995 recommended that all potentially abusable household products should be labelled to alert retailers and parents to the danger.[1] Many products manufactured in the UK are now labelled with the warning: 'Solvent abuse can kill instantly' (Figure 10.1), although not all manufacturers comply with the recommendation and there is no commitment to a similar labelling policy in the rest of Europe.[2] The warning does of course also enable potential users to identify abusable products more easily.

It is difficult for shopkeepers, parents or teachers to identify a potential user; Table 10.2 summarises some key points that may help. Clearly some of these indicators could be confused with the normal process of teenage development. UK mortality data shows that most deaths from VSA occur in the home.[9]

References

1. Advisory Council on the Misuse of Drugs. *Volatile Substance Abuse*. London: HMSO, 1995.
2. *Seminar Report. Young People and Volatile Substance Abuse – Developing a Shared Approach*. London: Department of Health, November 2002.
3. Aust R, Sharp C, Goulden C. *Prevalence of Drug Use: Key Findings from the 2001/02 British Crime Survey*. Home Office Research Study 182. London: Home Office, 2002.

4. National Centre for Social Research/National Foundation for Educational Research. *Drug Use, Smoking and Drinking among Young People in England in 2003: headline figures*. London: Department of Health, 2004.

5. Department of Health. *Solvents – a Parent's Guide*. London: HMSO, 1992.

6. *Statistics on Drug Use in Australia 2002. Drug Statistics Series No. 12*. Cat no. PHE 43. Canberra: Australian Institute of Health and Welfare, February 2003.

7. *National Survey on Drug Use and Health*, Substance Abuse and Mental Health Services Administration (SAMHSA), Report ref. 30415. Rockville, MD: Office of Applied Studies, 2002.

8. Johnston L D, O'Malley P M, Bachman J G, *et al. Ecstasy Use Falls for Second Year in a Row, Overall Teen Drug Use Drops*. National press release, University of Michigan News and Information Services, Ann Arbor, 19 December 2003.

9. Field-Smith M E, Butland B K, Ramsey J D, *et al. Trends in Death Associated with Abuse of Volatile Substances*. Report No. 16. London: Department of Community Health Sciences, St George's Hospital Medical School, June 2003.

10. Hanson G R. Director's column: Rising to the challenges of inhalant abuse. *NIDA Notes* 2002; 17(4).

11. Watson J M. *Solvent Abuse – Adolescent Epidemic?* London: Croom Helm, 1996.

12. Chadwick O, Anderson R, Bland M, *et al.* Neuropsychological consequences of volatile substance abuse; a population based study of secondary school pupils. *BMJ* 1989; 298: 1679–1684.

13. Evans A C, Raistrick D. Phenomenology of intoxication with toluene based adhesives and butane gas. *Br J Psychiatry* 1987; 150: 769–773.

14. Reinhardt C F, Azar A, Maxfield M E, *et al.* Cardiac arrhythmias and aerosol sniffing. *Arch Environ Health* 1971: 22: 265–279.

15. Clark D G, Tinston D J. Acute inhalation toxicity of some halogenated and non-halogenated hydrocarbons. *Hum Toxicol* 1982; 1: 239–247.

16. Taylor G J, Harris W S. Cardiac toxicity of aerosol propellants. *JAMA* 1970; 214: 81–85.

17. White J, Carlson G. Epinephrine-induced cardiac arrhythmias in rabbits exposed to trichloroethylene: potentiation by ethanol. *Toxicol Appl Pharmacol* 1981; 60: 458–465.

18. McLeod A A, Marjot R, Monaghan M J, *et al.* Chronic cardiac toxicity after inhalation of 1,1,1-trichloroethane. *BMJ* 1987; 294: 727–729.

19. Shepherd R T. Mechanism of sudden death associated with volatile substance abuse. *Hum Toxicol* 1989; 8: 287–292.

20. Cunningham S R, Dalzell G W N, McGirr P, *et al.* Myocardial infarction and primary ventricular fibrillation after glue sniffing. *BMJ* 1987; 294: 739–740.

21. Wodka R M, Jeong E W S. Cardiac effects of inhaled typewriter correction fluid. *Ann Intern Med* 1989; 110: 91–92.

22. Gunn J, Wilson J, Mackintosh A F. Butane sniffing causing ventricular fibrillation. *Lancet* 1989; 333: 617.

23. Lolin Y. Chronic neurological toxicity associated with exposure to volatile substances. *Hum Toxicol* 1989; 8: 293–300.

24. Rosenberg N L, Grigsby J, Dreisbach J, *et al*. Neuropsychologic impairment and MRI abnormalities associated with chronic solvent abuse. *J Toxicol Clin Toxicol* 2002; 40: 21–34.

25. Aydin K, Sencer S, Demir T, *et al*. Cranial MR findings in chronic toluene abuse by inhalation. *Am J Neuroradiol* 2002; 23: 1173–1179.

26. Miyagi Y, Shima F, Ishido K, *et al*. Tremor induced by toluene misuse successfully treated by a Vim thalamotomy. *J Neurol Neurosurg Psychiatry* 1999; 66: 794–796.

27. Byrne A, Kirby B, Zibin T, *et al*. Psychiatric and neurological effects of chronic solvent abuse. *Can J Psychiatry* 1991; 36: 735–738.

28. Crowe A V, Howse M, Bell G M, *et al*. Substance abuse and the kidney. *Q J Med* 2000; 93: 147–152.

29. Baerg R D, Kimberg D V. Centrilobular hepatic necrosis and acute renal failure in "solvent sniffers". *Ann Intern Med* 1970; 73: 713–720.

30. Mee A S, Wright P L. Congested (dilated) cardiomyopathy in association with solvent abuse. *J R Soc Med* 1980; 73: 671–672.

31. Wiseman M N, Banim S. 'Glue sniffer's' heart? *BMJ* 1987; 294: 739.

32. Merry J, Zachariadis N. Addiction to glue sniffing. *BMJ* 1962; 2: 1448.

33. American Psychiatric Association. *DSM-IV, Diagnostic and Statistical Manual of Mental Disorders*, 4th edn. Washington, DC: APA, 2000.

34. Tenenbein M, Casiro O G, Seshia M M K, *et al*. Neonatal withdrawal from maternal volatile substance abuse. *Arch Dis Child* 1996; 74: F204–207.

35. Wills S. Street drugs. In: Lee A, *et al*., eds. *Therapeutics in Pregnancy and Lactation*. Oxford: Radcliffe Medical Press, 2000, 227–246.

36. Scheeres J J, Chudley A E. Solvent abuse in pregnancy: a perinatal perspective. *J Obstet Gynaecol Can* 2002; 24: 22–26.

37. Goodwin T M. Toluene abuse and renal tubular acidosis in pregnancy. *J Obstet Gynecol* 1988; 71: 715–718.

11

Performance-enhancing drugs

Man is a gaming animal. He must always be trying to get the better in
something or other.
Charles Lamb (1775–1834), 'Essays of Elia'

The taking of prohibited drugs to improve physical attributes and performance in competition is also called doping. A huge range of drugs has been used to enhance athletic and gymnastic ability, to increase strength, assist in training, boost stamina or promote a lean and more muscular physique. Drugs such as amfetamines, cocaine, over-the-counter (OTC) sympathomimetics, gamma hydroxybutyrate (GHB) and caffeine have been used widely to enhance performance in endurance sports, and to increase stamina and 'fat-burning' during training, but these drugs are the subject of other chapters in this book. Similarly, cannabis has been used to promote calmness and relaxation for events where this is desirable. The remaining substances discussed below range from simple molecules to complex naturally occurring proteins. Many of the preparations used are nutritional supplements and a detailed discussion of these is beyond the scope of this book. Some medicines are banned in athletes by the World Anti-doping Agency and these are described in Box 11.1.

Anabolic-androgenic steroids

These are usually known simply as anabolic steroids and are used medicinally to treat male hypogonadism and certain haematological disorders. They are, however, infamous as the classic performance-enhancing drugs: associated with Soviet Bloc athletes in the Cold War, allegations of cheating in international sporting events, and the periodic banning of individual athletes following positive urine tests. They are particularly linked to a range of characteristic and unpleasant side-effects. The infamy of anabolic steroids is such that the generic term 'steroid' – which technically incorporates a wide range of drugs used therapeutically from vitamin D to oral contraceptives – has become synonymous with anabolic steroids in the minds of many.

> **Box 11.1**   Main categories of prohibited substances identified by the World Anti-Doping Agency in 2004.
>
> Athletes and others engaged in sports should consult up-to-date lists of **banned substances** for their specific sports, some of which may be allowed for certain medical conditions. However, at the time of writing the main categories of prohibited substances identified by the World Anti-Doping Agency in 2004 were:
>
> - Stimulants (including amfetamine derivatives, cocaine, ephedrine, etc.)
> - Narcotics (including heroin, methadone, morphine, etc.)
> - Cannabinoids
> - Anabolic agents (including anabolic steroids and clenbuterol)
> - Peptide hormones (including erythropoietin, growth hormone, chorionic gonadotrophin, insulin, etc.)
> - Beta-2 agonists
> - Agents with anti-estrogenic activity in men (e.g. tamoxifen)
> - Masking agents (including diuretics, probenecid, plasma expanders, etc.)
> - Glucocorticosteroids
> - Alcohol (in competition only – some sports)
> - Beta-blockers (in and out of competition – some sports only)

Reference: World Anti-Doping Agency. The World Anti-Doping Code – The 2004 Prohibited List: International Standard. Updated 25 November 2003; came into effect 1 January 2004.

National legal controls vary widely. For example, in the USA, both the possession and supply of these drugs was declared illegal in 1990. In the UK, the situation is more complex. It is not illegal to import anabolic steroids from outside the UK as long as these are for personal use. Consequently, possession of anabolic steroids in the form of a medicinal product is also not illegal. However, possession of anabolic steroids in the form of raw materials (i.e. unformulated) was made a criminal offence in 1996. An offence is also committed if anabolic steroids are supplied in any form to another private individual within the UK without a prescription.

Effects sought

Anabolic steroids are taken with the aim of increasing skeletal muscle mass and physical strength, and decreasing body fat. Users may also hope to produce increased stamina, decreased fatigue, aggression and even a mild euphoria. Such effects are particularly important because they enable users to train longer and harder. Perhaps surprisingly, the effectiveness of anabolic steroids plus exercise in increasing physical strength compared to exercise alone is open to doubt. Some studies show a beneficial effect,[1] while others do not.[2] It is a difficult subject to study: placebo-controlled trials are needed because there can be a high placebo response.[3] Standardising an anabolic steroid and exercise regimen, selecting appropriate trial participants, and providing authentic placebos, may not be easy. In placebo-controlled crossover studies where subjects act as their own control, athletes are likely to easily distinguish active drug from placebo.[4] So, although those who train intensively and take anabolic steroids do increase their muscle mass, the exact roles that steroids and exercise play separately in this process, and the precise benefits to the user, have not been clearly elucidated.

The abuse of anabolic steroids, mainly by international athletes, began in the 1950s but rapidly increased. However, by 1976, anabolic steroids were banned in the Olympic games. Over the past 30 years there has been a dramatic increase in the variety of users, which has extended to include those outside of high-level competitive sports, although estimating the true extent of anabolic steroid use is difficult. Bodybuilders, aspiring athletes and 'keep-fit' enthusiasts are some of the more obvious groups involved, but anabolic steroids are increasingly taken by those who desire a more muscular physique for cosmetic purposes or who seek to assert themselves. Many of these people also engage in weight training or intensive regular exercise.

In Australia in 2001, 0.3% of the adult population admitted to use of anabolic steroids at some time in their lives; the mean age at initiation was 23 years.[5] In the UK, a survey of population use of anabolic steroids in 2001/02 showed that 0.1% of adults aged 16–59 had used steroids in the past 12 months.[6] A UK survey in 11- to 15-year-olds in 2003 reported no use of anabolic steroids in the previous year.[7] These low figures contrast with prevalence rates in communities where anabolic steroid use is more accepted. Research involving 1649 UK gym attenders in 1992/93 found that 7.7% had used anabolic steroids at least once (9.1% of men and 2.3% of women); 5% were current users at the time of the survey.[8] However, the number of users at individual gyms ranged from zero to 46% of respondents. A similar survey of 160 attenders at gymnasia in Wales in 1992 reported that nearly 40% had used anabolic steroids.[9]

In the USA, there is greater use amongst schoolchildren than in the UK: a national survey of school pupils aged 12, 14 and 16 years in 2003 showed that 2.5%, 3.0% and 3.5% respectively had ever used anabolic steroids[10] This compares with figures of 1.6%, 1.7% and 2.0% from 1993. A large study from Norway involving 8508 youths aged 15–22 showed that 0.8% had used anabolic steroids at least once.[11] In all studies, a significantly greater proportion of users are male.

Administration

The drugs used are basically analogues of testosterone and examples are listed in Table 11.1. There are many drugs available, in a variety of formulations, some of which are marketed as veterinary preparations. Many have similar generic or brand names and to add to the confusion there are many counterfeit varieties available.

Administration is mainly via the oral or intramuscular route, but topical formulations are also available. Injection is the most popular method of administration, but frequently more than one route is used simultaneously. Testosterone cannot be given orally because the high rate of first-pass metabolism in the liver results in inadequate plasma concentrations; the intramuscular route is therefore mandatory. Anabolic steroid injections are formulated in oil, which allows a sustained release of drug from the intramuscular site over a period of weeks or days. A certain amount of discomfort or pain after injection is

Table 11.1 Some of the more common anabolic steroid preparations

Generic name	Example proprietary names	Routes
Boldenone	Boldenon, Equipoise	Injection
Drostanolone	Masteril, Masteron, Drolban	Injection
Mesterolone	Proviron	Oral
Metandienone (methandrostenolone)	Anabol, Anabolin, Dianabol, D-Bol	Oral, injection, topical
Metenolone	Primobolan, Primobolan Depot	Oral, injection
Methyltestosterone	Android, Oreton Methyl, Virilon	Oral, sublingual
Nandrolone (vars salts)	Anadur, Durabolin, Deca-Durabolin, Dynabol, Laurabolin	Injection
Oxandrolone	Anavar	Oral
Oxymetholone	Anapolon, Anadrol	Oral
Stanozolol	Stromba, Winstrol	Injection, oral
Testosterone (vars salts)	Androderm, Sustanon, Omnadren, Primoteston Depot, Testoject, Virormone	Topical, injection, implant

common, the various muscles differing in terms of the maximum volume of injection that each will accommodate comfortably. For the big muscles of the buttocks this is around 4 mL. However, users often attempt to boost the size of specific muscles by injecting into them specifically, often dividing a dose into several small injections spread over the area of the muscle.

The doses employed are usually far in excess of those used therapeutically, and it is common for more than one anabolic steroid to be used at the same time. This practice is referred to as 'stacking'. There is a belief amongst users that combinations of anabolic steroids are more effective. Sometimes different anabolic steroids are even mixed in the same syringe before administration, and this is called 'blending'. Steroids are often taken intensively for 6–12 weeks. There is then a 'recovery' period before the course is repeated, a process known as 'cycling'. At the beginning of a course it is common to start with a low dose of each steroid, before building up to a maximum halfway through the course and then tapering off towards the end – a technique known as 'pyramiding'. If a particular drug appears to become ineffective after a period of time ('plateauing') then users usually switch to another.

Adverse effects

Testosterone, the hormone on which other anabolic steroids are based, has both androgenic and anabolic actions. It is the anabolic effect that is desired, but none of the synthetic derivatives are devoid of androgenic effects, and these are responsible for a high proportion of the side-effects seen in users. It has not proved possible to synthesise an anabolic steroid that is devoid of these masculinising qualities. Almost all of the side-effects of anabolic steroids are dose-dependent and are also more likely when prolonged administration occurs.

It is difficult to obtain clear information on the range, prevalence and presentation of anabolic steroid side-effects. There are obviously no large-scale double-blind clinical trials comparing anabolic steroids with placebo in the context of performance enhancement. Consequently, much of the available data are derived from case reports, case series and surveys of users. These methods provide limited information, which may have the potential for bias in favour of the negative and/or most dramatic impact of anabolic steroids. It is also possible that the various anabolic steroids have differing adverse-effect profiles, yet there have been no adequate comparative studies to assess this. The results of three surveys of anabolic steroid users carried out to gather information on the prevalence of side-effects are shown in Table 11.2.

In men, the large doses of anabolic steroids used commonly depress the pituitary–testicular axis, giving rise to testicular atrophy and oligospermia or azoospermia.[15–17] Sperm that are produced are more likely to be abnormal and there is also less semen produced. Increased or decreased libido may occur. Impotence is quite common but priapism is rare and tends to be associated with very high doses. Usually all these gonadal effects are reversible upon discontinuation, although fertility may take months or years to return. Male-pattern baldness is accelerated.

Anabolic steroids can be metabolised to female sex hormones by the liver, which may subsequently produce feminising effects in men in the presence of suppressed testosterone production. For example, gynaecomastia is a recognised effect and the breasts are often painful or tender. In some cases, surgical correction may be necessary.[18] 'Hot flushing' is another potential problem. The prostate gland may enlarge and existing prostate problems could be made worse: these effects may result in impaired micturition.[19]

In women, anabolic steroids tend to cause irregular, smaller, infrequent menstruations or amenorrhoea, and reduced fertility. Virilisation may occur, with increased growth of hair on the body and face, male-pattern baldness, deepening of the voice, enlargement of the clitoris, increased libido and reduced breast size. Anabolic steroids may make it impossible to breastfeed. Unfortunately, most of these effects are permanent and do not improve when anabolic steroids are stopped. Although these effects are well known, most surveys of anabolic steroid users do not include very many women, so the incidence of these female-specific effects is not clear. The Welsh survey in Table 11.2 included eight women: six of these suffered from menstrual problems, three described smaller breasts and one reported clitoral enlargement.[14] Six women were involved in one of the Australian surveys, and all of them reported clitoral enlargement and deepening of the voice; four described menstrual irregularities.[12]

There have been no studies of anabolic steroid abuse in human **pregnancy**.[20] When therapeutic drugs such as testosterone or danazol are used inadvertently in human pregnancy, each can be associated with virilisation of the genitalia of female fetuses.[20] These drugs are related to anabolic steroids but therapeutically are used in much smaller amounts than anabolic steroids. No adverse effects have been described in male fetuses.

Table 11.2 Side-effects reported from three surveys of anabolic steroid users

Study 1[12] (Australia, 100 participants, 94% male)		Study 2[13] (Australia, 44 participants, 100% male)		Study 3[14] (Wales, 70 participants, 89% male)	
Side-effect	% reporting	Side-effect	% reporting	Side-effect	% reporting
Fluid retention	64	Change in libido	61	Sleeplessness	64
Painful injection site	57	Mood changes	57	Frequent colds	54
Acne	54	Testicular atrophy	46	Acne	50
Testicular atrophy	55 (of men)	Acne	43	Fluid retention	49
More aggression	42	Hypertension	34	Nosebleeds	46
Gynaecomastia	34 (of men)	Gynaecomastia	27	Sexual performance problems	30
Hypertension	18	Erectile dysfunction	21	Increased body hair	24
		Headaches	9	Gynaecomastia	19 (of men)
		Increased body hair	5	Alopecia	16
		Fluid retention	5	Tendon injury	16
		Sleeplessness	2	Muscle damage	16
				Liver problems	13
				Testicular atrophy	11 (of men)

The abuse of anabolic steroids in **breastfeeding** has not been studied. However, they are known to reduce breast size when taken chronically and androgenic drugs have also been used therapeutically in the past to suppress lactation.[20] These effects may make breastfeeding impossible. Anabolic steroids are lipid-soluble, but also highly plasma-protein bound, so the extent of milk penetration is difficult to estimate. They might theoretically cause virilisation of girls exposed to them via breast milk.

Dermatological side-effects are very common. Acne is a frequently reported side-effect in both sexes, as is an oily skin, cutaneous striae, and increased growth of body hair. Alopecia, taking the form of male-pattern hair loss, is also widely documented in men and women.

The **cardiovascular effects** of anabolic steroids have excited concern but inadequate systematic clinical study. They cause sodium (fluid) retention, which could cause hypertension or exacerbate an existing condition.[12,13,21] Raised blood pressure might theoretically worsen existing medical problems such as heart and kidney disorders. Research suggests that anabolic steroids could be both thrombogenic and atherogenic because, amongst other actions, they promote platelet aggregation, alter vascular reactivity, and promote an unfavourable plasma-lipid balance – they reversibly increase the blood concentrations of low-density lipoprotein cholesterol and decrease beneficial high-density lipoprotein levels.[21–23] Consequently, there have been numerous reports linking anabolic steroid use to acute myocardial infarction (MI) in young men.[21,24–29] Other reports have suggested an association with pulmonary embolus.[30,31] Anabolic steroids may also cause histological changes in the heart that have been linked to cardiac hypertrophy, cardiomyopathy and heart failure.[21,32–34]

Cancer caused by anabolic steroids is rare. However, abuse has been suggested as a rare cause of cancer of the liver,[35–37] and other cancers have been reported in users, including those of the prostate[38] and kidney.[39] It has been suggested that these cancers may arise because of the relatively higher levels of tumorigenic circulating oestrogen and the hypertrophic effects of synthetic androgens.[39]

Apart from cancer, anabolic steroids have been linked to other adverse effects affecting the **liver**. Steroids that are 17-alpha-methyl derivatives of testosterone seem more likely to be associated with liver-related side-effects. In particular, cholestatic hepatitis has been described, caused by a dose-dependent ability to inhibit bile production.[40,41] The condition appears to be reversible in almost all cases.

Peliosis hepatis has also been reported in patients taking anabolic steroids for medical reasons.[40] However, in looking for evidence of steroid-induced liver damage it should be noted that plasma levels of enzymes associated with liver impairment should be assessed carefully. In one study, the liver function test results from four groups were compared: bodybuilders using anabolic steroids ($n = 15$), bodybuilders not using steroids ($n = 10$), patients with viral hepatitis ($n = 49$) and medical students ($n = 592$).[42] Levels of creatine kinase (CK), aspartate aminotransferase (AST) and alanine aminotransferase (ALT) were elevated in bodybuilders whether they used anabolic steroids or not, although steroid users had bigger increases. Gamma-glutamyltranspeptidase (GGT) levels were not elevated in either group. AST and ALT were much more markedly elevated in those with viral hepatitis but they also showed significantly increased plasma levels of GGT, which was not seen in any of the bodybuilders; CK levels were not raised. As a result, when assessing potential hepatotoxicity, the more liver-specific enzyme GGT should always be assessed in anabolic steroid users, because exercise alone may cause AST, ALT and CK to be released from muscle.

The adverse **mental effects** of anabolic steroids have been the subject of some controversy. Relatives and friends of an anabolic steroid user may feel that an individual's personality has changed since commencing abuse. As a result of observations such as these, the effects of anabolic steroids on the mind have been investigated in some detail.[40,43–46] Initially, use of anabolic steroids may produce stimulatory effects such as increased confidence, decreased fatigue, heightened motivation, agitation, irritability and insomnia. This may progress so that users become argumentative, impetuous, moody, suspicious and aggressive. Not uncommonly, violent periodic outbursts of temper are reported ('roid rages'), particularly when large doses are taken for a long time. Dangerous and antisocial behaviour may occur, resulting in impetuous actions that have been linked to deaths.[45,47] However, a confounding factor to bear in mind when assessing published research and case reports is that it is not clear whether aggressive personality types, or those with personality disorders, are more attracted to the use of anabolic steroids.[44,46] Another important potential confounding factor is that weight-training itself may cause some personality and mood changes, and increased assertiveness.[48] These confounding factors are not always taken into consideration in studies or reports of the effects of anabolic steroids on personality.

Anabolic steroid use may also cause frank psychiatric problems such as depression (particularly as part of withdrawal – see below), severe paranoia and psychosis.[40,45]

Injecting any drug carries the risk of injection-site **infection** as well as systemic infection such as septicaemia. In one study, 13% of users acknowledged that they had shared injecting equipment or loaned it to someone else, thus increasing the risk of infections such as human immunodeficiency virus (HIV) and viral hepatitis.[9] Another study showed an incidence of 16%.[14] Cases of HIV infection and AIDS (acquired immunodeficiency syndrome) have been described in those injecting anabolic steroids.[49,50] Concern has been expressed that this population is not as well informed as other parenteral drug users concerning the risks of HIV transmission via shared needles. The chances of sharing may be increased because the large-bore needles needed for intramuscular injection of these viscous solutions may not be as easily available as the narrower-gauge intravenous varieties. Joint infection caused by inadequate aseptic technique and incorrect siting of a needle was described in one user: knee-joint sepsis developed after he inadvertently injected into the suprapatellar pouch while attempting to inject into a thigh muscle.[51]

A link between regular anabolic steroid use and **immunosuppression** has been suggested by some authors, but has not been proven. For example, two cases of infections characteristic of immunosuppression in otherwise healthy anabolic steroid users led to speculation that the link might go unnoticed because of failure to identify anabolic steroid use. One case involved sight-threatening *Candida albicans* endophthalmitis[52] and the other severe chickenpox pneumonitis.[53] A survey of 70 anabolic steroid users in North Wales discovered that 54% of those questioned reported 'frequent colds' as a side-effect, but there was no control group to assess the effects of regular exercise or gym attendance on the frequency of colds.[14] Interestingly, a 16-week study of high-dose nandrolone to increase lean body mass and strength in 30 immunosuppressed HIV-positive men did not lead to a decrease in CD4 lymphocyte counts or to any opportunistic infections during the course of the study.[54]

Musculoskeletal side-effects are relatively well known. Reduced growth and short stature is likely in children and young teenagers who use anabolic steroids, due to premature closure of long-bone epiphyses. At all ages, the use of anabolic steroids may increase the risk of tendon damage during exercise, which is detrimental to the desired effects because it prevents further training while healing occurs. This is probably due to over-exercise, rather than an innate ability of anabolic steroids to damage tendons.[55] Over-exercise can also trigger rhabdomyolysis and its sequelae.[56,57] Poor administration technique may give rise to injection injury to nerves, resulting in muscle weakness. One patient experienced mild wrist weakness, paraesthesia and other sensation changes as a result of radial nerve damage sustained while injecting into the forearm.[51] These effects spontaneously resolved after 1 month. Two patients have also been described who suffered probable sciatic nerve damage arising from intra-gluteal injection.[58] They experienced lower limb weakness and ill-defined anaesthesia and paraesthesia below the knee. Both patients were lost to follow-up, so resolution could not be determined.

Anabolic steroids can cause **dependence** in some individuals who continue to use them despite negative consequences such as adverse reactions, unpleasant lifestyle effects, and the expense of obtaining them.[12,59,60] A withdrawal reaction may even develop upon discontinuation with features including mood swings, fatigue, loss of appetite, depression, insomnia, weakness, headache, reduced interest in sex, diminished satisfaction with body image, and craving for steroids. However, these drugs do not seem to cause the Addisonian-like withdrawal reactions akin to those produced by glucocorticosteroids such as hydrocortisone.

Accessory drugs associated with anabolic steroid use

A whole range of other drugs may be used by athletes to counteract the side-effects of anabolic steroids or to augment their effects. Some common examples are highlighted below.

* *Acne treatments*. Antibiotics and retinoids may be taken to counteract the acne-inducing side-effects of anabolic steroids.
* *Captopril*. Some believe that captopril helps the body lose fat and to become more sensitive to insulin. There may also be a mild diuretic effect.
* *Chorionic gonadotrophin*. Human chorionic gonadotrophin (HCG) stimulates the Leydig cells of the testis to increase secretion of testosterone, thus theoretically reversing the adverse gonadal effects of a depressed pituitary–testicular axis in men. It is given intramuscularly, often upon completion of a course of anabolic steroids, to restore testicular size and function. It is an expensive drug to buy, and some varieties sold to users may be counterfeit.
* *Diuretics*. Diuretics counteract the fluid retention caused by anabolic steroids and may sharpen the definition of skeletal muscle contours.
* *Finasteride*. Taken to prevent male-pattern alopecia (and sometimes acne), particular in those using testosterone-based steroids.

- *Growth hormone (somatropin).* There is little evidence that growth hormone has any beneficial effects on muscle mass or athletic performance,[61] but athletes take it to promote muscle growth and fat loss, and to strengthen tendons. Growth hormone may even have detrimental effects upon exercise performance.[61] As with HCG, supplies from illicit sources may be of poor quality and very expensive. Concern has been expressed in the past that illicit growth hormone with a cadaveric source has increased the risk of users developing Creutzfeldt–Jakob disease.[62,63] However, modern legitimate varieties are synthetic. Acute side-effects include fluid retention, carpal tunnel syndrome and possibly an increased risk of cardiac arrhythmias.[61] Prolonged excessive use of growth hormone could cause adverse reactions reminiscent of acromegaly. Clonidine, levodopa and vasopressin can all stimulate growth hormone production and each of them has been abused for this effect.
- *Hypnotics.* Anabolic steroids may cause insomnia, as can many of the drugs taken with them (e.g. ephedrine, amfetamines, clenbuterol, thyroid hormones).
- *Insulin.* Used to promote muscle growth, the potency of this drug gives great cause for concern. Hypoglycaemia can arise as a result of inadvertent overdose, the choice of the wrong formulation, or failure to maintain a high enough calorific intake after injection.
- *Levothyroxine and liothyronine.* Levothyroxine increases the rate of metabolism, which might theoretically increase the ability of anabolic steroids to boost physical strength. Levothyroxine also encourages rapid utilisation of a high-calorie diet and helps to reduce body fat.
- *Oestrogen antagonists.* Drugs such as tamoxifen, clomifene and anastrozole help to reduce the gynaecomastia that may develop as a side-effect of anabolic steroid use in men. Gynaecomastia is not only unsightly but can also be painful.

Androgenic-anabolic steroid precursors

In an attempt to gain the benefits of anabolic steroids more 'naturally', and allegedly without the side-effects, some people engaged in regular gym training may utilise steroid precursors. Compounds such as dehydroepiandrosterone (DHEA, prasterone), androstenedione (ADN) and androstenediol (ADL) are taken in the belief that they will be converted into testosterone by the body. These three compounds occur naturally in human plasma as sex-steroid precursors, being produced mainly by the adrenal glands and gonads. One US survey of 334 male gym attenders in 2001 discovered that 18% had taken one of these substances in the last 3 years compared with only 5% who had taken anabolic steroids.[64] Although they have little androgenic action

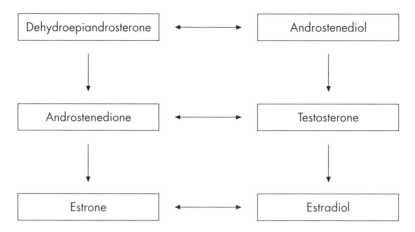

Figure 11.1 Metabolic relationship between sex-hormone precursors and testosterone/estradiol. Adapted from references 65 and 66.

themselves, DHEA, ADN and ADL are converted to sex steroids by the testes and various peripheral tissues (Figure 11.1). They may be taken with, or more usually instead of, anabolic steroids because in many countries they are not subject to the same legal restrictions.

The steroid precursors are claimed to have effects similar to anabolic steroids but there is little scientific evidence available to support these alleged benefits. An analysis of published human studies suggests that steroid precursors such as DHEA, ADN and ADL do not increase plasma levels of testosterone in the main target population, i.e. healthy young men, and do not increase muscular strength or lean body mass.[65,66]

There is limited information on potential side-effects, but doubts have been cast on their safety because precursors are known to decrease the plasma levels of beneficial high-density lipoprotein (HDL) cholesterol and to increase oestrogen plasma levels in men.[65,66] Whether they have the potential to cause any of the other side-effects of conventional anabolic steroids is unknown.

Analgesics

For reasons that are not entirely clear, the partial opioid receptor agonist **nalbuphine** has particular popularity among those undertaking intense physical training. Most of the users described in the medical liteature also utilised injectable anabolic steroids, so the fact that nalbuphine is an injectable analgesic may add to its appeal. In many countries, unlike other injectable opioids, it is not controlled under substance-misuse legislation, which is another attraction to users. Those who regularly use anabolic steroids may be reluctant to seek medical advice if a sports injury occurs and it may be easier to self-medicate with an analgesic obtained from 'underground' sources if an injury occurs, and this seems to be a common reason for initiation of nalbuphine. However, nalbuphine is also used to prevent pain during intense exercise such that training can continue 'through the pain barrier' for longer periods, to dull soreness after training, or to promote post-exercise relaxation. Nalbuphine has been claimed to have 'anti-catabolic' effects by users, but this has not been substantiated and seems unlikely. It may also be used to promote calmness before competitions, or just to give a 'high' during or after exercise.

Many cases of nalbuphine dependence have been documented,[67–69] characterised by high-dose regular intravenous use more than once per day at doses up to 200 mg in 24 hours. This is accompanied by tolerance, a typical opioid-withdrawal reaction upon cessation, and other signs of dependence. Methadone has been successfully used to wean patients off nalbuphine.[69] Those who become dependent on nalbuphine often have a history of abuse of illicit substances.

Non-steroidal anti-inflammatory drugs (NSAIDs) are also used to treat sports injuries and to train through the pain barrier. NSAIDs have a range of side-effects, but particular attention has focused upon their potential for renal toxicity, because intense exercise can also impose a strain on the kidneys by causing hypovolaemia, hyperthermia and muscle catabolism. One author has proposed four principles for doctors when prescribing NSAIDs to athletes:[70]

1. Avoid NSAIDs when hyperthermia, hypovolaemia or dehydration might occur.
2. Recognise the potential gastrointestinal and renal side-effects.
3. The risks associated with injectable NSAIDs do not justify their use: try rapidly absorbed oral varieties.
4. Educate sportsmen on first aid measures for musculoskeletal injuries (e.g. compression, ice and rest).

Beta-blockers

These can decrease tremor, pulse and other feelings of anxiety in sports where intense concentration and a steady hand are a necessity, e.g. archery, shooting, snooker.

Clenbuterol

This drug is a long-acting beta-2 adrenoceptor agonist that has been used medicinally in some European countries as an oral bronchodilator. Clenbuterol is not licensed as a medicine for human use in the UK or USA. It is used by bodybuilders and athletes because it supposedly has anabolic-like effects: promoting muscle build-up and fat loss. Some refer to clenbuterol as a 'repartitioning' agent because the mode of action is not the same as that of anabolic steroids. It is taken by itself or with anabolic steroids.

In several species of animal, clenbuterol increases the bulk of certain groups of skeletal muscles and reduces the amount of subcutaneous fat.[71,72] The doses required for this effect are greater than those needed for bronchodilation. These experiments in animals have been extrapolated to humans by proponents of the use of clenbuterol. However, it is often the case that drugs which produce one effect in animals do not produce the same effects in humans, and these actions of clenbuterol have not been studied in humans or any closely related species such as primates. Another limitation of the laboratory work available is that, unlike the human athletes who take it, the animal species involved were not engaged in regular heavy exercise and were studied under controlled conditions. Animal work also shows that skeletal muscles are affected unequally and the importance of this observation to the hopeful athlete or bodybuilder is not clear.

The typical dose taken for an anabolic effect in humans is 40–160 mcg daily, usually in the form of 20-mcg tablets. Interestingly, clenbuterol has occasionally been reported as an adulterant of anabolic steroid injections in sufficient quantities (2 mg) to cause toxicity after injection.[73]

The mechanism of action is not clearly understood, but the drug may produce an initial increase in the rate of skeletal muscle protein synthesis that is then followed by a drug-induced decrease in the rate of protein breakdown.[74] This has led to interest in the therapeutic potential of clenbuterol for treating conditions where muscle wastage can occur as a result of sepsis or immobility, for example.

Tachycardia, tremor and insomnia are common acute side-effects, but longer-term effects in humans have not been studied.

Diltiazem

Diltiazem is not a drug that would be expected to enhance performance in a healthy adult. However, a report in 1993 described a man who took

480 mg of diltiazem each day and developed severe abdominal cramps as a result.[75] He revealed that the drug was widely abused amongst bodybuilders and rugby players locally to augment training, but the exact benefits that he anticipated from the drug were not made clear.

Diuretics

As has been noted, diuretics may be used with anabolic steroids (see above). They may also be used to promote a rapid, short-lasting weight loss prior to 'weighing in' before competitions where exceeding a maximum weight could result in disqualification. A third potential use of diuretics is as masking agents, to give false-negative urine tests for prohibited substances.

Incautious use of diuretics can cause electrolyte disturbances. This is particularly important if large changes in plasma potassium occur: either hypokalaemia or hyperkalaemia can occur depending upon the diuretics used. One case has been described of a bodybuilder who developed diuretic-induced hyperkalaemia and hypotension as a result of using diuretics and potassium supplements.[76] He took bumetanide, with spironolactone and potassium supplements. An admission to the intensive care unit was required but the patient survived. Another athlete died as a consequence of hyperkalaemia caused by spironolactone with potassium supplements.[77]

Diuretics carry the risk of dehydration, which may affect athletic performance, and this also increases the risk of thromboembolsim and heat exhaustion.

Erythropoietin

Increasing plasma haemoglobin, and thence the oxygen-carrying capacity of the blood, is believed to be beneficial to muscular function during sustained physical exercise. Blood transfusions rich in red blood cells can be given to achieve this, a practice called 'blood doping', but erythropoietin is also used because it is a glycoprotein that increases the rate of production of red blood cells. It is produced in the human body mainly by the kidneys in response to hypoxia.

Synthetic varieties are available, known as epoietin and darbepoietin, which are given by subcutaneous injection. They increase plasma haemoglobin levels in normal healthy individuals and seem to increase maximal aerobic power during exercise, as well as increasing the time to exhaustion.[78]

However, there are dangers involved in this practice. Strenuous exercise is known to promote haemoconcentration because of loss of fluid and this in turn results in increased blood viscosity. This effect might be further potentiated by diuretics. Elevating the red blood cell concentration has a similar effect on viscosity so erythropoietin administration in this setting may increase the risk of thrombosis during exercise.

Nutritional supplements

A survey of advertisements for nutritional supplements in five UK body-building magazines in 1993 identified 145 products with 66 different ingredients.[79] Of these, 53% contained vitamins and/or metal cations and 19% disclosed no ingredients at all. The most popular claim, made by one-third of advertisements, was that of enhanced performance. Other common claims were assisting muscle gain, promoting weight reduction and a 'general supplement'. The author of the report highlighted that, in the UK, as long as no medicinal claims are made, the manufacturers of nutritional products can make any claims they wish about the benefits of using their preparations. No scientific evidence is necessary to back them up.

Many preparations are simply mixtures of proteins, amino acids, carbohydrate, fats, minerals and/or vitamins, in varying proportions. Others contain more specific, unusual or exotic ingredients. Whatever the formulation, any claims of efficacy that are made are often unreasonable extrapolations from animal studies or from unrepresentative or limited human exposure. Sometimes evidence for benefits is conflicting. Table 11.3 lists some of the ingredients that have been identified in such products.[66,80–82] Vitamins are not included in this table although most of them can be found in various guises in such products. Vitamins C, B_{12} and E are probably the most popular. Although certain ingredients have been studied in some detail, none of them has been tested adequately enough in humans to fully support the claims made for them.

The precise identity, purity and quality of some supplements are open to doubt. Some products could even contain banned substances, and so athletes entering competitions should be aware that use of these products from unreliable sources might put them at risk of failing drug tests. For example, one study revealed the existence of the anabolic steroid metandienone in three dietary supplements.[83]

Table 11.3 Selected ingredients found in natural or nutritional products used by athletes and bodybuilders

Ingredient	Claimed beneficial effects
Animal organs	Extracts of these are found in some preparations, with a variety of claims; liver, testes, pituitary and pancreas are examples
Arginine	Amino acid claimed to increase release of growth hormone
Bee pollen	Increased speed of recovery after exercise
Boron	Augments action of testosterone
L-carnitine	Promotes loss of body fat; decreased lactic acid production; sparing of muscle glycogen
Choline	Promotes loss of body fat
Chromium	Anabolic compound, usually supplied as picolinate salt
Citrus aurantium ('bitter' or 'sour' orange)	Contains phenylephrine (*m*-synephrine) a mild stimulant that stimulates metabolic rate and weight loss
Co-enzyme Q10	Increased performance, increased oxidative metabolism
Creatine	Sustained power output with delayed fatigue
Diosgenin	Substitute for anabolic steroids, because of similar structure
Ephedra	Natural plant source of ephedrine, a stimulant
Ferulic acid	Anabolic effect
Gamma-oryzanol	Anabolic effect
Ginseng	Improved and/or prolonged performance in endurance events
Inosine	Energy enhancer; increased oxygen release to muscle
Medium chain triglycerides	Increased energy and reduced body fat
Octacosanol	Ergogenic effects – decreased recovery time after training
Ornithine	As for arginine
Phosphate	Enhanced energy utilisation
Smilax spp.	Natural source of testosterone or testosterone enhancer
Yohimbine	Testosterone enhancer

In summary, these products are marketed with no, very little, or conflicting evidence for efficacy, and limited safety data. Often details of dosage or contraindications are lacking, and quality assurance procedures may be suspect.

References

1. Bhasin S, Storer T W, Berman N, *et al*. The effects of supraphysiologic doses of testosterone on muscle size and strength in normal men. *N Engl J Med* 1996; 335: 1–7.

2. Hervey G R, Hutchinson I, Knibbs A V, *et al*. 'Anabolic' effects of methandienone in men undergoing athletic training. *Lancet* 1976; 2: 699–702.

3. Ariel G, Saville W. Anabolic steroids: the physiological effects of placebos. *Med Sci Sports* 1972; 4: 124–126.

4. Freed D L J, Banks A J, Longson D, *et al*. Anabolic steroids in athletics: crossover double-blind trial on weightlifters. *BMJ* 1975; 2: 471–473.

5. *Statistics on Drug Use in Australia 2002. Drug Statistics Series No. 12*. Cat no. PHE 43. Canberra: Australian Institute of Health and Welfare, February 2003.

6. Aust R, Sharp C, Goulden C. *Prevalence of Drug Use: Key Findings from the 2001/02 British Crime Survey*. Home Office Research Study 182. London: Home Office, 2002.

7. National Centre for Social Research/National Foundation for Educational Research. *Drug Use, Smoking and Drinking among Young People in England in 2003: headline figures*. London: Department of Health, 2004.

8. Korkia P, Stimson G V. *Anabolic Steroid Use in Great Britain: an Exploratory Investigation*. The Centre for Research on Drug Health Behaviour. London: HMSO, 1993.

9. Perry H M, Wright D, Littlepage N C. Dying to be big: a review of anabolic steroid use. *Br J Sports Med* 1992; 26: 259–261.

10. Johnston L D, O'Malley P M, Bachman J G, *et al. Ecstasy Use Falls for Second Year in a Row, Overall Teen Drug Use Drops*. National press release, University of Michigan News and Information Services, Ann Arbor, 19 December 2003.

11. Wichstrom L, Pedersen W. Use of anabolic-androgenic steroids in adolescence: winning, looking good or being bad? *J Stud Alcohol* 2001; 62: 5–13.

12. Copeland J, Peters R, Dillon P. A study of 100 anabolic-androgenic steroid users. *Med J Aust* 1998; 168: 311–312.

13. O'Sullivan A J, Kennedy M C, Casey J H, *et al*. Anabolic-androgenic steroids: medical assessment of present, past and potential users. *Med J Aust* 2000; 173: 323–327.

14. Burton C. Anabolic steroid use among the gym population in Clwyd. *Pharm J* 1996; 256: 557–559.

15. Knuth U A, Maniera H, Nieschlag E. Anabolic steroids and semen parameters in bodybuilders. *Fertil Steril* 1989; 52: 1041–1047.

16. Torres-Calleja J, Gonzalez-Unzaga M, DeCelis-Carrillo R, *et al*. Effect of androgenic anabolic steroids on sperm quality and serum hormone levels in adult male bodybuilders. *Life Sci* 2001; 68: 1769–1774.

17. Lloyd F H, Powell P, Murdoch A P. Lesson of the week: anabolic steroid abuse by body builders and male subfertility. *BMJ* 1996; 313: 100–101.

18. Babigian A, Silverman R T. Management of gynecomastia due to use of anabolic steroids in bodybuilders. *Plast Reconstr Surg* 2001; 107: 240–242.

19. Wemyss-Holden S A, Hamdy F C, Hastie K J. Steroid abuse in athletes, prostatic enlargement and bladder outflow obstruction – is there a relationship? *Br J Urol* 1994; 74: 476–478.

20. Wills S. Street drugs. In: Lee A, *et al.*, eds. *Therapeutics in Pregnancy and Lactation*. Oxford: Radcliffe Medical Press, 2000, 227–246.

21. Sullivan M L, Martinez C M, Gennis P, *et al.* The cardiac toxicity of anabolic steroids. *Prog Cardiovasc Dis* 1998; 41: 1–15.

22. Glazer G. Atherogenic effects of anabolic steroids on serum lipid levels. *Arch Intern Med* 1991; 151: 1923–1933.

23. Urhausen A, Torsten A, Wilfried K. Reversibility of the effects on blood cells, lipids, liver function and hormones in former anabolic-androgenic steroid abusers. *J Steroid Biochem Mol Biol* 2003; 84: 369–375.

24. Kennedy M C, Lawrence C. Anabolic steroid abuse and cardiac death. *Med J Aust* 1993; 158: 346–348.

25. Ment J, Ludman P F. Coronary thrombus in a 23 year old anabolic steroid user. *Heart* 2002; 88: 342.

26. Varriale P, Mirzai-Tehrane M, Sedighi A. Acute myocardial infarction associated with anabolic steroids in a young HIV-infected patient. *Pharmacotherapy* 1999; 19: 881–884.

27. Hourigan L A, Rainbird A J, Dooris M. Intracoronary stenting for acute myocardial infarction (AMI) in a 24-year-old man using anabolic androgenic steroids. *Aust N Z J Med* 1998; 28: 838–839.

28. Fisher M, Appleby M, Rittoo D, *et al.* Myocardial infarction with extensive intracoronary thrombus induced by anabolic steroids. *Br J Clin Pract* 1996; 50: 222–223.

29. Ferenchick G S. Are androgenic steroids thrombogenic? *N Engl J Med* 1991; 322: 476.

30. Montine T J, Gaede J T. Massive pulmonary embolus and anabolic steroid abuse. *JAMA* 1992; 267: 2328–2329.

31. Robinson R J, White S. Misuse of anabolic drugs. *BMJ* 1993; 306: 61.

32. Nieminen M S, Ramo M P, Viitasalo M, *et al.* Serious cardiovascular side effects of large doses of anabolic steroids in weight lifters. *Eur Heart J* 1996; 17: 1576–1583.

33. Madea B, Grellner W. Long-term cardiovascular effects of anabolic steroids. *Lancet* 1998; 352: 33.

34. Ferrera P C, Putnam D L, Verdile V P. Anabolic steroid use as the possible precipitant of dilated cardiomyopathy. *Cardiology* 1997; 88: 218–220.

35. Farrell G C. *Drug-induced Liver Disease*. London: Churchill Livingstone, 1994, 177, 334.

36. Overly W L, Dankoff J A, Wang B K, *et al.* Androgens and hepatocellular carcinoma in an athlete. *Ann Intern Med* 1984; 100: 158–159.

37. Goldman B. Liver carcinoma in an athlete taking anabolic steroids. *J Am Osteopath Assoc* 1985; 85: 56.

38. Roberts J T, Essenhigh D M. Adenocarcinoma of prostate in 40-year-old body-builder. *Lancet* 1986; 2: 742.

39. Brygden A A G, Rothwell P J N, O'Reilly P H. Anabolic steroid abuse and renal-cell carcinoma. *Lancet* 1995; 346: 1306–1307.

40. Smith D A, Perry P J. The efficacy of ergogenic agents in athletic competition Part I: Androgenic-anabolic steroids. *Ann Pharmacother* 1992; 26: 520–528.
41. Lowdell C P, Murray-Lyon I M. Reversal of liver damage due to long term methyltestosterone and safety of non-17 alpha-alkylated androgens. *BMJ* 1985; 291: 637.
42. Dickerman R D, Pertusi R M, Zachariah N Y, *et al.* Anabolic steroid-induced hepatotoxicity: is it overstated? *Clin J Sport Med* 1999; 9: 34–39.
43. Parrott A C, Choi P Y L, Davies M. Anabolic steroid use by amateur athletes: effects upon psychological mood state. *J Sports Med Phys Fitness* 1994; 34: 292–298.
44. Cooper C J, Noakes T D, Dunne T, *et al.* A high prevalence of abnormal personality traits in chronic users of anabolic-androgenic steroids. *Br J Sports Med* 1996; 30: 246–250.
45. Corrigan B. Anabolic steroids and the mind. *Med J Aust* 1996; 165: 222–226.
46. Midgley S J, Heather N, Davies J B. Levels of aggression among a group of anabolic-androgenic steroid users. *Med Sci Law* 2001; 41: 309–314.
47. Thiblin I, Lindquist O, Rajs J. Cause and manner of death among users of anabolic androgenic steroids. *J Forensic Sci* 2000; 45: 16–23.
48. Bahrke M S, Yesalis C E. Weight training – a potential confounding factor in examining the psychological and behavioural effects of anabolic-androgenic steroids. *Sports Med* 1994; 18: 309–318.
49. Scott M J, Scott M J Jr. HIV infection associated with injections of anabolic steroids. *JAMA* 1989; 262: 207–208.
50. Sklarek H M, Mantovani R P, Erens E, *et al.* AIDS in a bodybuilder using anabolic steroids. *N Engl J Med* 1984; 311: 1701.
51. Evans N A. Local complications of self administered anabolic steroid injections. *Br J Sports Med* 1997; 31: 349–350.
52. Widder R A, Bartz-Schmidt K U, Geter H, *et al. Candida albicans* endophthalmitis after anabolic steroid abuse. *Lancet* 1995; 345: 330–331.
53. Johnson A S, Jones M, Morgan-Capner P, *et al.* Severe chickenpox in anabolic steroid user. *Lancet* 1995; 345: 1447–1448.
54. Sattler F R, Jaque S V, Schroeder E T, *et al.* Effects of pharmacological doses of nandrolone decanoate and progressive resistance training in immunodeficient patients infected with human immunodeficiency virus. *J Clin Endocrinol Metab* 1999; 84: 1268–1276.
55. Evans N A, Bowrey D J, Newman G R. Ultrastructural analysis of ruptured tendon from anabolic steroid users. *Injury* 1998; 29: 769–773.
56. Shotliff K, Asante M. Misuse of anabolic drugs. *BMJ* 1993; 306: 61–62.
57. Braseth N R, Allison E J Jr, Gough J E. Exertional rhabdomyolysis in a body builder abusing anabolic androgenic steroids. *Eur J Emerg Med* 2001; 8: 155–157.
58. Perry H M. An unusual cause of abnormal gait. *Br J Sports Med* 1994; 28: 60.
59. Pärssinen M, Seppälä T. Steroid use and long-term health risk in former athletes. *Sports Med* 2002; 32: 83–94.
60. Korkia P. Anabolic-androgenic steroids series: part II. Psychological effects of anabolic steroid use – a review. *J Subst Misuse* 1998; 3: 106–113.

61. Rennie M J. Claim for the anabolic effects of growth hormone: a case of the Emperor's new clothes? *Br J Sports Med* 2003; 37: 100–105.

62. Deyssig R, Frisch H. Self-administration of cadaveric growth hormone in power athletes. *Lancet* 1993; 341: 768–769.

63. Perry H M. Risk of Creutzfeldt-Jakob disease in bodybuilders. *BMJ* 1993; 307: 803.

64. Kanayama G, Gruber A J, Pope H G Jr, *et al*. Over-the-counter drug use in gymnasiums: an underrecognized substance abuse problem? *Psychother Psychosomat* 2001; 70: 137–140.

65. Powers M E. The safety and efficacy of anabolic steroid precursor: what is the scientific evidence? *J Athletic Training* 2002; 37: 300–305.

66. Congeni J, Miller S. Supplements and drugs used to enhance athletic performance. *Pediatr Clin North Am* 2002; 49: 435–461.

67. McBride A J, Williamson K, Peteren T. Three cases of nalbuphine hydrochloride dependence associated with anabolic steroid use. *Br J Sports Med* 1996; 30: 69–70.

68. Wines J D Jr, Gruber A J, Pope H G, *et al*. Nalbuphine hydrochloride dependence in anabolic steroid users. *Am J Addictions* 1999; 8: 161–164.

69. Williams H, Remedios A, Rooney J, *et al*. Nalbuphine dependence: a brief report from the UK. *Ir J Psychol Med* 2000; 17: 20–21.

70. Gerrard D F. Renal abuse from non-steroidal anti-inflammatory agents in sport. *N Z Med J* 1998; 111: 107–108.

71. Prather I D, Brown D E, North P, *et al*. Clenbuterol: A substitute for anabolic steroids? *Med Sci Sports Exerc* 1985; 27: 1118–1121.

72. Spann C, Winter M E. Effect of clenbuterol on athletic performance. *Ann Pharmacother* 1995; 29: 75–77.

73. Lenehan P. *Warning: Counterfeit Anabolic Steroid Health Risk – Anabol*. Liverpool: The Drugs and Sport Information Service, 1996.

74. Anonymous. Muscling in on clenbuterol. *Lancet* 1992; 340: 403.

75. Richards H, Grocutt M, McCabe M. Use of diltiazem in sport. *BMJ* 1993; 307: 940.

76. Al-Zaki T, Talbot-Stern J. A bodybuilder with diuretic abuse presenting with symptomatic hypotension and hyperkalaemia. *Am J Emerg Med* 1996; 14: 96–98.

77. Kennedy M C, Lawrence C H, Duflou J. Drug related cardiac death in sport. *Clin Exp Pharmacol Physiol* 1992; Suppl 21: 35.

78. Ekblom B. Erythropoietin. In: Karch S B, ed. *Drug Abuse Handbook*. Boca Raton, FL: CRC Press, 1998, 710–720.

79. Timmins A J. Survey of advertisements for nutritional supplements in bodybuilding magazines. *Pharm J* 1994; 253: 894–895.

80. Beltz S D, Doering P L. Efficacy of nutritional supplements used by athletes. *Clin Pharm* 1993; 12: 900–908.

81. Grunewald K K, Bailey R S. Commercially marketed supplements for bodybuilding athletes. *Sports Med* 1993; 15: 90–103.

82. Barron R L, Vanscoy G J. Natural products and the athlete: facts and folklore. *Ann Pharmacother* 1993; 27: 607–615.

83. Geyer H, Bredehoft M, Mareck-Engelke U, *et al*. High doses of the anabolic steroid metandienone found in dietary supplements. *Eur J Sports Sci* 2003; 3: 1–5.

12

Prescription drugs

The medicine increases the disease.
Virgil (70–19 BC), 'The Aeneid'

This chapter highlights prescription drugs that may be abused. Cocaine and anabolic steroids are prescription medicines in many countries but they have been the subject of earlier chapters. Similarly, a variety of prescription opioids (e.g. oxycodone) and amfetamine derivatives (e.g. methylphenidate) are abused and these are also discussed in other chapters. Finally, some 'smart drugs' and certain preparations used in association with anabolic steroids are prescription medicines and the reader is again referred to the appropriate sections of this book for a description of them.

The prevalence of prescription drug abuse is hard to estimate. Notwithstanding the drugs that are considered in other chapters (see above), there are still many other medicines that can be abused. Occasionally data are available to give some indication of the extent of abuse, but such information is rare. For example, a study in France in 1993 revealed that 392 prescriptions presented to nearly 100 pharmacies over the course of a year were forged.[1] This was estimated as 0.04% of all prescriptions, and most were for medicines subject to abuse.

Although some of those abusing prescription drugs are healthcare professionals who exploit their privileged access to medicines, many are patients, some of whom undoubtedly become dependent. Features of dependence may include the patient continuing to take the drug despite deriving no medical benefit from it (and even suffering side-effects), tolerance, withdrawal reactions, preoccupation with the drug, and drug-seeking behaviour (see Box 12.1).

Anaesthetics

Many gaseous anaesthetics have been subject to abuse, but in practice these all have a comparatively low abuse potential because, although

---

Box 12.1 Examples of drug-seeking behaviour in patients dependent on prescribed drugs.

Patients who become dependent upon prescription medicines may exhibit drug-seeking behaviour, which can take various forms but some examples are given below:

1. Faking or exaggerating withdrawal symptoms when further supplies of the drug are refused or the dose reduced.
2. Faking or exaggerating an exacerbation of the underlying medical condition if a prescription is refused or dose reduced.
3. Claiming that alternative medicines without abuse potential, or non-pharmacological treatment options, do not work or cannot be tolerated.
4. Asking for a prescription to be re-issued because it has been lost; claiming that supplies have run out early; altering the quantity or identity of drugs to be supplied on a prescription; approaching a second doctor in order to obtain supplies if the first one refuses.
5. Stealing medication or prescriptions; buying supplies of medication from illicit domestic sources, from abroad, or via the Internet.
6. Making threats, or offering bribes, to prescribers or those supplying medication.

---

they may produce pleasurable effects, they are not easily available and are inconvenient to use, even for healthcare professionals with access to them. Ketamine is different because it can be taken by mouth or injected and is thus more portable. Abuse of ketamine has consequently become a well-described problem at street level.

Ketamine

Therapeutically, ketamine is used by the intravenous or intramuscular routes to induce or maintain anaesthesia. It also has analgesic and amnesic properties, and is in many ways similar to phencyclidine, to which it is structurally related. The two drugs have a similar mode of action, affecting a range of central neurotransmitters, but, significantly, both are antagonists of glutamate at NMDA (N-methyl-D-aspartate) receptors in the brain.

Ketamine was developed in the 1960s and is now used mainly in children, but it has also found a place in the treatment of some types of chronic pain in adults, and is even employed as a battlefield anaesthetic. Ever since its first use as an anaesthetic, it has been known that patients may experience curious psychotropic reactions after ketamine anaesthesia. These effects, which occur during recovery ('emergence' phenomena), commonly include feelings of mind–body dissociation (so-called 'out-of-body experiences'), sensations of floating, severe disorientation, vivid dreams and even, occasionally, delirium. Any of these effects may be subjectively pleasant or unpleasant. Children seem to be less susceptible to them.

Abuse by healthcare professionals has been reported,[2–7] but unlike the other anaesthetic agents described below ketamine is readily available on the street in Europe, Australia and the USA and has been since the 1970s. Much ketamine is obtained by domestic diversion of hospital and particularly veterinary preparations, although supplies from non-European and non-US pharmaceutical or illicit manufacturers may be used. It is simply a prescription drug in most countries, but the prevalence of abuse amongst certain populations is such that a move to a more restricted legal status for non-medical use has been advocated, or in some cases actually invoked (e.g. the USA).

Street names for ketamine included 'K', 'vitamin K', 'super K', 'special K' and 'kit-kat'. It is also known under its most common medical brand name, Ketalar. A mixture with cocaine is known as 'CK' or 'Calvin Klein'.

Effects and administration

Ketamine is abused in a variety of settings. Although it is an anaesthetic, at the lower doses used recreationally it may have some stimulant properties. It is popular as a 'rave' or club drug, where it may be taken in public with friends and in association with other substances, but ketamine is also used by itself in a quieter setting for pleasure or to facilitate self-exploration. Ketamine has been used to 'spike' drinks in clubs and bars, and as a 'date rape' drug.

Commercially, ketamine is only available in a parenteral formulation. It is abused by injection – both intravenously and intramuscularly – but this is not the most common means of administration. A powder can be easily created by evaporating water from the injection solution, and crushing the resulting crystals. Inhalation of the powder into the nose ('bumping') is the most popular method of delivering the drug, as its lipophilicity aids rapid absorption by this route. Another method of administration is smoking. The powder can also be packed into capsules for oral administration, and the injection solution can be taken by mouth, although it has an unpleasant taste. Ketamine is a well-known substitute for, and adulterant of, ecstasy tablets.

The doses used for psychedelic effects are 10–25% of the anaesthetic dose by the same route.[8] Hence, those taking ketamine typically remain alert or rousable during their intoxication. Common experiences include a dreamy sensation, visual hallucinations, illusions, spiritual or mystic revelations, and enhanced enjoyment of sensory experiences.[8,9] One reason that some users give for continued use is the finding of a specific mental state that they find pleasurable. This is termed a 'K-hole'.[10] Precise descriptions vary, but during the period of intoxication there seems to be a sense of profound detachment from everyday life, with physical immobility, time and spatial distortions, and engagement in an alternative perception of the world that to some extent may be controlled or created by the user.

A survey of 20 users in Scotland in 1996[9] reported the following as the most common experiences in a relaxed, private setting:

Absence of sense of time	90%
Unusual distortions of body consistency (e.g. being made of wood, plastic, etc.)	85%
A sensation of light through the body	70%
Distorted shape or size of body parts	70%
An experience of leaving the body	65%
Insight into riddles of existence, or of self	60%

A survey of 100 long-term users in Australia gave similar results.[11] The following were described as the most common effects ever experienced:

Absence of time	74%
Unusual thought content	60%
Separated from body	57%
Euphoria	55%
Altered body perceptions	53%
Visual hallucinations	49%

When inhaled nasally, the effects of ketamine begin within a few minutes, and administration of small doses may be repeated to reach or maintain a satisfactory mental state. After a single dose, the acute phase of psychotropic effects is not long and typically lasts about an hour,[9] but a return to full 'normality' may take longer. After intravenous use, acute psychedelic effects may last for as little as 10 minutes, but oral use may produce effects lasting 4 hours.[8] The half-life of ketamine is about 2–4 hours, but it is metabolised to norketamine by cytochrome P450 isoenzyme CYP3A4, and this metabolite has about one-sixth of the potency of the parent compound.[12]

Adverse effects

Side-effects include a peripheral numbness with difficulty in moving, incoordination, dizziness, myoclonus, slurred speech, inability to speak, blurred vision, hypertension, vomiting, increased body temperature, nosebleeds, tachycardia, palpitations and chest pains.[2,5,8,9,11,13–15] Some users become incoherent or semi-conscious if they take too much.

Confusion, agitation and anxiety have been described, and can be severe.[13] Ketamine can also give rise to 'flashbacks'.[8,15] Frequent use of ketamine may cause persisting memory impairment[16,17] and measurement of dissociative and schizotypal effects suggest that these may persist for days after use as well.

Two cases of mild rhabdomyolysis have been reported.[13] There has also been one case report of a prolonged tongue and neck dystonia in a young male patient after abusing intravenous ketamine.[18]

An interview survey of 100 ketamine users in Australia provided a list of the commonest reactions to the drug that users had ever experienced.[11] Although these might conventionally be termed adverse events, some of these were rated as positive effects by certain users:

Lack of coordination	77%	Impaired memory	32%
Blurred vision	61%	Nausea or vomiting	27%
Feeling no pain	49%	Dizziness	26%
Confusion	45%	Anxiety	24%
Pyrexia	41%	Temporary paralysis	23%
Inability to speak	39%	Difficulty breathing	21%
Increased heart rate	38%		

The frequency of nosebleeds when ketamine is snorted has led to a warning that there could be an increased risk of blood-borne **infections** such as HIV (human immunodeficiency virus) and viral hepatitis in users who share administration devices ('bumpers') such as straws.[14] The results from one US study where 25 young injectors were interviewed has also led to concern that those injecting ketamine may be at particularly high risk of blood-borne infections because frequent repeat injection in a group setting is common.[10] The same study also showed that 44% of injectors had begun their injecting career with ketamine.

Although an anaesthetic agent, ketamine only causes significant respiratory depression after high doses, and those who abuse it usually employ lower doses than are used by anaesthetists. The risk of respiratory depression is greater after intravenous use. The main danger from abuse arises from **accidents** subsequent to the peculiar changes in mental state that ketamine can produce without loss of consciousness. Individuals may become so divorced from reality that the surrounding environment is perceived completely differently: he or she may experience a 'different world'. In this respect, ketamine intoxication has some similarities to the effects of phencyclidine, although ketamine is much shorter-acting (see Chapter 9). Amongst other actions, the drug can also affect movement and has analgesic properties; there is thus obvious potential for harm to those who are intoxicated in certain circumstances.

Some users become **dependent** on ketamine. There may be an urge to repeatedly experience the drug's short-lived psychedelic effects; there may also be tolerance and an escalation of dose, evidence of harm, drug-seeking behaviour, neglect of important personal matters, and a preoccupation with the drug and its effects.[3,5–7,19] Despite use of high doses, no withdrawal reaction has been reported. To some extent the advent of dependence may be limited by the availability of ketamine, which is still mainly derived from pharmaceutical and veterinary sources.

Nitrous oxide

The euphoric and analgesic properties of nitrous oxide were first described by Sir Humphrey Davy in 1800. Since the 19th century it has been used therapeutically to induce anaesthesia and analgesia, and has found particular favour with dentists because of its short-lasting effects. In the medical or dental setting it is usually mixed with oxygen and is available commercially under brandnames such as Entonox. It is not a prescription medicine in all countries (e.g. the UK).

Effects and administration

Healthcare personnel who use nitrous oxide in the workplace have easy access to it and are familiar with its effects. Many cases of abuse involve dentists, anaesthetists and operating theatre staff. There are no recent data on the prevalence of abuse amongst medical staff, but a US survey of 524 medical and dental students conducted between 1976 and 1978 showed that up to 20% of those questioned had abused nitrous oxide socially on at least one occasion.[20] However, most students did not obtain the gas from operating theatres: nitrous oxide is available to the non-medical community as the propellant in canisters of pressurised whipped cream. The experienced user is able to release the gas into containers, allowing subsequent gas inhalation with minimum cream contamination. Inhalation is usually via a plastic bag, balloon or similar device.

Acute exposure to nitrous oxide can produce a short-lasting pleasurable intoxication: an initial rush of euphoria accompanied by flushing, then relaxation, feelings of detachment, auditory hallucinations and merriment (hence the alternative name of 'laughing gas'). The mechanism behind these central nervous system (CNS) effects is not fully understood but research suggests that it may be, to a greater or lesser extent, the result of an agonist action at central opioid receptors. This could be a direct action on opioid receptors, augmentation of the effects of endogenous opioids, or stimulation of their release.[21,22] The cognitive impairment produced usually lasts only a few minutes because the gas is rapidly excreted via the lungs. However, there may be a lingering sense of well-being for some time after inhalation stops.

Adverse effects

Inhalation of the pure gas without oxygen can cause acute hypoxia, either via oxygen insufficiency during inhalation or by nitrous oxide displacement of oxygen from alveoli during the excretion of the gas from the body. This latter mechanism – diffusion hypoxia – can be fatal. Other reported acute side-effects have included dizziness, fainting, and frostbite or pneumomediastinum due to inhaling directly from a pressurised gas cylinder.[23,24,25]

As with volatile substance abuse, intoxication is a potentially dangerous cause of accidents in the disorientated user. Nitrous oxide can sometimes cause nausea or vomiting; consequently there is a risk of aspirating vomit if the individual becomes unconscious. Unlike many chemicals subject to volatile substance abuse, nitrous oxide is not flammable and it also does not itself seem to cause 'sudden death' in the same manner as volatile substances (see Chapter 10). However, some fresh cream aerosol canisters with a nitrous oxide propellant may contain other propellants, such as chlorofluorocarbons, and nitrous oxide itself may produce degrees of hypoxia, as mentioned above. These two factors theoretically increase the risk of arrhythmia.

In a review of 11 fatal cases of abuse the cause of death, when it could be determined, was attributed to asphyxiation, fatal accident or aspiration of vomit.[26]

Chronic use has been associated with two problems believed to result from nitrous oxide accelerating vitamin B_{12} breakdown. A range of severe neurological disorders (mostly myeloneuropathies and neuropathies) have been described after chronic administration.[27-34] These are believed to occur because nitrous oxide prevents vitamin B_{12} involvement in the production of methionine, which is necessary for the production of the protective myelin sheaths surrounding nerves. The typical pattern of neurological damage begins with numbness or tingling, which is initially confined to the extremities but spreads if abuse continues. This in turn progresses to reduced muscle power in the areas affected. It may ultimately result in inability to walk unaided or loss of manual dexterity, and can be associated with impotence, urinary incontinence and disrupted bowel function. Neurological damage is usually at least partly reversible but recovery is often slow and incomplete. The second problem related to accelerated vitamin B_{12} breakdown is bone marrow depression. This is more quickly and completely reversible and does not seem to have been described as a result of nitrous oxide abuse, but has proved a serious complication in acutely ill patients administered long-term, continuous nitrous oxide for therapeutic reasons.[33,35,36]

A case of psychosis has been attributed to long-term use of the gas,[37] as well as depression in patients with myeloneuropathy[27] and delirium in one patient.[38] Dependence can occur: several case reports describe patients becoming preoccupied with abuse, increasing the amounts taken, and persisting with abuse despite knowledge of it harming them. A withdrawal reaction on cessation has not been described.

Other gaseous anaesthetics

Historically, anaesthetic ether was subject to abuse in the same way as many volatile liquids have been. Ether is no longer used as an anaesthetic in the developed world and supplies are difficult for the potential user to obtain. Some of the simple chlorinated alkanes (e.g. 1,1,1-trichloroethane) abused as solvents today have also been employed as anaesthetics in the past. There are occasional reports of abuse of more modern gaseous anaesthetics, e.g. enflurane,[39–41] cyclopropane,[42] halothane[43–46] and isoflurane.[47,48] In most cases those abusing these agents were operating theatre or laboratory workers with easy access; abuse is usually reported in the medical literature because the subject died as a result. Many inhalational anaesthetics are similar to the chemicals subject to volatile substance abuse – a well-known cause of sudden death (see Chapter 10). Ethyl chloride has also been abused by inhalation;[49] this product is sometimes used as a topical anaesthetic.

Chronic halothane abuse has been cited as a cause of hepatitis, a rare idiosyncratic side-effect when the drug is used an anaesthetic.[43]

Antidepressants

All antidepressants serve to increase the concentration of certain neuro-transmitters in the brain: principally serotonin, noradrenaline and dopamine. Illicit drugs such as cocaine and amfetamines also boost the concentrations of these substances in the CNS and this property is known to be important for producing psychotropic effects. It is not surprising therefore that antidepressants have been the subject of abuse. However, the total number of cases reported over the past 30 years is very small. Consequently, it has been argued that patients should not be informed of this abuse potential, because the benefits of warning about the tiny chance of abuse are outweighed by the risk of the warning causing non-compliance with a medication that can be life-saving (by preventing suicide).[50] However, other authors feel that the patient should be warned in a non-alarmist way.[51]

Monoamine oxidase inhibitors

Tranylcypromine is the most commonly abused monoamine oxidase inhibitor (MAOI). It has an amfetamine-like structure and has been abused for its stimulant-like effects. Most reported cases have involved patients with a history of depression who discover that taking 100–300 mg of tranylcypromine per day resolves depression and produces a sense of well-being similar to hypomania.[52–60] Many of those involved have a history of substance abuse, especially for amfetamine. In one case a dose of up to 600 mg was taken daily for 6 weeks;[60] in another case 440 mg was taken daily for 2 years.[58] During high-dose use, thrombocytopenia has been described.[53,60]

Some patients become dependent, and there may be a withdrawal reaction with features such as anxiety, restlessness, sleep disturbance, various aches, gastrointestinal upset, and even delirium or convulsions.[53,54,56–58,60] Abuse of **phenelzine** has also been reported at a dosage of 90–150 mg per day.[56] As with tranylcypromine, patients reported stimulant effects from these high doses and withdrawal effects upon discontinuation have been described in some cases.

Moclobemide, a selective inhibitor of CNS monoamine oxidase A, has been abused to produce euphoria in combination with citalopram or clomipramine.[61] The authors of a report describing five cases do not provide details of the doses used or the source of supply, but do suggest that all those involved in this practice died from the serotonin syndrome.

Selective serotonin reuptake inhibitors

The medical literature primarily describes abuse of fluoxetine, the fore-most selective serotonin reuptake inhibitor (SSRI) in the world, although sertraline abuse has also been described. SSRIs are abused in two different ways, described below.

Abuse alone for amfetamine-like effect

Two cases of fluoxetine abuse have been described in which known street drug users discovered that high doses of fluoxetine produced an amfetamine-like stimulant effect.[62] The first of these initially discovered the effect when taking 80 mg of fluoxetine and two cans of beer on an empty stomach. This produced 'increased energy, talkativeness, mood elevation and slight jitters' but she reported that it was unlike amfet-amine because she also felt 'numb and calm'. The second patient took 80–140 mg of fluoxetine per day initially but later increased this to a 'handful'. He also experienced an amfetamine-like effect and used trazodone and later diazepam to sedate him at night. Both patients' lives eventually became dominated by the taking of the drug, leading to hos-pital admission. Neither patient experienced a withdrawal reaction upon discontinuation.

One published account described a patient with anorexia who took up to 120 mg fluoxetine per day on account of the appetite-suppressing effects she experienced at high doses.[63] No psychotropic effects were reported.

Another patient – a former intravenous drug user – injected 20 mg fluoxetine several times each day.[64] The exact reasons for his habitual use were unclear, although he said it gave him 'a boost' and he had found it difficult to stop. The lack of a clear description of psychotropic effects is important, as another case in the medical literature makes clear. This describes an ex-drug polysubstance user who ritually took 1 mg of fluoxetine by mouth every day as a powder obtained by divid-ing the contents of a capsule and sucking it into her mouth.[65] She had previously found that a 10–20 mg dose prescribed for dysthymia caused over-stimulation, but the 1 mg dose was 'similar to "speeding"'. In both of these cases, it is possible that the patients experienced a placebo effect, reinforced by preparing and administering fluoxetine in a similar way to the way in which they formerly prepared their street drugs.

A single case describes a young man who regularly took 56 sertra-line 100-mg tablets twice daily.[66] His description of the effects produced suggest an amfetamine-like effect. The experience started with relaxation and euphoria, progressed to a feeling of excitement, and was followed by a period of hallucinations and mental hyperactivity lasting for more than a day. He experienced tremor and insomnia as side-effects and knew of two other people who abused sertraline in the same way.

Use with ecstasy

Fluoxetine has been used at street level in an attempt to help users cope with the aftermath of acute ecstasy intoxication, particularly the hangover effect and acute depression, which may be mediated by a depletion in central serotonin levels. Fluoxetine is taken in the belief that it will prevent or reduce long-term ecstasy-induced damage to serotonergic nerves[67] (see chapter 6). Animal studies have shown that fluoxetine may prevent the excessive loss of brain serotonin that has been associated with destruction of nerves by ecstasy and that behavioural changes linked to this depletion may also be prevented,[68,69] but whether this translates into reduced nerve damage in humans is unknown.

However, the psychotropic effects of ecstasy can be blocked by SSRIs.[70] Ecstasy users are aware of this potential problem and typically take fluoxetine some hours after an ecstasy dose in an attempt to avoid the blunting of psychotropic effects that may otherwise take place.

Tricyclic and related antidepressants

There have been several case reports of the abuse of amitriptyline.[71-74] This is a drug with significant antimuscarinic effects and the abuse potential may derive solely from this pharmacological property. A study in New York in 1978 reported that 25% of 346 participants in a methadone maintenance programme admitted to taking non-prescribed amitriptyline.[71] These 86 patients abused amitriptyline mostly to attain a 'sedative type of high'. Although precise details of dose were not provided, 'the number of pills taken at any one time ranged from one to 20'. These observations led to a second study in which 533 methadone maintenance patients were screened for non-prescribed amitriptyline use via urine analysis. A total of 115 (22%) had a positive urine test. In some cases, dependency was attested to by patients' attempts to forge prescriptions, to seek higher doses of amitriptyline, and to the existence of a local black market in amitriptyline.

In one documented case, amitriptyline abuse led to the onset of repeated grand mal convulsions and a diagnosis of epilepsy; these symptoms abated when amitriptyline was withdrawn.[72] The patient took up to 750 mg of amitriptyline per day. In a similar case, the chronic administration of 800 mg of amitriptyline daily led to convulsions and toxicity suggestive of overdose.[73] Another patient took up to 2 g per day.[74] The three patients described here were all female and all claimed a calming and/or euphoric effect from high-dose amitriptyline.

Abuse of dosulepin (dothiepin) has been reported from Ireland, where this has been a particularly popular antidepressant.[75] A questionnaire of 83 attenders at a Drug Treatment Centre in Dublin revealed that 38 had taken dosulepin for the purpose of abuse. Urine analysis of 99 other attenders who were not taking prescribed antidepressants showed that 19 had positive tests for tricyclics. The total amount taken per day varied from 150 to 600 mg orally and was reported to cause euphoria, sedation and various hallucinations (auditory and visual).

Two psychiatric patients with a history of alcohol dependence were reported to abuse mianserin at doses of up to 150 mg per day.[76] Both patients identified the rapid anti-anxiety action at high dose as the reason for abuse. Trazodone has also been abused. A case report describes a patient who took large doses of fluoxetine during the day as a substitute for amfetamine and up to 250 mg of trazodone at night for its sedative effects.[62]

Venlafaxine

One case report has described the oral abuse of venlafaxine.[77] The patient, an ex-amfetamine user, reported an amfetamine-like 'high'. He exhibited a range of drug-seeking behaviour in order to secure supplies and progressively increased his daily dose, eventually reaching 4050 mg per day. At this dose level he was forced to visit an emergency department because of chest pain, which was probably secondary to a raised pulse and blood pressure.

Antimuscarinic drugs

Trihexyphenidyl (benzhexol), orphenadrine, benzatropine and procyclidine are examples of antimuscarinic agents that have been abused to produce euphoric, and sometimes hallucinogenic, effects. Those who take antimuscarinics for these effects are often psychiatric patients who have been prescribed the drugs to counteract the extrapyramidal side-effects of neuroleptic medication. A large number of cases have been described, and several reviews published.[78-82] The prevalence of antimuscarinic drug abuse in psychiatric patients varies widely, but may be increasing: a study of 50 patients with serious mental illness in Australia in 2000 revealed a 34% incidence – the highest figure ever described at the time of writing.[83] Abuse by those who have not been prescribed them is less common in most countries, but has been reported. However, there are exceptions: in Jordan, for example, trihexyphenidyl has been described as the most commonly abused drug amongst youths.[84]

Effects and administration

These drugs are usually taken orally. Their psychotropic effects include euphoria, increased energy, relaxation, hallucinations and perceptual distortions. Trihexyphenidyl seems to be the most popular drug abused, either because it is widely prescribed or because it may have more stimulant properties than the others. Doses up to 60 mg per day have been taken.

As a group, prescription antimuscarinic drugs are not widely available on the street in most countries, although illegal purchasing of supplies is occasionally reported.[85,86] Psychiatric patients abusing their own prescribed antimuscarinic drugs may go to great lengths to obtain further quantities. They may, for example, claim to have lost prescribed supplies,[86] demand more supplies from healthcare professionals,[87] claim resistance to dosage reduction,[87] deny receipt of doses, steal or buy from other patients,[88] and even fake extrapyramidal symptoms.[88,89]

Identifying abuse amongst psychiatric patients may be difficult because antimuscarinic intoxication may mimic some of the symptoms of deterioration in an underlying psychotic condition, e.g. bizarre behaviour, hallucinations, paranoia and disorientation. To further complicate the picture, neuroleptics may blunt some of the pleasurable effects of antimuscarinic drug abuse and so patients may stop taking their regular medication. There is also the risk that some patients will swap antimuscarinics for other, illicit, drugs of abuse, so further confusing their own clinical presentation and introducing antimuscarinics onto the local street scene.

While many patients simply seek a 'high' or entertaining hallucinations from antimuscarinic medication, for others with schizophrenia it is harder to classify this problem as 'abuse' because the effects sought are an increased sociability and contentment or a relief from chronic symptoms of schizophrenia and its treatment.[82,90]

Adverse effects

Large doses of antimuscarinics carry the risk of severe intoxication. The exact presentation of the intoxicated patient depends on the dose taken but some of the symptoms are listed in Table 12.1. These effects usually subside within 24–72 hours but the diagnosis can be missed because symptoms may resemble those of a patient's existing psychiatric illness. Withdrawal symptoms have been described in some chronic users and include rebound cholinergic effects, dysphoria, fatigue, insomnia, headache, myalgia, various forms of gastrointestinal upset, and sleep disturbance.[79,81]

The antimuscarinic properties of certain other medications may, wholly or partly, account for their abuse potential. Examples include amitriptyline (see above) and antihistamines (Chapter 13). Plants with antimuscarinic properties are discussed in Chapter 17. Opioids, alcohol and cannabis can also produce antimuscarinic-like effects and, perhaps because of this, those abusing opioids can be peculiarly sensitive to antimuscarinic drugs – hence the prevalence of amitriptyline abuse amongst opioid users discussed above, and the dramatic toxicity of hyoscine (scopolamine) when found as an adulterant in heroin supplies.[91]

Table 12.1 Potential signs and symptoms of antimuscarinic intoxication

- Dilated pupils, dry eyes
- Dry mouth and hot, dry skin
- Tachycardia
- Incoherence, impaired concentration and memory, confusion, disorientation, hallucinations, paranoia, anxiety, euphoria, excitement
- Ataxia
- Constipation
- Urinary retention

Sedatives

Barbiturates

The abuse of barbiturates on the street is now a relatively small problem. For example, a national household survey in Australia in 2001 showed that while 0.9% of the population had abused barbiturates for non-medical purposes at some point in the past, only 0.2% had abused them within the past 12 months.[92] Barbiturates are abused for the purposes of producing relaxation and increased sociability. Sometimes the oral formulations are injected for much the same reasons as benzodiazepines.

Barbiturates are more likely than benzodiazepines to cause unpleasant side-effects. Even small doses can produce aggression, confusion, depression or anxiety and, unlike benzodiazepines, the drugs are quite likely to depress mental acuity. Barbiturates also commonly precipitate sedation, incoherence and incoordination. These effects are all dose-dependent. Large doses can cause potentially fatal respiratory depression and this effect is potentiated by alcohol and other CNS depressants such as opioids. In the heyday of barbiturate prescribing for insomnia, this was the usual cause of death when barbiturates were taken in overdose. In the absence of pre-existing lung disease, benzodiazepines are less likely to cause respiratory depression even when enormous doses are taken. The number of fatal toxicities per million prescriptions dispensed in the UK from 1983 to 1999 gives a figure of 146.2 for barbiturates and 7.4 for sedating benzodiazepines (deaths were in patients who took a single drug with or without alcohol).[93]

Barbiturates can cause dependence, and affected individuals exhibit both tolerance to the effects of these drugs and a withdrawal syndrome upon cessation, which can include convulsions and death. Consequently, barbiturates should be withdrawn slowly in the chronic user. This has been done by changing the patient to phenobarbital first, and equivalent doses are given in Table 12.2.

Barbiturates are now less easily obtainable on the black market than benzodiazepines and so are more expensive; any illicit manufacture is probably very limited.

Table 12.2 Phenobarbital equivalents for prescribing as cited by UK Department of Health and Social Security in 1984[94]

Drug	Oral sedative dose (mg)	Equivalent phenobarbital dose (mg)
Amalobarbital	100	30
Butobarbital	100	30
Secobarbital	100	30

Benzodiazepines

The inappropriate use of benzodiazepines has three different aspects:

1. Over-prescribing of hypnotic and anxiolytic benzodiazepines has resulted in large numbers of people becoming dependent upon them. These patients, who were originally prescribed benzodiazepines for a medical indication, might be termed 'benzodiazepine dependents'.
2. Abuse of benzodiazepines occurs on the street, often by intravenous injection of formulations designed for oral administration. This group is largely composed of known users of a range of illicit substances. For ease of discussion, these will be referred to as 'benzodiazepine abusers'.
3. Benzodiazepines have been used to sedate individuals in order for them to be subjected to sexual intercourse against their will – so-called 'date rape'.

1. Benzodiazepine dependents

In 2002, family doctors in England wrote 12.7 million prescriptions for benzodiazepines.[95] This compares with 15.8 million in 1992, and over 30 million in the late 1970s, suggesting that doctors are gradually acting to combat the problem of benzodiazepine dependence. Benzodiazepines are very useful and, on the whole, safe drugs, but prescribing practice still needs to be more rational in many cases. For example, the Department of Health in England has noted that about a third of benzodiazepine prescriptions are still written for 56 or more doses, suggesting that many doctors are not heeding advice to use these drugs for short periods.[95] Doctors in primary and secondary care are jointly responsible for starting patients on benzodiazepine, failing to review treatment regularly, and not stopping treatment when it is no longer required.

However, as Hallström has argued, it can be very difficult to specify why patients should not take these drugs chronically.[96] He suggests that the main reasons are as follows:

- Benzodiazepines are often prescribed to blot out psychological stresses and so do not enable the affected individual to learn how to adapt to stress and thereby mature.
- Patients and doctors can be tempted into thinking there is a 'pill for every ill' and rely too much on pharmacological approaches to treatment when other approaches might be more appropriate.
- A large proportion of prescriptions are made out by male doctors for female patients. Where the unequal role of women in society is a cause of stress, then benzodiazepines are not the answer.

- Side-effects, although sometimes difficult to identify, include memory loss and psychomotor incoordination. Benzodiazepines also impair driving ability.
- Insomnia and anxiety are generally self-limiting; taking benzodiazepines helps resolve symptoms but at the risk of taking tablets daily for years as a result of dependency. Once dependent, the effects of stopping treatment (i.e. prolonged withdrawal) can be worse than continuing with it.
- The long-term efficacy of benzodiazepines is unproven.

Because the best form of management of benzodiazepine dependence is prevention, healthcare communities should produce guidelines on benzodiazepine prescribing and withdrawal to support prescribers. Some key points are given in Table 12.3. It is important that new patients are warned of the risk of dependence and that steps are taken to prevent it happening. Elderly patients are particularly at risk of becoming dependent. In England in 2002, 56% of all prescriptions for the three commonest benzodiazepines were for patients over 65 years old.[95] This is of concern because of the link between benzodiazepines and falls in the elderly.

Educating the patient about the best means to acquire a good night's sleep may be beneficial, and can obviate the need for a benzodiazepine prescription. Box 12.2 gives some helpful tips.

Box 12.2 Factors likely to improve sleep at night.

1. Try to establish a regular pattern of waking and rising.
2. Avoid taking naps during the day as this is deducted from the night-time quota of sleep.
3. Do not retire to bed until tired.
4. Regular daily exercise helps to encourage sleep.
5. Ensure appropriate treatment for any medical conditions causing sleeplessness (e.g. pain).
6. Avoid caffeinated drinks and large amounts of alcohol or food before going to bed.
7. Some medicines may cause insomnia (e.g. fluoxetine). Try alternatives, or avoid them at bedtime if possible.
8. Relaxation before going to bed may help, e.g. a walk, reading, meditation.
9. Avoid a hot room or bed, or a very hot bath just before going to bed.
10. Try to avoid stressful events near bedtime (e.g. dwelling on worrying events).

Table 12.3 Avoiding benzodiazepine dependence or abuse – guidance on prescribing

Benzodiazepine dependents
- Use benzodiazepines only for anxiety or insomnia that seriously disrupts the patient's lifestyle, not for minor complaints
- There are non-drug alternative treatment strategies for both conditions that should be considered, e.g. elimination of underlying causes, lifestyle changes, counselling
- Warn the patient of tolerance, dependence potential and the difficulty of withdrawal if treatment is prolonged
- Limit the supply of medication provided, e.g. an initial prescription for insomnia could be 7 doses, for anxiety 14 days
- Write 'when required' on the prescription and make sure the patient understands that daily dosing is usually not mandatory for beneficial effects. Generally, intermittent use (by this method or by prescribing occasional short courses) is efficacious and is less likely to cause dependence in the long term
- Use the smallest dose possible
- Regularly review the need for medication and discontinue as soon as possible

Benzodiazepine abusers
- Avoid prescribing to those with a history of drug abuse
- Do not prescribe benzodiazepines to temporary residents and be cautious concerning supply to new patients of a practice
- Remember that non-abusers may sell their medication to abusers, so review all benzodiazepine prescriptions regularly and limit quantities prescribed
- Document known history of benzodiazepine abuse so that any other doctor will be aware of the problem
- Where street abuse is suspected, refuse to supply; or supply low-concentration elixir, which is much more difficult to abuse intravenously

Cessation of long-term benzodiazepines is associated with a withdrawal syndrome in about a third of patients on chronic therapy, but it is impossible to determine in advance which patients will experience the problem.[97] The symptoms are varied, but include anxiety, irritability, dysphoria, decreased concentration, insomnia, nausea, malaise, muscle twitching, tremors, depersonalisation, perceptual distortions, sweating and headaches. Convulsions occur infrequently. Symptoms usually peak a few days after stopping chronic benzodiazepines abruptly. However, some symptoms may last for months afterwards.[98] Where practicable, existing dependents should be withdrawn slowly over several weeks, usually following conversion to oral diazepam, which has a very long half-life and thus may render withdrawal easier. Equivalent doses are given in Table 12.4. A common regimen is to withdraw a small proportion of the dose every fortnight,[99] but the extent and speed of

Table 12.4   Appropriate dosages of common benzodiazepines equivalent to 5 mg of diazepam[99]

Drug	Dose
Chlordiazepoxide	15 mg
Diazepam	5 mg
Loprazolam	500 mcg
Lorazepam	500 mcg
Oxazepam	15 mg
Temazepam	10 mg
Nitrazepam	5 mg

withdrawal should be titrated to the patient's feelings of comfort. The symptoms of withdrawal must be explained to the patient, as these are often very similar to the original complaint for which benzodiazepines were prescribed.

2. Benzodiazepine abusers

In Australia, a 2001 survey showed that 3.2% of the adult population had abused tranquillisers or sleeping pills other than barbiturates for non-medical reasons.[92] In the USA, a similar survey in 2002 identified that 4.2% of the adult population had taken prescription 'sedatives' for a non-medical reason, and 8.2% had used prescription 'tranquilizers' in the same way; presumably a substantial proportion of both of these categories was benzodiazepine abuse.[100] However, abuse amongst users of illicit drugs is much higher. In England in 2004 an estimated 14% of illicit substance users attending drug treatment centres reported benzodiazepine abuse subsidiary to their main drug use.[95] Table 12.5 lists some of the reasons for benzodiazepine abuse.

The main benzodiazepines involved in abuse vary according to geographical location, and to some extent reflect differences in local availability, preference, and established patterns of use, because benzodiazepines are often obtained via diversion of legitimate pharmaceuticals. The benzodiazepines that figure most prominently in published medical literature seem to be diazepam, temazepam, nitrazepam, chlordiazepoxide and flunitrazepam.

Although sometimes taken by mouth, it is common for users to inject oral preparations intravenously. The doses used can be very large. One UK study cited 3600 mg as the maximum daily dose of temazepam encountered, with 600 mg as the average.[101] Liquid-filled capsules were

Table 12.5 Reasons for benzodiazepine abuse 'on the street'

- 'Rush' or 'buzz' after rapid injection
- CNS depressant properties (e.g. sedative, relaxant, anxiolytic, confidence-boosting and disinhibitive effects)
- Increase in the intensity and duration of the effect of heroin when the two are used concurrently. Street heroin may be very impure and over-'cut' with bulking agents. Use of temazepam is claimed partially to counteract this
- Suppression of opioid withdrawal symptoms
- Assistance with 'coming down' after use of stimulant drugs such as cocaine or amfetamine; to induce sleep when using any stimulant drug

withdrawn from sale in many countries in 1990 because the formulation enabled easier abuse by injection, but users still injected the contents of gel-filled capsules after liquefying the contents, or tablets after crushing and dispersing them in water. Often quite elaborate preparation is required. Injection of preparations intended for oral use can clearly have a range of deleterious consequences, which are discussed in more depth in Chapter 2. In the case of temazepam, the effects are exacerbated by the irritant nature of the drug.

Temazepam and diazepam oral liquid formulations are often low-concentration viscous formulations. Parenteral administration of such preparations would require injection of very large quantities of a thick, sticky liquid, which is obviously difficult. Consequently, a switch to prescribing of liquid formulations has been advocated as a means of reducing temazepam abuse.[102] This would undoubtedly be a useful measure, but might simply encourage the preferential abuse of the other benzodiazepines, which are available in tablet form.

Supplies of benzodiazepines are obtained by purchase on the black market or from legitimate receivers of benzodiazepine prescriptions. Theft from health centres and pharmacies may also play a part. Some users obtain prescriptions by deception, claiming temporary resident status or giving false names. There is significant manufacturing of temazepam and diazepam oral formulations in eastern Europe and parts of Asia, and such products, including temazepam liquid-filled capsules, are imported into western Europe for illicit use.

Apart from the problems detailed above, abuse of temazepam clearly could cause sedation in potentially dangerous circumstances. The high doses may be associated with blackouts, risk-taking behaviour and personality disorders (e.g. paranoia, violent behaviour) and benzodiazepine withdrawal symptoms may sometimes occur in the chronic user when regular administration is interrupted.

In the UK, the prevalence of temazepam abuse persuaded the government to impose tighter legal controls on its supply in 1996. However, legal restrictions of this nature – even when successful in limiting access – may only focus users' attentions onto other benzodiazepines not controlled by this legislation. For example, a seven-city UK survey of 208 patients attending drug clinics in 1992 found that 89% of 208 respondents had abused benzodiazepines and 50% had injected them.[103] Although temazepam was most popular, 75% of respondents had abused diazepam tablets, 52% had used nitrazepam tablets and 35% lorazepam.

3. Benzodiazepines and date rape

Benzodiazepines, particularly flunitrazepam, have been used to incapacitate victims before a sexual assault. Benzodiazepines are not only sedative: intoxication tends to promote disinhibition and there is also an amnesic effect, which means that victims may not be able to remember clearly what has happened. One brand of flunitrazepam, Rohypnol, has been reformulated to make dissolution harder – it also releases a blue colour as it dissolves.

A police operation in Essex, UK, in 2002 revealed that 8 out of a total of 200 drinks randomly sampled from mainly women drinkers at a nightclub had been 'spiked' with drugs.[104] Of the eight drinks involved, seven contained benzodiazepines. Although it is not clear whether the sole motivation for attempting to drug individuals was sexual assault, a 4% incidence is remarkably high.

Zopiclone and zolpidem

Although chemically unrelated to benzodiazepines, both of these short-acting hypnotics act via the benzodiazepine/GABA (gamma-aminobutyric acid) receptor complex. They have both been subject to abuse.[105–110] Daily doses of zopiclone abused in cases reported in the medical literature have ranged up to 380 mg, and for zolpidem up to 1200 mg.[107]

Zopiclone has been used mainly to produce sedative or tranquillising effects, but also to produce euphoria with alcohol.[105] There are at least three reports of intravenous use.[105–107] Advantages over benzodiazepines reported by users include the fact that zopiclone does not show up on routine urinalysis and that it does not cause amnesia.

Interviews with 100 consecutive methadone maintenance patients in Liverpool, UK, in 1996 found that six abused zopiclone, although these six knew of many others who were abusing zopiclone.[108] All of them were former temazepam users, who initially took zopiclone to help them sleep but they developed tolerance to its effects, and a withdrawal reaction characterised by insomnia, edginess and a very strong craving 6–8 hours after the last dose. The speed of onset of craving led them to take zopiclone in two or three divided doses throughout the day. Common side-effects during abuse included drowsiness, dry mouth, bitter taste, nausea, ataxia, and psychomotor slowing.

A report from Eire described a survey of 55 methadone maintenance patients.[106] A total of 38 (69%) had abused zopiclone at least once. Of these, 12 took zopiclone to induce sleep, 16 used it to experience tranquillising effects, and 10 reported no effects.

Physical dependence on zopiclone in patients prescribed the drug for insomnia has also been described with signs of tolerance and withdrawal reactions.[111–113] In most cases these were patients with a history of substance abuse or psychiatric problems, and in the latter cases self-medication with zopiclone as an anxiolytic seems to have been part of the motivation. Patients generally increased the dose themselves to levels greater than those prescribed for insomnia. Withdrawal symptoms included anxiety, insomnia, tremor, palpitations and sweating. In a pooled analysis of clinical studies involving 441 patients who took zopiclone for 28 days or less, withdrawal reactions were seen in only 2.7% of patients.[114] However, some of these patients were taking 15 mg daily, which is greater than the dose of 7.5 mg used therapeutically in many countries.

Clomethiazole

Clomethiazole abuse has been described. A 1979 study provided details on 17 users.[115] All but four of these were alcoholics, ex-alcoholics or heavy drinkers of alcohol. Data on dosage is only provided for three patients and each took up to 10 g clomethiazole daily when available. Seven patients were identified by urine-screening alone, so few data are available on these, but the remaining ten patients all showed drug-seeking behaviour of one kind or another – mostly by manipulating extra supplies from doctors. Symptoms of withdrawal were described in two patients in whom dosage reduction was attempted; these were similar to those seen with other sedatives.

The intravenous injection of the contents of clomethiazole capsules is unlikely to be attractive because the drug is dissolved in lipid. The lipid would break into small globules in plasma from which the drug would diffuse slowly. There would not be the desired rapid rise in plasma concentrations of clomethiazole.

Other drugs

Many other prescription medicines have been abused. Often there are only a very small number of cases reported in the literature. Some of these are described below.

Antibiotics

Five women were said to have enjoyed 'giddiness and excitement' from the intentional abuse of metronidazole plus alcohol.[116] This combination is known to produce a disulfiram-like reaction in some recipients, but this is the only report of intentional abuse. Another report highlighted a case of tetracycline and penicillin abuse in association with alcohol.[117] The combination was said, rather dubiously, to produce euphoria.

Carbamazepine

Three reports have together described eight cases of carbamazepine abuse orally for its euphoric effects.[118–120] Sometimes the drug was taken with alcohol or benzodiazepines. The authors of one of the papers stated that they were aware of other cases.[118]

The doses ranged from 1 to 8 g, the higher doses tending to cause plasma carbamazepine levels within the toxic range. Five of the eight cases described in the medical literature seem to represent a 'one-off' recreational exposure,[119] whereas three cases involved a chronic habit lasting 4 months or more.[118,120]

Clonidine

Two reports have identified clonidine abuse amongst patients on methadone maintenance programmes.[121,122] The reasons for abusing clonidine were an ability to boost the effects of methadone; to reduce symptoms associated with insufficient methadone; for clonidine's own psychotropic effects (euphoria, sedation, relaxation). In two cases, the average daily dose was 1–2 mg per day but one patient had occasionally taken up to 15 mg per day.[121] Both patients experienced a withdrawal reaction upon discontinuation, although the symptoms of this were completely different in each case. Each patient was aware of others maintained on methadone who abused clonidine.

A survey of 48 consecutive applicants to join a methadone maintenance patients in Baltimore in 1992 revealed that 46% of them had used clonidine at some point in their lives.[122] A separate series of interviews with 30 self-confessed clonidine users already on methadone maintenance showed clonidine to be the current drug of choice in 13, and 17 reported physical withdrawal symptoms upon cessation. In both applicants and existing patients, doses ranged from 0.1 to 2.4 mg at a time, but some patients took these doses several times a day. Most patients abused clonidine regularly, and were able to buy it easily 'on the street' or to obtain it by deception from doctors.

A study of 90 pregnant, opiate-abusing women in Baltimore discovered 30 who either had a positive urine test for clonidine, or who volunteered their abuse within the preceding 30 days.[123] Interestingly, only 20% of positive cases could be identified by self-report alone. A polydrug user who took up to 3 mg of clonidine per day described the effects of clonidine as a sleepy dreamland 'similar to what he had experienced with morphine'.[124] He said that clonidine was better than heroin because it did not cause nausea and the effects lasted up to half a day.

Side-effects of clonidine that might be seen in those abusing it could include low blood pressure, tiredness and depression.

Diuretics

Abuse of diuretics has been attempted as a misguided method of quick weight loss. They are also used in various ways by sportsmen and bodybuilders (see Chapter 11).

Levodopa

Five patients taking levodopa plus carbidopa ('Sinemet') for Parkinson's disease were reported to have derived psychotropic effects from taking the preparation.[125] All of those involved were male and younger than the average sufferer from this condition (46–60 years of age). Patients reported effects such as feelings of optimism, increased mental power, a sense of well-being, increased sexual energy and animation. However, relatives noticed a range of unpleasant personality changes, including paranoia and aggression. Larger doses than prescribed were taken for this purpose – up to 2500 mg of levodopa per day – despite patients experiencing severe dystonias and other movement-related side-effects of levodopa at this dosage. When the drug was discontinued, both the adverse effects and psychotropic effects disappeared, but these were often replaced by depression, craving for the drug, drug-seeking behaviour and covert administration. In each case Parkinsonian symptoms were later controlled with lower doses of levodopa.

Two similar cases have also been described in which patients with Parkinson's disease persistently elevated their intake of levodopa–benserazide combinations to give higher doses of levodopa than were necessary to control their symptoms.[126] Daily doses of 1500 and 2000 mg per day respectively caused euphoria, hyperkinesia and hypomania. One patient also experienced hallucinations. Doses were reduced to lower levels with difficulty.

Neuroleptics

Occasionally reports appear in the medical literature of patients who obtain neuroleptics on the street and take them either as an experiment or because they believe them to be some other drug. Haloperidol is the most commonly involved,[127–129] and reported side-effects include, most notably, dramatic extrapyramidal symptoms, which are the usual reason for abuse coming to medical attention. Two cases have also been described of patients with schizophrenia who injected themselves with prescribed neuroleptic tablets for their sedative properties.[130] One patient, an ex-intravenous drug user, had been prescribed high doses of chlorpromazine tablets but frequently requested additional doses, which he injected. The second patient was not known to have used intravenous drugs before, but injected himself on a number of occasions with crushed haloperidol tablets.

Oestrogens

Although no cases of abuse have been described *per se*, oestrogens are psychoactive. It has been proposed that women taking this group of drugs for therapeutic reasons could exhibit tolerance and dependence during prolonged administration after the menopause.[131]

Pergolide

A single case report describes abuse of a 10-mg oral dose to experience disassociation and visual hallucinations, which subsided after 2 hours and had finished within 6 hours.[132]

Salbutamol

Abuse of salbutamol has been reported. In most cases the individuals involved were children. Infants and children may be more susceptible to the psychotropic effects of salbutamol. Brennan reported a variety of anecdotes connected with salbutamol abuse, including that of a non-asthmatic schoolboy who used salbutamol rotacaps because they 'made him feel good'.[133] This is unusual because most cases of salbutamol abuse involve the use of aerosol devices. Abuse of salbutamol and other available medications by the inhalation of large amounts of aerosol inhalers may be attributable to intoxication with the chlorofluoro-carbon propellant as a form of volatile substance abuse. The eight patients described in four published papers were all from 4 to 17 years old and in many cases a whole inhaler (200 puffs) or more was used each day,[134–137] sometimes producing a discernible euphoria or hallu-cinations. Anecdotally, the sale of salbutamol inhalers in association with glue sniffing has also been reported,[133] and in one reported case of abuse replacing a salbutamol inhaler with a placebo one gave the sub-ject the same euphoric effect.[134] In cases where patients were changed from an aerosol inhaler to a dry powder inhaler, abuse promptly stopped. One report described abuse in a 24-year-old man who used up to 90 puffs of salbutamol aerosol per day and exhibited drug-seeking behaviour to ensure that he had a constant supply of inhalers. However, no psychotropic effects were reported by the patient, who had a history of psychiatric illness. The patient seems more likely to have suffered from an obsessive–compulsive disorder.[138]

Salbutamol inhalers have also been employed by some who regu-larly use cannabis to counteract increased airways resistance secondary to the irritant smoke.

Sildenafil

Within a few weeks of being launched, sildenafil (Viagra) was available to purchase as a recreational drug.[139] Although licensed as a treatment for erectile dysfunction, the main recreational use may be different. A survey of 519 attenders at an English nightclub in October 1998 dis-covered that 3% reported buying the drug in the club. The positive effects seen included enhanced sexual desire and feelings during sex, and a feeling of warmth. The drug is taken by men and women. Some men may take sildenafil to counteract impotence caused by certain street drugs (e.g. cocaine). A survey of 837 gay and bisexual men in San

Francisco in 2003 showed that a third had used sildenafil at least once, and most of these had not obtained it via a doctor's prescription.[140] Use of sildenafil may be associated with a heightened incidence of sexual behaviour that facilitates the transmission of the human immuno-deficiency virus.

Sumatriptan

Daily use of sumatriptan for migraine may be associated with intense withdrawal migraines upon discontinuation.[141,142] This could encourage excessive regular use.

References

1. Baumevieille M, Haramburu F, Begaud B. Abuse of prescription medicines in southwestern France. *Ann Pharmacother* 1997; 31: 847–850.
2. Ahmed S N, Petchkovsky L. Abuse of ketamine. *Br J Psychiatry* 1980; 137: 303.
3. Moore N N, Bostwick J M. Ketamine dependence in anaesthesia providers. *Psychosomatics* 1999; 40: 356–359.
4. Rosenberg M. Drug abuse in oral and maxillofacial training programs. *J Oral Maxillofac Surg* 1987; 44: 458–462.
5. Kamaya H, Krishna P R. Ketamine addiction. *Anesthesiology* 1987; 67: 861–862.
6. Hurt P H, Ritchie E C. A case of ketamine dependence. *Am J Psychiatry* 1994; 151: 779.
7. Jansen K L R, Darracot-Cankovic R. The nonmedical use of ketamine part two: a review of problem use and dependence. *J Psychoactive Drugs* 2001; 33: 151–158.
8. Jansen K L R. A review of the nonmedical use of ketamine: use, users and con-sequences. *J Psychoactive Drugs* 2000; 32: 419–433.
9. Dalgarno P J, Shewan D. Illicit use of ketamine in Scotland. *J Psychoactive Drugs* 1996; 28: 191–199.
10. Lankenau S E, Clatts M C. Ketamine injection among high risk youth: pre-liminary findings from New York city. *J Drug Issues* 2002; 32: 893–905.
11. Dillon P, Copeland J, Jansen K. Patterns of use and harms associated with non-medical ketamine use. *Drug Alcohol Depend* 2003; 69: 23–28.
12. Dollery C, ed. *Therapeutic Drugs*, 2nd edn. Edinburgh: Churchill Livingstone, 1999, K3–7.
13. Weiner A L, Vieira L, McKay C A Jr, *et al.* Ketamine abusers presenting to the emergency department: a case series. *J Emerg Med* 2000; 18: 447–451.
14. Tellier P-P. Club drugs: is it all ecstasy? *Pediatr Ann* 2002; 31: 550–556.
15. Jansen K L R. Non-medical use of ketamine. *BMJ* 1993; 306: 601–602.
16. Curran H V, Morgan C. Cognitive, dissociative and psychotogenic effects of ketamine in recreational users on the night of drug use and 3 days later. *Addiction* 2000; 95: 575–590.

17. Curran H V, Monaghan L. In and out of the K-hole: a comparison of the acute and residual effects of ketamine in frequent and infrequent ketamine users. *Addiction* 2001; 96: 749–760.

18. Felser J M, Orban D J. Dystonic reaction after ketamine abuse. *Ann Emerg Med* 1982; 11: 673–675.

19. Pal H R, Berry N, Kumar R, *et al*. Ketamine dependence. *Anaesth Intensive Care* 2002; 30: 382–384.

20. Rosenberg H, Orkin F K, Springstead J. Abuse of nitrous oxide. *Anesth Analg* 1979; 58: 104–106.

21. Berkowitz B A, Ngai S H, Finck A D. Nitrous oxide 'analgesia': resemblance to opiate action. *Science* 1979; 194: 967–968.

22. Daras C, Cantrill R C, Gillman M A. [3H]Naloxone displacement: evidence for nitrous oxide as opioid receptor agonist. *Eur J Pharmacol* 1983; 89: 177–178.

23. LiPuma J P, Wellman J, Stern H P. Nitrous oxide abuse: a new cause for pneumomediastinum. *Radiology* 1982; 145: 602.

24. Rowbottom S J. Nitrous oxide abuse. *Anaesth Intensive Care* 1988; 16: 241–242.

25. Hwang J C F, Himel H N, Edlich R F. Frostbite of the face after recreational misuse of nitrous oxide. *Burns* 1996; 22: 152–153.

26. Suruda A J, McGlothlin J D. Fatal abuse of nitrous oxide in the workplace. *J Occup Med* 1990; 32: 682–684.

27. Layzer R B. Myeloneuropathy after prolonged exposure to nitrous oxide. *Lancet* 1978; ii: 1227–1230.

28. Pema P J, Horak H A, Wyatt R H. Myelopathy caused by nitrous oxide toxicity. *Am J Neuroradiol* 1998; 19: 894–896.

29. Nevins M A. Neuropathy after nitrous oxide abuse. *JAMA* 1980; 244: 2264.

30. Iwata K, O'Keefe G B, Karanas A. Neurologic problems associated with chronic nitrous oxide abuse in a non-healthcare worker. *Am J Med Sci* 2001; 322: 173–174.

31. Butzkueven H, King J O. Nitrous oxide myelopathy in an abuser of whipped cream bulbs. *J Clin Neurosci* 2000; 7: 73–75.

32. Brett A. Myeloneuropathy from whipped cream bulbs presenting as conversion disorder. *Aust N Z J Psychiatry* 1997; 31: 131–132.

33. King M, Coulter C, Boyle R S, *et al*. Neurotoxicity from overuse of nitrous oxide. *Med J Aust* 1995; 163: 50–51.

34. Lai N Y, Silbert P L, Erber W N, *et al*. 'Nanging': another cause of nitrous oxide neurotoxicity. *Med J Aust* 1997; 166: 166.

35. Jastak J T. Nitrous oxide and its abuse. *J Am Dent Assoc* 1980; 122: 48–52.

36. Sando M J H, Lawrence J R. Bone marrow depression following treatment of tetanus with protracted nitrous oxide anaesthesia. *Lancet* 1958; i: 588.

37. Brodsky L, Zuniga J. Nitrous oxide: a psychotogenic agent. *Compr Psychiatry* 1975; 16: 185–188.

38. Sterman A B, Coyle P K. Subacute toxic delirium following nitrous oxide abuse. *Arch Neurol* 1983; 40: 446–447.

39. Lingenfelter R W. Fatal misuse of enflurane. *Anesthesiology* 1981; 55: 603.

40. Jacob B, Heller C, Daldrup T, *et al*. Case report: fatal accidental enflurane intoxication. *J Forensic Sci* 1989; 34: 1408–1411.

41. Musshoff F, Junker H, Madea B. An unusual case of driving under the influence of enflurane. *Forensic Sci Int* 2002; 128: 187–189.

42. Krause J G, McCarthy W B. Case report: sudden death by inhalation of cyclopropane. *J Forensic Sci* 1989; 34: 1011–1012.

43. Kaplan H G, Bakken J, Quadracci L, *et al*. Hepatitis caused by halothane sniffing. *Ann Intern Med* 1979; 90: 797–798.

44. Spencer J D, Raasch F O, Trefny F A. Halothane abuse in hospital personnel. *JAMA* 1976; 235: 1034–1035.

45. Block S, Rosenblatt R. A halothane abuse fatality. *Anesthesiology* 1980; 52: 524.

46. Hiroki T, Teruuchi T, Kuroda T, *et al*. Two fatal cases of poisoning due to abuse of halothane. *Jpn J Legal Med* 1973; 27: 243–247.

47. Pavlic M, Haidekker A, Grubwieser P, *et al*. Fatal accident caused by isoflurane abuse. *Int J Legal Med* 2002; 116: 357–360.

48. Kuhlman J J, Magluilo J Jr, Smith M L. Two deaths involving isoflurane abuse. *J Forensic Sci* 1993; 38: 968–971.

49. Hersch R. Abuse of ethyl chloride. *Am J Psychiatr* 1991; 148: 270–271.

50. Siris S G. Do antidepressants have any meaningful potential for abuse? *CNS Drugs* 1995; 4: 253–255.

51. Pagliaro L A, Pagliaro A M. Abuse potential of antidepressants: Does it exist? *CNS Drugs* 1995; 4: 247–252.

52. Mielczarek J, Johnson J. Tranylcypromine. *Lancet* 1963; i: 388–389.

53. Griffin N, Draper R J, Webb M G T. Addiction to tranylcypromine. *BMJ* 1981; 283: 346.

54. Ben-Arie O, George G C W. A case of tranylcypromine (Parnate) addiction. *Br J Psychiatr* 1979; 135: 273–274.

55. Le Gassicke J. Tranylcypromine. *Lancet* 1963; i: 270.

56. Baumbacher G, Hansen M S. Abuse of monoamine oxidase inhibitors. *Am J Drug Alcohol Abuse* 1992; 18: 399–406.

57. Briggs N C, Jefferson J W, Koenecke F H. Tranylcypromine addiction: a case report and review. *J Clin Psychiatry* 1990; 51: 426–429.

58. Vartzopoulos D, Krull F. Dependence on monoamine oxidase inhibitors in high dose. *Br J Psychiatry* 1991; 158: 856–857.

59. Brady K T, Lydiard R B, Kellner C. Tranylcypromine abuse. *Am J Psychiatry* 1991; 148: 1268–1269.

60. Davids E, Roschke J, Klawe C, *et al*. Tranylcypromine abuse associated with delirium and thrombocytopenia. *J Clin Psychopharmacol* 2000; 20: 270–271.

61. Neuvonen P J, Pohjola-Sintonen S, Tacke U, *et al*. Five fatal cases of serotonin syndrome after moclobemide-citalopram or moclobemide-clomipramine overdoses. *Lancet* 1993; 342: 1419.

62. Tinsley J A, Olsen M W, Laroche R R, *et al*. Fluoxetine abuse. *Mayo Clin Proc* 1994; 69: 166–168.

63. Wilcox J A. Abuse of fluoxetine by patient with anorexia nervosa. *Am J Psychiatry* 1987; 144: 1100.

64. Pagliaro L A, Pagliaro A M. Fluoxetine abuse by an intravenous drug user. *Am J Psychiatry* 1993; 150: 1898.

65. Goldman M J, Grinspoon L, Hunter-Jones S. Ritualistic use of fluoxetine by a former substance abuser. *Am J Psychiatry* 1990; 147: 1377.

66. D'Urso P. Abuse of sertraline. *J Clin Pharm Ther* 1996; 21: 359–360.

67. Dotinga R. Ecstasy-Prozac: a dangerous cocktail. *USA Today*, 24 February 2002.

68. Sanchez V, Camarero J, Esteban B, *et al*. The mechanisms involved in the long-lasting neuroprotective effect of fluoxetine against MDMA ('ecstasy')-induced degeneration of 5-HT nerve endings in rat brain. *Br J Pharmacol* 2001; 134: 46–57.

69. Virden T B, Baker L E. Disruption of the discriminative stimulus effects of S(+)-3,4-methylenedioxymethamphetamine (MDMA) by (+/-)-MDMA neurotoxicity: protection by fluoxetine. *Behav Pharmacol* 1999; 10: 195–204.

70. Stein D J, Rink J. Effects of 'ecstasy' blocked by serotonin reuptake inhibitors. *J Clin Psychiatry* 1999; 60: 485.

71. Cohen M J, Hanbury R, Stimmel B. Abuse of amitriptyline. *JAMA* 1978; 240: 1372–1373.

72. O'Rahilly S, Turner T H, Wass J A H. Factitious epilepsy due to amitriptyline abuse. *Ir Med J* 1985; 78: 166–167.

73. Wohlreich M M, Welch W. Amitriptyline abuse presenting as acute toxicity. *Psychosomatics* 1993; 34: 191–193.

74. Delisle J D. A case of amitriptyline abuse. *Am J Psychiatry* 1990; 147: 1377–1378.

75. Dorman A, Talbot D, Byrne P, *et al*. Misuse of dothiepin. *BMJ* 1995; 311: 1502.

76. Theret L, Bertholon F, Germain M C. Two cases of mianserin abuse in psychiatric out-patients. *Eur Psychiatry* 1992; 7: 143–144.

77. Sattar S P, Grant K M, Bhatia S C. A case of venlafaxine abuse. *N Engl J Med* 2003; 348: 764–765.

78. Anon. Managing abuse of anticholinergic medication in patients with psychotic disorders. *Drug Ther Perspect* 1996; 8: 11–13.

79. Dilsaver S C. Antimuscarinic agents as substances of abuse: a review. *J Clin Psychopharmacol* 1988; 8: 14–22.

80. Hidalgo H A, Mowers R M. Anticholinergic drug abuse. *Ann Pharmacother* 1990; 24: 41–42.

81. Marken P A, Stoner S C, Bunker M T. Anticholinergic drug abuse and misuse: epidemiology and therapeutic implications. *CNS Drugs* 1996; 5: 190–199.

82. Dose M, Tempel H D. Abuse potential of anticholinergics. *Pharmacopsychiatry* 2000; 33(Suppl 1): 43–46.

83. Buhrich N, Weller A, Kevans P. Misuse of anticholinergic drugs by people with serious mental illness. *Psychiatr Serv* 2000; 51: 928–929.

84. Al-Nsour T S, Hadidi K A. Investigating the presence of a common drug of abuse (benzhexol) in hair; the Jordanian experience. *J Clin Forensic Med* 2002; 9: 119–125.

85. McGucken R B, Caldwell J, Anthon B. Teenage procyclidine abuse. *Lancet* 1985; i: 1514.

86. Shariatmadari M E. Orphenadrine dependence. *BMJ* 1975; 271: 486.

87. Marriott P. Dependence on antiparkinsonian drugs. *BMJ* 1976; 272: 152.

88. Pullen G P, Best N R, Maguire J. Anticholinergic drug abuse: a common problem? *BMJ* 1984; 289: 612–613.

89. Rubinstein J S. Abuse of antiparkinsonian drugs: feigning of extrapyramidal symptoms to obtain trihexyphenidyl. *JAMA* 1978; 238: 2365–2366.

90. Wells B G, Marken P A, Rickman L A, *et al.* Characterizing anticholinergic abuse in community mental health. *J Clin Psychopharmacol* 1989; 9: 431–435.

91. Centers for Disease Control and Prevention. Scopolamine poisoning among heroin users – New York City, Newark, Philadelphia, and Baltimore, 1995 and 1996. *JAMA* 1996; 276: 92–93.

92. *Statistics on Drug Use in Australia 2002. Drug Statistics Series No. 12.* Cat no. PHE 43. Canberra: Australian Institute of Health and Welfare, February 2003.

93. Buckley N A, McManus P R. Changes in fatalities due to overdose of anxiolytic and sedative drugs in the UK (1983–1999). *Drug Saf* 2004; 27: 135–141.

94. *Report of the Medical Working Group on Drug Dependence. Guidelines of Good Clinical Practice in the Treatment of Drug Misuse.* London: Department of Health and Social Security, 1984, 20.

95. Department of Health. *Benzodiazepines Warning. CMO's Update 37.* January 2004. http://www.benzo.org.uk/cmo.htm (accessed 28 November 2004).

96. Hallstrom C. Can GPs really manage without benzodiazepines? *Prescriber* 1995; 6: 81–85.

97. Russell J, Lader M, eds. *Guidelines for the Prevention and Treatment of Benzodiazepine Dependence.* London: The Mental Health Foundation, 1993.

98. Ashton H. Protracted withdrawal syndromes from benzodiazepines. *J Subst Abuse Treat* 1991; 8: 19–28.

99. Department of Health UK, Scottish Office Department of Health, Welsh Office, Department of Health and Social Services Northern Ireland. *Drug Misuse and Dependence – Guidelines on Clinical Management.* London: The Stationery Office, 1999.

100. *National Survey on Drug Use and Health*, Substance Abuse and Mental Health Services Administration (SAMHSA), Report ref. 30415. Rockville, MD: Office of Applied Studies, 2002.

101. Ruben S M, Morrison C L. Temazepam misuse in a group of injecting drug users. *Br J Addiction* 1992; 87: 1387–1392.

102. Drake J, Ballard R. Misuse of temazepam. *BMJ* 1988; 297: 1402.

103. Strang J, Griffiths P, Abbey J, *et al.* Survey of use of injected benzodiazepines among drug users in Britain. *BMJ* 1994; 308: 1082.

104. Sapsted D. Date rape drug found in 4pc of nightclub drinks. *The Daily Telegraph*, 11 November 2003, 11.

105. Sullivan G, McBride A J, Clee W B. Zopiclone abuse in South Wales: three case reports. *Hum Psychopharmacol* 1995; 10: 351–352.

106. Rooney S. Zopiclone, a current drug of misuse. *Addiction* 1998; 93: 925.

107. Hajak G, Muller W E, Wittchen H U, *et al.* Abuse and dependence potential for the non-benzodiazepine hypnotics zolpidem and zopiclone: a review of case reports and epidemiological data. *Addiction* 2003; 98: 1371–1378.

108. Sikdar S, Ruben S M. Zopiclone abuse among polydrug users. *Addiction* 1996; 91: 285–286.

109. Anonymous. Zolpidem and zopiclone: dependence. *WHO Drug Information* 1999; 13: 92.
110. Walter H, Samtani A. Misuse of zopiclone. *J Clin Forensic Med* 1998; 5: 95.
111. Jones I R, Sullivan G. Physical dependence on zopiclone: case reports. *BMJ* 1998; 316: 117.
112. Ayonrinde O, Sampson E. Physical dependence on zopiclone: risk of dependence may be greater in those with dependent personalities. *BMJ* 1998; 317: 146.
113. Thakore J, Dinan T G. Physical dependence following zopiclone usage: a case report. *Hum Psychopharmacol* 1992; 7: 143–145.
114. Bianchi M, Musch B. Zopiclone discontinuation: review of 25 studies assessing withdrawal and rebound phenomena. *Int Clin Psychopharmacol* 1990; 5(Suppl 2): 139–145.
115. Gregg E, Akhter I. Chlormethiazole abuse. *Br J Psychiatr* 1979; 134: 627–629.
116. Giannini A J, DeFrance D T. Metronidazole and alcohol – potential for combinative abuse. *J Toxicol Clin Toxicol* 1983; 20: 509–515.
117. Reed F S. Antibiotics for kicks. *BMJ* 1976; 1: 835.
118. Stuppaeck C H, Whitworth A B, Fleischhacker W W. Abuse potential of carbamazepine. *J Nerv Ment Dis* 1993; 181: 519–520.
119. Crawford P J, Fisher B M. Recreational overdosage of carbamazepine in Paisley drug abusers. *Scott Med J* 1997; 42: 44–45.
120. Sullivan G, Davis S. Is carbamazepine a potential drug of abuse? *J Psychopharmacol* 1997; 11: 93–94.
121. Lauzon P. Two cases of clonidine abuse/dependence in methadone-maintained patients. *J Subst Abuse Treat* 1992; 9: 125–127.
122. Beuger M, Tommasello A, Schwartz R, *et al.* Clonidine use and abuse among methadone program applicants and patients. *J Subst Abuse Treat* 1998; 15: 589–593.
123. Anderson F, Paluzzi P, Lee J, *et al.* Illicit use of clonidine in opiate-abusing pregnant women. *Obstet Gynecol* 1997; 90: 790–794.
124. Dy E C, Yates W R. Atypical drug abuse: a case report involving clonidine. *Am Fam Physician* 1996; 54: 1035–1038.
125. Nausieda P A. Sinemet 'abusers'. *Clin Neuropharmacol* 1985; 8: 318–327.
126. Spigset O, von Scheele C. Levodopa dependence and abuse in Parkinson's disease. *Pharmacotherapy* 1997; 17: 1027–1030.
127. Hoffman A S, Schwartz H I, Novick R M. Catatonic reaction to accidental haloperidol overdose: an unrecognized drug abuse risk. *J Nerv Ment Dis* 1986; 174: 428–430.
128. Doenecke A L, Heuermann R C. Treatment of haloperidol abuse with diphenhydramine. *Am J Psychiatry* 1980; 137: 487–488.
129. Jack R A. Unintentional haloperidol abuse. *Am J Psychiatry* 1982; 139: 258.
130. Duffett R, Laker M. Intravenous neuroleptic misuse. *Psychiatric Bull* 1995; 19: 324–325.
131. Bewley S, Bewley T H. Drug dependence with oestrogen replacement therapy. *Lancet* 1992; 339: 290–291.
132. Wilcox J A. Psychoactive properties of pergolide mesylate. *J Psychoactive Drugs* 1995; 27: 181–182.

133. Brennan P O. Inhaled salbutamol: a new form of drug abuse? *Lancet* 1983; ii: 1030–1031.

134. Thompson P J, Dhillon P, Cole P. Addiction to aerosol treatment: the asthmatic alternative to glue sniffing. *BMJ* 1983; 287: 1515–1516.

135. Brennan P O. Addiction to aerosol treatment [letter]. *BMJ* 1983; 287: 1877.

136. Wickramasinghe H, Liebeschuetzz H J. Addiction to aerosol treatment [letter]. *BMJ* 1983; 287: 1877.

137. O'Callaghan C, Milner A D. Aerosol treatment abuse. *Arch Dis Child* 1988; 63: 70.

138. Edwards J G, Holgate S T. Dependency upon salbutamol inhalers. *Br J Psychiatr* 1979; 134: 624–626.

139. Aldridge J, Measham F. Sildenafil (Viagra) is used as a recreational drug in England. *BMJ* 1999; 318: 669.

140. Chu P L, McFarland W, Gibson S, *et al*. Viagra use in a community-recruited sample of men who have sex with men, San Francisco. *J AIDS* 2003; 33: 191–193.

141. Osborne M J, Austin R C T, Dawson K J, *et al*. Is there a problem with long term use of sumatriptan in acute migraine? *BMJ* 1994; 308: 113.

142. Gaist D, Hallas J, Sindrup S H, *et al*. Is overuse of sumatriptan a problem? A population-based study. *Eur J Clin Pharmacol* 1996; 50: 161–165.

13

Over-the-counter products

A hundred doses of happiness are not enough: send to the drug store for
another bottle – and, when that is finished, for another . . .
Aldous Huxley (1894–1964), 'Brave New World Revisited'

Over-the-counter (OTC) medicines are those that are available without prescription. The range of OTC products available varies around the world, but in many countries there has been a trend towards the increasing deregulation of medicines, such that greater numbers are now available to purchase from retail pharmacies or shops. This has distinct advantages for the customer in that he or she is empowered to assume greater responsibility for personal health. Buying a medicine is also more convenient for the patient than visiting a doctor. However, with these advantages come a number of potential disadvantages and foremost amongst them is the 'improper' use of OTC medicines, which takes various forms.

As is the case with prescribed medicines (see Chapter 12), it is important to be clear about what OTC medicine abuse means in the context of this book, as well as in the wider world. Even so, defining the nature of the problem is difficult because potentially a wide range of disparate behaviours is involved, and to some extent these behaviours may overlap.

It has been proposed that the term OTC 'abuse' be used to describe the taking of medicines for non-medical purposes (e.g. mind-altering effects), while the term 'misuse' be reserved for the improper use of an OTC medicine for a medical indication (e.g. incorrect dose).[1] Although it is helpful to separate 'non-medical use' from 'medical use', this simple classification is misleading in that it fails to reflect the full range of incorrect use, abuse and dependence associated with OTC medicines. It also adds an undesirable complication, in that an artificial distinction has been created between the terms 'abuse' and 'misuse', which outside the field of OTC medicines tend to be used synonymously. This has the potential to create confusion.

A more complete categorisation of the 'improper' use of OTC medicines would be as follows:

1. **Inappropriate medical use.** This occurs when OTC medicines are used to treat a medical condition, but incorrectly. 'Incorrectly' means that they are used with medicinal intent for a purpose or in a manner that is not supported by the manufacturer's instructions, the advice of a healthcare professional, or a reasonable body of published medical evidence. In the simplest examples, products are taken at the wrong dose or for excessively long periods of time. However, this behaviour also incorporates self-medication for inappropriate medical conditions or where there is little evidence of therapeutic benefit (e.g. taking vitamin C to treat the common cold). Purchasers falling into this category generally have insufficient or incorrect knowledge about the medicines they are buying or the medical condition that they hope to treat.

2. **Medication dependence.** Some patients begin to take an OTC medicine for medical reasons, but eventually abuse it chronically or even become dependent. Sometimes individuals may discover a pleasurable mind-altering effect while self-medicating with certain preparations. Such patients may escalate the dosage as they become tolerant to this effect and so become dependent. Particularly with certain cough and cold preparations, the inability to stop may be fuelled in some cases by psychiatric problems, which can sometimes be caused by the drugs themselves.

3. **Altered body image.** Various OTC medicines are abused in an attempt to lose weight (e.g. laxatives), to increase stamina during training (e.g. sympathomimetics) or to build body muscle (various dietary supplements). Chronic abuse of certain preparations may sometimes lead to dependence.

4. **Intentional psychotropic abuse.** This occurs when OTC medicines are taken not for medical reasons, but to produce psychotropic effects. Much intentional abuse is probably undertaken by existing users of street drugs. Sometimes OTCs are used to 'top up' or augment the effects of an illicit substance, and it is common for those dependent on street drugs to obtain OTC medicines to stave off withdrawal when supplies of illicit substances are not available (e.g. OTC sympathomimetics in amfetamine users). These substances may also be purchased in order to attempt self 'detoxification'. Various OTC products are employed by street drug users to produce psychoactive effects in their own right and users may experiment with different preparations to try to find an effect to their liking. Rumours among the drug culture may alert illicit drug users to a cheap, ready source of an alternative to street drugs. Sometimes they may cause dependence.

5. **Abuse support.** Various preparations assist with abuse, but are not themselves abused. Examples include citric acid and other OTC acids used to

convert base heroin, cocaine or amfetamines into a more soluble salt; preparations that are purchased to help relieve the side-effects of street drugs; and various OTC products used for the clandestine manufacture of illicit drugs.

This classification has the merit of providing convenient motivation-related 'pigeonholes', yet many OTC medicines could be accommodated into more than one category, depending on an individual's reasons for purchasing that medicine. The chronic user of laxatives, for example, could be purchasing them to maintain a regular bowel habit in lieu of attention to diet, exercise and other easily correctable factors: this is inappropriate medical use. Laxatives are also abused to assist with weight loss, or by patients with eating disorders such as bulimia. This is category 3 above (altered body image). They are also taken by some chronic users of illicit opioids to counteract the constipating effect of these drugs (category 5: abuse support).

In terms of motivation, the first of these categories – inappropriate medical use – is widely recognised and is the result of a combination of factors, but poor public education is perhaps the major determinant. However, the subject of inappropriate medical use is beyond the scope of this book. The remaining categories above are more akin to the abuse and dependence described in earlier chapters, and a detailed discussion of the manifestation of these problems will form the basis of the rest of this chapter.

Extent of the problem

A number of studies have attempted to assess the scale of the problem of OTC medicines abuse in relatively small geographical areas. Almost all of these studies have been conducted in the UK. The medication involved and the prevalence of the problem is likely to vary widely from country to country, depending upon the drugs that are available OTC and the prevailing drug culture. A major problem in all such research is the identification of abuse, because this can only rely upon confession from users or the highly subjective judgement and memory of community pharmacists. A failure to define abuse or a lack of consistency between researchers in defining the nature of abuse/misuse is also not helpful when attempting to estimate the size of the problem by comparing studies.

The studies that have been conducted are summarised in Table 13.1. There are obvious limitations to these, which have in part already

Table 13.1 Summary of studies of OTC medicines abuse in the general population in the UK

Geographical area of UK (year)	Study design	Pharmacist participation rate	Reported incidence of abuse	Products involved	Ref.
Belfast, Northern Ireland (2002)	A preliminary study enabling 8 selected community pharmacies to prospectively identify OTC medicine 'abusers' (non-medical use), as opposed to 'misusers' (incorrect medical use), on a daily basis.	100%	Over 7 weeks, an average of 1.0 abusers per pharmacy per week was identified, and 0.7 misusers per pharmacy per week.	Opioids, then antihistamines, then laxatives were most abused.	2
West Central Scotland (2001)	Postal survey of community pharmacies (n = 110) asking pharmacists to identify the nature and extent of OTC misuse.	79% (n = 87)	All pharmacies reported some misuse, but it was more frequent in urban areas. The average number of patients per pharmacy suspected of misusing medicines in a typical week was 5.6.	The medicines most commonly identified were antihistamines, opioid-containing products, laxatives and sympathomimetics.	3

Location (year)	Method	Response rate	Findings	Products	Ref
South Wales (2000)	Hand-delivered questionnaire survey of community pharmacists (n = 180) seeking estimation of the extent and nature of OTC medicine misuse in their shops over the past month.	89% (n = 161)	66% of respondents believed that OTC medicines misuse occurred during the study. The average number of attempts to buy medicines to be misused was 4.5 per pharmacist per month (range 0–60 attempts).	Opioid-containing products were identified most commonly, followed by sleep aids (mostly antihistamines) and then laxatives.	4
Scotland (1995 + 2000)	Two postal surveys of community pharmacists 5 years apart in 1995 (n = 1091) and in 2000 (n = 1162). Pharmacists were asked to identify the nature of OTC medicines misuse.	79% (n = 864) + 83% (n = 969)	Approximately 68% of pharmacists said OTC medicines were misused in both years. There was significantly more suspected misuse in urban and city centre areas, than in rural communities. The number of customers involved was not estimated.	Antihistamines and opioid-containing products were identified most commonly	5
Northern Ireland (1997)	A postal questionnaire survey of community pharmacists (n = 509) asking them to identify the number of suspected abusers in the past 3 months, and the products involved. Abuse was defined as non-medical use.	50% (n = 253)	The cases of suspected abuse in the past 3 months ranged from 0 to 700, with a median of 10 and a mode of 6. Postal code analysis revealed no link between reported estimates of abuse and pharmacy location.	Opioid-containing products were identified most frequently, followed by antihistamines and then laxatives.	1

Table 13.1 continued

Geographical area of UK (year)	Study design	Pharmacist participation rate	Reported incidence of abuse	Products involved	Ref.
Northumberland, England (1994)	A postal questionnaire survey of community pharmacists (n = 60) asking them to quantify attempts by customers to buy medicines for possible misuse in the past month, and identify the products involved.	65% (n = 39)	67% of pharmacists reported attempts by individuals to purchase OTC medicines for misuse in the month before the survey. 56% of pharmacists reported 1–5 people attempting to buy medicines for possible misuse; 10% reported 6 or more people.	Opioid-containing products predominated. Possible misuse of laxative, antihistamine and sympathomimetic preparations was reported with similar, but lower, frequency.	6
West Cumbria, England (1989)	A telephone survey of community pharmacists (n = 25) asking them to identify OTC medicines that they suspected were misused.	96% (n = 24)	The number of customers was not estimated.	Opioid-containing medicines were most frequently suspected as being abused.	7

been alluded to, but in drawing the results together to form general conclusions it appears that:

*   The majority of community pharmacists in the UK believe that OTC medicines abuse takes place.
*   Abusing, or dependent, customers are likely to represent a small minority of the thousands of visitors to community pharmacies each day.
*   Opioid-containing products, antihistamines and laxatives have been consistently perceived as the OTC medicines with the biggest abuse problem.

The probable small scale of OTC abuse and dependence does not mean that it is unimportant, particularly because, in the UK at least, it appears to be widespread. However, it should be kept in perspective and neither ignored nor sensationalised. In particular, community pharmacists, their professional bodies, and manufacturers need to develop strategies to identify, treat, prevent and advise on OTC medicines abuse to respond to their own concerns and those of customers.

The various studies summarised in Table 13.1 highlight particular ways in which pharmacists attempt to minimise abuse. These techniques include:

*   The pharmacist educating counter staff on the abuse potential of selected products so that sales can be scrutinised appropriately by a pharmacist. In some cases standard operating procedures are used.
*   Stocking the preparations most likely to be abused out of sight of customers.
*   The pharmacist challenging or advising those suspected of abuse, and those who purchase certain products regularly.
*   Refusing to sell particular medicines if abuse is suspected, particularly if large quantities are requested.
*   Pharmacists sharing suspicions about abuse of specific products with other pharmacists locally.
*   Keeping a register of sales of particular abusable products.
*   No longer stocking certain products.
*   Having a written policy to guide all staff.

Finally, it is worth adding to these studies a unique piece of research involving street drug users. Structured interviews with 53 'heavy' amfetamine and opioid intravenous drug users in Hull, UK, in 1992 identified that two-thirds of them had abused an OTC medicine at some point in their drug-using career.[8] Fifty per cent of the amfetamine users and 19% of the opiate users had abused OTC sympathomimetics, whereas 45% of opioid users had abused OTC opioid-containing products.

Sympathomimetics

The principal OTC sympathomimetic agents that are abused are pseudo-ephedrine, ephedrine and phenylpropanolamine, and this section will focus on these three drugs. They are closely related to each other structurally, as well as to amfetamine and the endogenous neurotransmitter noradrenaline (norepinephrine). They may be psychoactive if taken in large doses and probably act in a similar way to amfetamine.

The three sympathomimetics have both direct and indirect actions at adrenergic receptors. In other words they act by direct receptor stimulation, as noradrenaline does, and via an increased release of natural receptor agonists (such as dopamine and noradrenaline). This latter mechanism is the same means by which amfetamine exerts its pharmacological effects. Phenylephrine is an example of an OTC sympathomimetic that may be less susceptible to abuse because it has a more selective adrenergic action (primarily alpha-1 receptor agonism).

Many OTC cough and cold products throughout the world contain sympathomimetics. The preparations are usually taken by mouth, and sympathomimetics have good oral bioavailability.

Effects and administration

Sympathomimetics have weak amfetamine-like psychotropic effects but large doses in adults can produce pleasant perceptual changes, euphoria and mental stimulation. Children may be particularly sensitive to the psychoactive effects of sympathomimetics: visual hallucinations, agitation, nightmares and night terrors have been reported in children under 5 years of age given normal therapeutic doses.[9–11]

In adults, sympathomimetics may be deliberately abused in their own right to experience these mind-altering effects – either because the effects are found to be pleasant or in order to counteract pre-existing morbidity such as depression or social anxiety.[12–16] At street level, knowledge of the abuse potential of OTC products is passed from person to person, giving novices the chance to experiment with them. Although mostly taken orally, two cases of acute intravenous abuse have been described in the medical literature.[17,18] One of these involved the deliberate injection of a crushed pseudoephedrine tablet and caused acute psychosis in an 18-year-old man.[17] The other case of intravenous use concerned a 25-year-old man who injected a powder that he believed to be amfetamine, but which was later discovered to be ephedrine. He developed an acute myocardial infarction (MI).[18] OTC sympathomimetics are also used as a cheap substitute for amfetamine by illicit drug users, and human research has suggested that 75–150 mg/kg ephedrine by subcutaneous injection may elicit similar subjective effects to 15–30 mg/kg amfetamine.[19] A UK study in 1992 showed that 11 out of 22 intravenous amfetamine users had used OTC sympathomimetics in the past year to avoid or reduce cravings for amfetamine.[8] These were mostly taken intermittently, but two subjects took them on a daily basis with regular amfetamine for 2 years or more (see Box 13.1).

Abuse can have its origins in self-medication for approved indications. Sometimes the process starts by patients casually taking bigger doses, presumably in the belief that larger amounts should be more effective. Historically, abuse has been reported in patients taking escalating amounts of OTC ephedrine products for asthma.[20–22] Furthermore, it is well known, for example, that patients commonly exceed the recommended dose in countries such as Australia and the USA where sympathomimetics can be purchased to treat obesity.[23,24] If taken regularly in large enough doses, sympathomimetics can theoretically promote weight loss by suppressing appetite, as can amfetamines. However, these drugs are not very effective.[25,26] Despite this, cases of chronic abuse and dependence have been reported, including cases in which patients suffered from eating disorders such as bulimia or anorexia nervosa.[27,28]

Sympathomimetics may also help to combat fatigue via central nervous system (CNS) stimulation and OTC products are marketed for this purpose in some countries (e.g. USA). Some patients taking sympathomimetics for this reason have subsequently increased the dosage markedly and developed acute side-effects, or become chronic users or dependents.[20,21,27]

Box 13.1 Ways in which sympathomimetics can be abused.

- To elevate mood, produce euphoria and perceptual changes.
- As a substitute for amfetamine by regular users to alleviate craving.
- To cause weight loss [approved use in some countries].
- To combat fatigue in a similar way to caffeine [approved use in some countries].
- To enhance athletic stamina and performance.
- To manufacture more potent, illicit, amfetamine-like drugs.

Sympathomimetics are banned in competing athletes by the International Olympic Committee, although there is little evidence that these substances actually have any significantly useful effect in practice.[29–31] Nonetheless, sympathomimetics are widely used by athletes and those attending gymnasiums to assist them during training and performance. They are believed by users to increase stamina and reduce body fat. A US study of 36 female athletes who admitted to ephedrine use revealed that many had used the drug in high doses for years.[28] Seven of them were classified as ephedrine-dependent by the authors.

Although this discussion has concentrated on ephedrine, pseudoephedrine and phenylpropanolamine, abuse of preparations containing other sympathomimetics is occasionally reported. Agents such as oxymetazoline and phenylephrine have a more specific pharmacological action, and are primarily alpha-adrenergic sympathomimetics, but despite this they have both been abused.[32–35] The Chinese herbal preparation Ma Huang is prepared from the dried plant *Ephedra sinica* and related species. This naturally contains a quantity of ephedrine and has also been the subject of abuse (see Chapter 16).

Manufacture of illicit drugs

The use of OTC sympathomimetics as precursors for the clandestine manufacture of illicit drugs has been the cause of much concern, particularly in the USA and Australasia where there have been organised criminal raids on pharmacies and warehouses to seize supplies, as well as large-scale importing. Both ephedrine and pseudoephedrine can be used to synthesise more potent amfetamines such as metamfetamine and methcathinone (see Chapter 6). The scale of the illicit manufacturing process is illustrated by successful operations organised by the Drug Enforcement Agency in the USA. By January 2002, Operation 'Mountain Express' had resulted in the seizure of 30 tonnes of pseudoephedrine and the closure of nine metamfetamine manufacturing sites over the course of 2 years.[36] In Operation 'Northern Star' one supplier alone was criminally charged for supplying 108 million pseudoephedrine tablets.[37]

The sheer scale of the problem has forced further action. In the USA this has led to bulk suppliers of ephedrine and pseudoephedrine being required to register their activities, and the manufacturers of OTC products are obliged to keep transaction records. Pharmacists who wish to sell these products must also register with the Drug Enforcement Agency and keep records of sales. In Australia and New Zealand, pharmacists ask for identification before selling certain OTC sympathomimetics. Many manufacturers are considering reformulating their products to exclude ephedrine and pseudoephedrine.

Dependence

Tolerance can develop during chronic administration of sympathomimetics, such that progressively higher doses are taken. Withdrawal symptoms can also manifest during attempts at cessation. Full dependence may arise. The doses taken by individuals during chronic abuse, or when they are dependent, can be very large indeed and typically the patient is brought to medical attention because of side-effects arising from ingesting these large amounts. The daily dose ranges reported in the medical literature for cases of chronic abuse or dependence involving the three principal sympathomimetics are:

Pseudoephedrine	1800–4500 mg[12,13,14,27]
Phenylpropanolamine	500–2000 mg[16,27,38]
Ephedrine	240–6660 mg[15,20,21,27,39,40]

Cases of sympathomimetic dependence described in the medical literature indicate that escalating dosage due to tolerance is a common feature. Sometimes the quantities involved are so large that they cannot be estimated accurately. Withdrawal reactions in dependent persons have been inadequately described, but features appear similar to withdrawal from amfetamine and include weight gain, fatigue, sleepiness, difficulty concentrating, depression, lethargy and confusion.[13,15,27,31]

Adverse effects

The common side-effects of large doses of sympathomimetics include insomnia, agitation, anxiety, tremor, nausea and vomiting, tachycardia, palpitations, headache and anorexia.

A large number of case reports have described the advent of **psychosis** in association with abuse. In many ways, and not surprisingly, this is similar to 'amfetamine psychosis'. Symptoms can be paranoid in nature and are typically accompanied by bizarre delusions and hallucinations.[10,12,14,16,20–22,34,38,39,41] There may also be confusion. Psychosis may arise acutely after a single large dose or develop over long periods of time as a result of chronic high-dose administration. In either case, symptoms usually resolve within a few days of cessation, although long-lasting psychiatric problems can occur. It is unclear whether there are any residual effects in those suffering from pre-existing mental illness or with a predisposition to it. It has already been noted that young children can be particularly sensitive to the psychiatric side-effects of sympatho-mimetics,[9–11] but sometimes adults demonstrate a similar sensitivity. Small doses within the normal therapeutic range have provoked anxiety, agitation, hallucinations and even psychosis.[10,17,42]

Hypertension is a well-known dose-related effect of OTC sym-pathomimetics.[43] As with their psychiatric side-effects, there may be a wide variation in susceptibility to the hypertensive effects of sym-pathomimetics. For example, some cases of hypertension have been reported at normal OTC doses,[23,24] others in patients abusing higher doses than recommended.[23,24,44,45] Interestingly, most case reports of chronic high-dose abuse do not refer to blood pressure changes. It is inconceivable that this most common of medical procedures was not undertaken and this suggests that, perhaps, chronic exposure might encourage physiological adaptation to the drugs' presence. Nonetheless, when hypertension does occur it may be associated with headache, dizziness and/or gastrointestinal upset and can be dramatic enough to prompt urgent investigation and treatment.[44,45]

It is not surprising that sympathomimetics have been associated with **strokes**, haemorrhagic forms being the predominant variety and phenylpropanolamine the leading causative agent.[23,46,47] These strokes have not necessarily occurred in patients with known hypertension caused by these drugs. Once more the variation in susceptibility to sym-pathomimetic side-effects is revealed, in that strokes have been observed at normal OTC doses in some patients, as well as in situations where larger doses have been taken.

Renal adverse effects of high-dose sympathomimetic abuse have been reported rarely in the medical literature. Perhaps predictably – because amfetamines can cause the same reaction – rhabdomyolysis has been attributed to sympathomimetics, leading to renal failure.[48,49] A single case of nephrolithiasis has also been documented in which ephedrine was contained in the stone.[40]

It is worth noting that acute sympathomimetic overdose can be associated with hypokalaemia, arrhythmias and convulsions.

Dextromethorphan

Dextromethorphan was developed as a non-opioid cough suppressant. Although similar in structure to the opioids, it does not possess typical opioid properties. The main metabolite, dextrorphan, may be largely responsible for the drug's abuse potential because in animal studies it has similar actions to phencyclidine[50] (see Chapter 9). It also binds to similar parts of the brain as phencyclidine, antagonising at the NMDA (N-methyl-D-aspartate) receptor.[51]

Dextromethorphan is converted into dextrorphan by the cytochrome P450 isoenzyme known as CYP2D6. Around 5–10% of the Caucasian population is deficient in this enzyme. This has led to speculation that enzyme-deficient persons ('poor metabolisers') may be less able to experience the pleasurable psychoactive effects of dextromethorphan because the rate of production of dextrorphan will be very much reduced. This theory has some support from a small experimental study in both poor metabolisers and extensive metabolisers.[52] Despite this, known poor metabolisers may still become intoxicated.[53]

Effects and administration

Unlike sympathomimetics, dextromethorphan seems only to be abused for its mind-altering effects. Despite its similar structure to the opioids, dextromethorphan produces very different effects when it is abused. Excitation tends to occur, rather than the CNS depression characteristic of the opioids, and this is also a feature of overdose. The subjective effects are quite variable, users having likened the experience of intoxication to that of LSD (lysergide)[54] or cannabis.[55] However, the dissociative nature of many of the effects have most often led to comparisons with phencyclidine.[56,57] Reactions described by users typically include euphoria, hallucinations, illusions, increased perceptual awareness, hyperactivity, time distortions and synaesthesia.[54–62] These actions begin within an hour of oral ingestion and typically last a few hours. Abuse has been particularly prevalent amongst teenagers in some parts of the USA.[55,60,63,64] In Sweden, dextromethorphan was restricted to prescription-only status in 1986 because of abuse concerns.

The limited data on poor metabolisers of dextromethorphan suggest that they tend to experience different effects. A laboratory study comparing poor and extensive metabolisers revealed that poor metabolisers experienced greater dysphoric effects.[52] A case report of intoxication in a poor metaboliser showed an atypical clinical presentation for someone abusing dextromethorphan: the patient suffered from malaise, became semi-comatose, and experienced apnoea and fitting.[53] These data suggest that both dextromethorphan and its major metabolite dextrorphan can be abused but that they produce different effects: dextromethorphan predominates in poor metabolisers, dextrorphan in extensive metabolisers.

Dextromethorphan hydrobromide is usually taken orally in doses of 300 mg or more for its psychoactive effects. From case reports cited in the medical literature, the doses involved can exceed 1000 mg per day;[38,55–57,62–66] the highest dose recorded was 2160–2880 mg per day for up to 5 years.[61]

Although usually taken orally, one case of nasal inhalation ('snorting') of 500–750 mg of dextromethorphan powder per day has been described.[59]

Dependence

Several case reports describe chronic daily administration over periods of months or years, with escalation of dose and drug-seeking behaviour. After a single high dose, users may experience short-term depression and tiredness as the effects wear off. When abused daily for longer periods, but as little as 2 weeks, discontinuation may bring about more persistent withdrawal symptoms such as craving for the drug, insomnia, somnambulism, lethargy, dysphoria, depression and ataxia.[58,59,61,64]

Adverse effects

The most frequently reported side-effects of dextromethorphan when it is abused include tachycardia, hypertension, ataxia/dizziness, lethargy/sleepiness or insomnia, confusion, nausea/vomiting, restlessness, slurred speech, tremor, nystagmus and blurred vision.[55,58,61,63,66] As already noted above, those who are poor metabolisers of dextromethorphan may show a different range of side-effects.

The most serious reactions reported are psychiatric in nature. **Psychosis** has been described in four case reports where dextromethorphan was cited as the causative agent.[54,57,67,68] However, a number of cases of psychosis attributed to OTC sympathomimetics have involved patients who were also taking large amounts of dextromethorphan, and the contribution that this latter drug may have made to the aetiology of the condition has been overlooked by some authors.[16,38,41,56] The presentation of psychosis in published case reports is rather variable, but resolution occurs within a few days of stopping dextromethorphan.

Five cases of **mania** associated with high-dose dextromethorphan abuse have also been described.[62,64,65,69] In one of these cases a patient with a history of depression self-medicated with a dextromethorphan/phenylpropanolamine cough syrup to produce mania that helped him cope with his depression.[69] The authors attributed this mania-inducing effect mainly to phenylpropanolamine, and the potential role of high-dose dextromethorphan was downplayed. In another case report a 39-year-old male patient experienced repeated episodes of mania lasting 1 or 2 days after ingesting dextromethorphan.[65] The authors described progressive cognitive deterioration in this man and proposed that dextromethorphan was responsible. In all the cases described, manic symptoms resolved quickly once dextromethorphan administration ceased.

Two deaths as a result of ingesting large amounts of dextromethorphan have been described from Sweden.[70] In one of these cases the subject probably intended to commit suicide, but the other victim seems to have been a long-term dextromethorphan user and may have died from pulmonary aspiration.

Opioid-containing preparations

Codeine is the opioid that is most widely available OTC around the world. It is used as a painkiller and to suppress coughing. Some OTC analgesics contain dihydrocodeine, and morphine is available in very low concentration in some traditional pharmacy products, but codeine is the principal OTC agent that is abused. Much of codeine's abuse liability is probably mediated via its metabolic conversion to morphine in the body, a reaction catalysed by the cytochrome P450 isoenzyme CYP2D6. Inhibition of this enzyme with drugs may blunt codeine's subjective effects and abuse liability.[71] The analgesic effects of codeine are impaired in those who are genetically deficient in CYP2D6 and deficiency may also protect against codeine dependence.[72]

Illicit opioids are dealt with in more detail in Chapter 3, while prescription opioids are discussed in Chapter 12. Example OTC medicines that may be abused are given in Box 13.2.

Box 13.2 Examples of OTC preparations containing opioids.

- Codeine linctus or cough syrup.
- Cough mixtures containing codeine plus other ingredients.
- Analgesic products containing codeine or dihydrocodeine with aspirin or paracetamol [acetaminophen]. These products may contain other ingredients too.
- Traditional old pharmacy products such as kaolin and morphine mixture.

It is notable that opioid-containing OTC medicines have been identified consistently as key products subject to abuse in most research on this subject (see Table 13.1). However, three notes of caution should be sounded at the outset. Firstly, opioids suffer by reputation as 'dangerous substances' with a world-renowned propensity for being abused. The word 'opioid' instantly conjures up pictures of heroin 'addicts', morphine and opium. The research summarised in Table 13.1 relied on pharmacist identification of suspected substance abuse and it is possible, even likely, that there is a bias in favour of reports of suspected opioid abuse because all healthcare professionals know and expect opioids to be abused. A second problem is that, as already mentioned, published research does not usually differentiate between inappropriate medical use and the forms of abuse and dependence with which we are primarily concerned in this book.

The third note of caution when considering the abuse potential of OTC opioid-containing products is the most important: few of these medicines actually contain opioids alone. The UK formulation of codeine linctus is an exception in that it contains nothing else of pharmacological significance except codeine. Otherwise all OTC analgesics, for example, contain other significant ingredients. This fact is of vital importance when understanding how patients taking OTC opioids may become habitual users, may abuse them or even become dependent. The two commonest ingredients formulated with codeine are paracetamol or aspirin. These can both cause a form of dependence with chronic use, which causes a well-characterised withdrawal reaction. This is discussed in more detail under 'analgesics' below. Caffeine is another common ingredient in OTC analgesics and this too can produce withdrawal reactions (see below and Chapter 14). In the cocktails that comprise many OTC products, opioids can be formulated with sympathomimetics (see above), antihistamines (below), antimuscarinic drugs such as hyoscine (below and Chapter 12), and in the past they have even been mixed with barbiturates. All of these accessory, and possibly unnecessary, ingredients can be abused, and yet it is the opioid constituent that may attract the 'blame', even though the amount of opioid in most OTC analgesics is extremely small.

Effects and administration

OTC opioids are usually taken by mouth, although intravenous administration of a solution made from tablets containing codeine has been described.[73,74] In the USA, the dipping of cannabis cigarettes into codeine syrup before smoking them has also been reported.[75]

Many of those who abuse OTC opioids are established users of intravenous opioids. Abuse of codeine linctus by this group is well known: each 100 mL of the UK formulation comprises 300 mg of codeine (which is equivalent to about 25 mg of morphine). One study of 31 intravenous opioid users in the UK illustrates the reasons why OTC opioids are bought by injecting drug users.[8] In this cohort, 20 individuals had used OTC opioids; 16 used single large doses to avoid a withdrawal reaction when intravenous opioids were not available; 10 used OTC opioids in an attempt at self-detoxification; 5 used OTC products to supplement or augment the action of intravenous opioids. Codeine linctus was the most popular product and was named by 16 participants. Codeine has in fact been used successfully instead of methadone as a maintenance treatment for those dependent on heroin, particularly in Germany, where until the early 1990s methadone was not widely prescribed.[76]

Non-analgesic opioid-containing OTCs are also abused by people who are not intravenous drug users. Codeine syrup can be consumed as a recreational substance in its own right, largely on account of its mellowing, relaxing effect.[75] Products containing mixtures of potentially psychoactive ingredients may be particularly prone to abuse. Interestingly, a study of 46 patients dependent on a sympathomimetic-codeine cough mixture revealed that while the desired effects were mostly stimulant-like, withdrawal reactions were mainly opioid-like.[77]

Patients with recurring headaches who take OTC analgesics chronically – whether they contain opioids or not – may become dependent. This is discussed in more detail under 'analgesics' below.

The presence of paracetamol or aspirin limits the abuse potential of OTC opioid-containing analgesics for their opioid effects because the large doses needed for psychotropic effect will tend to cause paracetamol or aspirin toxicity. Observations originally from Denmark suggested that some users are able to separate codeine from certain compound analgesics containing aspirin using water and a filter system, without dissolving enough aspirin to cause toxicity.[74] A separation procedure that was known to be used in Scotland using water and a coffee filter[78] was initially shown to be unreliable.[79] However, the work from Denmark and further research in Northern Ireland suggests that codeine can be preferentially separated from other constituents depending upon the amount of water used and the precise nature of the formulation; there are notable differences in ease of separation between apparently similar products.[74,80] It has also been reported that in some compound tablet formulations codeine is added as a surface layer by the manufacturer and this can be scraped off easily.[81] The use of non-aqueous solvents may also facilitate separation of codeine from other tablet ingredients.[82]

OTC codeine has been used as a precursor for the manufacture of illicit opioids such as heroin and morphine, mainly for injection.[82,83] This is often referred to as 'homebake', and has been reported particularly from New Zealand and Australia. 'Homebake' is particularly popular in New Zealand, an island with a comparatively small population and limited access to conventional sources of heroin (see Box 13.3).

Dependence

Dependence upon OTC opioids is clearly possible if a product such as codeine linctus is ingested in large amounts, regularly, for a long enough period of time. However, as discussed above, for compound OTC analgesics it is often more likely that dependence occurs because of the effects of other pharmacologically active constituents in the product being taken, because within the recommended dose range the amount of opioid involved is so small.

Adverse effects

The adverse effects of OTC opioids are potentially the same as for all other opioids (see Chapter 3). Being dose-dependent effects, serious reactions are less likely to be seen than in, say, heroin users, because OTC opioids are much less potent, are generally taken orally and often in comparatively small doses. One problem that might be more specifically associated with chronic codeine use is depression. A Canadian study of 339 long-term users revealed that 41% met diagnostic criteria

---

Box 13.3 Ways in which opioids can be abused.

- For their psychotropic opioid effects, either by themselves or as an adjunct to other OTC or street drugs.
- To prevent opioid withdrawal in users of heroin who are temporarily unable to get supplies.
- As a method of detoxification in those using illicit opioids.
- To synthesise more-potent illicit opioids.

for abuse or dependence.[84] Two-thirds of all participants (n = 213) had sought help for mental health problems, most commonly depression (70%). This association could simply be due to depression arising from the chronic pain that many participants admitted to. Another explanation is that some psychiatric disorders predispose patients to chronic use of certain drugs as a form of self-medication. Alternatively, long-term exposure to codeine itself may cause dysphoric symptoms.

It is worth stressing once more that OTC opioid products contain other ingredients too, and one should assess the role of these when evaluating a patient's symptoms. Two specific examples are particularly noteworthy. In many countries traditional cough mixtures contain both an opioid and the extract of a plant called **squill** (*Urginea maritima*) as an expectorant. For example, APF Linctus Codeine (Australia) and Gee's Linctus (UK) both contain squill. High-dose, long-term use has been reported to cause a progressive muscle weakness resembling myasthenia gravis and even cardiac toxicity.[85–89] Squill contains glycosides that are thought to be responsible for these effects.

Prolonged administration of **kaolin and morphine mixture** in large doses may cause severe hypokalaemia.[90,91] Quantities such as 600–1400 mL per day have been taken (the UK product only contains 7 mg of morphine per 100 mL). Hypokalaemia probably arises as a result of potassium binding by kaolin in the gut and/or the mineralocorticoid action of the liquorice extract in the product. Both of these actions are likely to be exacerbated by the high sodium bicarbonate content, which can promote kaliuresis. Chronic hypokalaemia universally causes profound skeletal muscle weakness, which may be accompanied by muscle pain or paraesthesiae. One case report describing a chronic user attributed death to myocardial necrosis secondary to persistent hypokalaemia and/or intestinal obstruction.[90] Ventricular ectopic beats secondary to hypokalaemia were described in another case.[91] Hypertension may also occur in heavy users, perhaps caused by the high sodium content of the preparation.[92] Muscle weakness, arrhythmias and hypertension are all reversible when kaolin and morphine is stopped and hypokalaemia treated.

Analgesics

Aspirin, paracetamol and ibuprofen are the principal analgesics available OTC, although as discussed above these are frequently combined with other drugs with more well-known abuse potential such as opioids.

Discriminating between inappropriate medical use and other forms of abuse can be particularly difficult for this category of drugs.

Analgesic headache

The repeated use of analgesics for treating recurring headaches can develop into a long-term, regular habit. Paradoxically, this can then result in the analgesia becoming the cause of headaches. The continual presence of analgesics causes pain receptors to become over-sensitive such that they fire off spontaneously, or after minimal stimulation, and produce the sensation of pain more or less continuously. The patient continues to take analgesia to try to treat the pain, but this serves simply to keep the cycle going.

These drug-induced headaches occur every day, or at least every other day and, perhaps unsurprisingly, migraine sufferers are particularly at risk. Historically ergotamine, which is a prescription drug in most countries, is a well-documented cause of this problem. However, simple OTC analgesics such as paracetamol, aspirin and ibuprofen also cause this effect when taken by themselves or as compound preparations with other ingredients such as caffeine.[93–96] The problem has been described in both adults and children,[96] and is sometimes referred to by the generic term 'chronic daily headache', although more precise terms are 'analgesic headache', or 'medication overuse headache'.

The headache produced by analgesics is different in character to the headache for which the analgesic was originally taken – it typically occurs much more frequently, becoming virtually constant in some sufferers, and acts as a driving force for regular analgesic administration. The headache may be present as soon as the patient wakes up in the morning.[93] The pain may be a dull generalised daily headache, or a more intense rebound headache that occurs between doses as the effects of the analgesic wears off.[95] Sometimes both can occur. Usually normal or near normal doses of analgesics are taken. The key to identifying the problem is the frequency of analgesic use over a prolonged period, typically several years. Analgesic headache has only been described in patients who originally started taking long-term painkillers for headaches, not in those using analgesics for other indications.

The only way to treat analgesic headache is to stop all current analgesia. This is very difficult for most patients to do, and inpatient treatment has been advocated for difficult cases.[94,95] Stopping analgesia causes increased intensity 'rebound' headaches, and sleep and mood disturbances. This usually lasts up to 10 days, but may take longer.[95] It may take a further 6–12 weeks for headaches to resolve completely or for their frequency to be reduced to an acceptable level. Patients need support to enable this to happen and examples of information leaflets for patients have been published.[93] Prophylactic medicines such as amitriptyline and sodium valproate have been employed as a means of preventing headaches during the analgesic withdrawal period.[93]

Where possible, patients self-medicating with simple analgesics for recurrent headaches or migraine should be advised not to take painkillers frequently, and daily use must be avoided. This should help to prevent analgesic headache from developing.

Aspirin

In terms of psychoactive effects, it is sometimes claimed that ingestion of a mixture of one or two soluble aspirin with a fizzy cola drink or beer will produce a 'high'. There is no evidence that this is anything other than an unfounded rumour or a placebo effect.

Two cases have been described where individuals appeared to enjoy intoxication from dangerously high doses of aspirin.[97] Both patients described a pleasurable effect that could be accompanied by hallucinations. In one patient, 20–30 aspirin 300-mg tablets were taken, which 'produced an agreeable haze, with a disembodied feeling of detachment accentuated by deafness; tinnitus was "a gentle singing noise, very soothing" '. Salicylism produced a condition of 'isolation, relaxation, protection'. Clearly, these large doses of aspirin carry the potential for a fatal outcome.

Paracetamol

Paracetamol abuse has also been described in four female patients with eating disorders.[98] In each case, overdoses of paracetamol (between 8 and 30 tablets of 500 mg) were taken to induce vomiting after food binges or when subjects felt overweight. This occurred once every week or on alternate weeks. These large doses could be fatal if sufficient drug is absorbed before vomiting.

Antihistamines

Abuse and dependence have been reported in particular for three drugs of this class: cyclizine, dimenhydrinate and diphenhydramine. The reasons for the popularity of these three antihistamines in particular, rather than others, is unclear, but the antimuscarinic properties of anti-histamines become more prominent at high dose and this may be responsible for some or all of the abuse potential (see Chapter 12). Cyclizine also has some structural similarities to phencyclidine.

Cyclizine

Cyclizine is available OTC in many countries for treating travel sick-ness. In the UK, concern over cyclizine abuse is such that it has been the subject of a special statement from the Council of the Royal Pharmaceutical Society of Great Britain, advising that medicines con-taining cyclizine should be sold personally by a pharmacist.[99] Counsellors in drug dependency units have also found the problem of cyclizine abuse to be a major challenge.[100]

Effects and administration

Cyclizine has been abused via the oral route in doses of up to 1800 mg and is reported to cause euphoria and hallucinations.[101–103] In one series of 55 cases, the average dose taken by mouth was about 600 mg.[101] Many cases reported in the literature involve young people aged under 20 years experimenting with cyclizine abuse for its psychoactive effects.

Tablets may also be prepared for intravenous injection,[100,104,105] and this is more likely to be a chronic problem. Parenteral administra-tion may produce a 'rush' of exhilaration followed by general mental stimulation and hallucinations. Regular users may inject very frequently when using cyclizine, because of the intensity of the 'rush' and its short duration. As is also seen with repeated cocaine injection, users com-monly feel depressed as the effects of cyclizine wear off, and this may encourage repeat administration.[105]

The drug is more likely to be abused by those already using opioids, perhaps because cyclizine enhances or prolongs their effects.[104,105] In some countries, cyclizine–opioid combined formulations are available on prescription, and these have been very popular at street level when they can be obtained (e.g. the cyclizine–morphine combina-tion product 'Diconal' in the UK[100]). Of a total of 120 individuals main-tained on methadone by a UK regional drug dependency unit in 1989, 20 were found to be abusing intravenous cyclizine concurrently in doses of 50–800 mg per 'hit'.[105]

Dependence

A substantial proportion of the methadone recipients abusing cyclizine in the study above may have been cyclizine-dependent – demonstrating a compulsion to continue using it despite knowledge of its harmful effects, showing tolerance, craving for the drug, and depression or other more vague withdrawal-like symptoms.[105] Another report cites three cases in which patients prescribed opioids for chronic pain showed signs of dependency on both opioids and cyclizine.[106] These patients all had chronic pain for which no physical cause could be found, but attempts at withdrawing cyclizine met with complaints of increased pain, nausea and lowered mood.

Adverse effects

Adverse reactions to cyclizine abuse include tachycardia, hypertension, disorientation, mental confusion, agitation, fever, dysarthria, drowsiness, palpitations, ataxia, tremor, slurred speech and fits.[101,102,105] Dramatic acts of aggression, emotional lability and violent behaviour are sometimes seen.[103,105]

Dimenhydrinate and diphenhydramine

These are both available in various forms, and are popular in many countries as OTC antihistamines, hypnotics and as medication for preventing travel sickness. Dimenhydrinate consists of diphenhydramine coupled with 8-chlorotheophylline in approximately equal proportions.

Effects and administration

Both antihistamines are abused by the oral route. Effects reported by users include sedation, elevation of mood, euphoria and hallucinations.[107–116] Daily diphenhydramine doses in published cases of abuse range from 700 mg to 3 g.[107,108,117–119] For dimenhydrinate, the daily doses reported by those abusing it have ranged from 250 mg to as much as 5 g.[109–111,113–116]

   In the UK, a liquid-filled gel capsule formulation of diphenhydramine was injected by drug users in the Glasgow area, who rapidly learned to ask for the product by brand name in preference to tablet formulations.[119] This ultimately led to the withdrawal of this formulation by the manufacturer. However, a similar product is available in other countries and there are reports from Australia, for example, that injection of this formulation now occurs there.[120]

Dependence

A number of case reports have described chronic self-administration of dimenhydrinate or diphenhydramine, with tolerance and drug-seeking behaviour. Withdrawal symptoms have also been associated with either drug after chronic high-dose intake. Symptoms described have included craving for the drug, tremor, agitation, restlessness, insomnia, diarrhoea, abdominal cramps, vomiting, hypersalivation, akathisia-like symptoms, and elevated pulse, respirations and blood pressure.[107-111,117]

As has been observed with cyclizine, one small study suggested that patients prescribed diphenhydramine for medical purposes can exhibit signs of abuse and dependence.[121] All five of the subjects were inpatients, ranging in age from 8 to 20 years, and all had been receiving the drug intravenously. Behaviour included requesting the drug when it was not indicated, increasing the frequency of self-administration inappropriately, hoarding secret supplies of the drug and becoming upset when further supplies were refused. In order to minimise recurrence of this problem the authors recommended that oral diphenhydramine be used where possible, and when intravenous use was necessary that it be given slowly to minimise the intensity of any psychotropic effects.

Adverse effects

Side-effects from abuse of either dimenhydrinate or diphenhydramine include classic antimuscarinic effects such as dry mouth, tachycardia, urinary hesitancy, flushing and confusion; other reported reactions include sedation, vomiting, ataxia, slurred speech and hypotension.[107-110,113-115,119]

Laxatives

Many people who purchase OTC laxatives have short-term constipation caused by problems that are easily remedied, e.g. poor diet or lack of exercise. However, there are also patients who take laxatives when constipation does not exist, or who continue to take them long-term unnecessarily; these habits are more easily defined as abuse (see Box 13.4).

Box 13.4 Examples of abused laxatives.

Bisacodyl	Rhubarb
Dantron	Senna
Castor oil	Sodium citrate
Frangula	Sodium phosphate
Magnesium sulphate	Sodium picosulfate
Phenolphthalein	Syrup of figs

Laxatives are usually taken orally, but can also be administered rectally. Abuse can be very difficult to identify and relies upon the subject admitting it, or the performance of stool/urine analysis for laxatives. The majority of those abusing laxatives are female and the laxatives involved are commonly of the stimulant variety (e.g. senna, bisacodyl), although osmotic laxatives are also used (e.g. magnesium sulphate). An analysis of published studies in 1995 suggested that the lifetime occurrence of laxative abuse was about 4%; however in patients with bulimia this was 15%.[122] Those who abuse seem to fall into three groups:

1. **Eating disorders**. Patients with bulimia or anorexia nervosa may abuse laxatives. These are conditions where sufferers have a distorted image of their own bodies and a fear of obesity. Most sufferers are women between late teens and 30 years of age. Patients with anorexia drastically reduce their food intake, whereas those with bulimia display a binge/starvation pattern of food intake. Patients use a variety of other techniques to control their weight including vomiting and excessive exercise. They may believe that laxatives will reduce the calorific impact of food by inhibiting absorption and thus prevent weight gain, although this is not the case, as most of the nutrient from food is absorbed before it reaches the colon. Some ill-informed members of the public who do not suffer from eating disorders may also use laxatives in this way as an aid to dieting. Interestingly, studies suggest that laxative abuse by bulimics may cause an increase in anxiety that dissipates once abuse is discontinued.[123] Laxatives can be successfully withdrawn from these patients as an isolated intervention and this clearly prevents or remedies laxative-induced side-effects, but it does not necessarily by itself lead to an improvement in eating behaviour.[124]

2. **Bowel obsession**. These patients tend to be older than those in the previous group. They have a determination to defaecate regularly at the same time of day and/or to produce stools of a certain precise appearance. These beliefs may have arisen from training instilled in childhood, from a

previous experience of constipation, a lack of understanding of the nature and causes of constipation, or from a belief that a very regular bowel habit is necessary for bodily cleanliness. Indeed two words formerly used to describe laxatives – cathartics and purgatives – are derived from Greek and Latin words meaning cleansing. The elderly are prone to this problem, and laxatives are commonly overused by this group.[125] Individuals may suffer from real constipation initially, but persistent use of stimulant laxatives causes a degree of tolerance to their effects and consequently dosage tends to be progressively increased.[126] This pattern of behaviour can be difficult to interrupt.

3. **Factitious diarrhoea**. In this condition patients take high doses of laxatives secretly, and present for medical assessment with chronic diarrhoea of unknown cause. They continue to take enormous doses of laxatives surreptitiously, despite being subjected to extensive medical investigations and even surgery.[126] It is a form of Munchausen syndrome, sometimes called the laxative abuse syndrome. Patients appear emotionally detached from their ordeal and typically deny laxative abuse even when confronted with proof of it. Although not suffering from an eating disorder, these patients often have an associated psychiatric condition. Urine and stool analysis of 47 patients from Denmark with diarrhoea of uncertain origin, who denied laxative use, revealed that 15% of them were actually taking laxatives.[127] A study from Scotland reported a 4% incidence in unscreened patients reporting to a gastroenterology department with diarrhoea for the first time, but a 20% incidence in patients who had already been extensively investigated for chronic diarrhoea of unknown origin.[128]

    Parents have been reported to deliberately administer laxatives to infants in order to produce factitious diarrhoea.[129]

Adverse effects[126]

Not surprisingly, many people who abuse laxatives suffer from chronic diarrhoea. There may be nocturnal diarrhoea, blood in the stool and the frequency of motions may reach 20 per day. Defaecation is often associated with rectal and/or abdominal pain. Chronic diarrhoea results in dehydration, with resulting hypotension, tachycardia and postural dizziness, even fainting. Hypokalaemia is an important symptom, caused by potassium loss in the faeces. It manifests typically as muscle weakness and fatigue, but can lead to more severe complications such as cardiac arrhythmias or renal impairment. Metabolic alkalosis, hypocalcaemia and hypomagnesaemia can also occur. There have been rare reports of steatorrhoea.

For many years long-term use of stimulant laxatives was suggested to result in atonic or cathartic colon, characterised by damage to enteric nerves and loss of normal colonic function. This would be expected to cause intractable constipation, an inability to defaecate and periodic faecal impaction. However, convincing published evidence to support this finding in humans is lacking, the assertion being based on small uncontrolled studies and conflicting animal research.[130]

Miscellaneous OTC preparations

Alcohol

Some OTCs contain ethanol in high concentration, which alcoholics may be attracted to. Examples include mouthwashes, surgical spirit, methylated spirits, aftershave and some cleaning products. They have an unpleasant taste, which should deter all but the most desperate alcoholics, but for those afraid of imminent withdrawal symptoms, mouthwashes and similar products may be a more economical way – or the only way – to purchase alcohol in some circumstances.[131,132] The adverse effects associated with consuming large amounts of the various additives in these products is unknown.

Anabolic compounds

A range of products available OTC are claimed to have anabolic properties. These are often referred to collectively as dietary supplements, and include arginine, ornithine, carnitine and inosine. However, in most cases these claims are founded on poor-quality evidence (see Chapter 11).

Antimuscarinics

The abuse of prescription antimuscarinic medicines has been discussed (Chapter 12) but note that the antimuscarinic hyoscine (scopolamine) hydrobromide is widely available OTC for travel sickness. A Scottish survey revealed that the OTC analgesic that pharmacists suspected most of abuse was Feminax.[5] This painkiller contains paracetamol, codeine and caffeine, but is also the only UK analgesic to contain hyoscine.

Menthol and camphor

In large enough quantities, camphor and menthol seem to cause psychotropic effects. One case report describes two men who ingested 6–10 g of camphor as a stimulant.[133] Both became intoxicated, with anxiety, psychomotor agitation and hallucinations. An elderly woman who had been ingesting a camphor/menthol product for 5 years showed signs of delirium characterised by euphoria, confusion, agitation, hallucinations and odd behaviour.[134] A range of mental symptoms developed in another patient dependent on mentholated cigarettes, including irritability, restlessness, confusion and intoxication.[135] In other cases it is not clear what part aromatic amines played in causing psychotropic effects. For example, one patient discovered that Vicks VapoRub and nasal spray gave her 'a pleasant psychological lift' when applied intranasally throughout the day.[32] Although the spray contains oxymetazoline (a sympathomimetic) both spray and rub also contain large amounts of camphor and menthol.

Vaporisation of certain camphor and menthol products may also be used to extend the euphoric effects of illicit drugs or to smooth the aftermath of a 'trip'. This behaviour has particularly been associated with ecstasy users.

Large doses of camphor have caused coma and death from respiratory failure or status epilepticus.[133]

Caffeine

In many countries caffeine-containing preparations are sold OTC for their stimulant effects. Although no more effective than caffeinated beverages, some members of the public are undoubtedly attracted by the 'medicine-like' format. Large doses have been taken for the purpose of abuse (see also Chapter 14). It is also noteworthy that some OTC analgesics contain caffeine. This undoubtedly makes cessation of chronic analgesic administration more difficult, because suddenly stopping caffeine can cause withdrawal effects, notably headaches.

Weak acids

In western Europe, ascorbic acid, citric acid, boric acid and a variety of others are commonly used to convert insoluble base heroin into a more water-soluble form for injection.

Illicit drug manufacture

The use of codeine and sympathomimetics as precursors for the manufacture of illicit substances has already been mentioned. Table 13.2 lists

Table 13.2 Chemicals used in clandestine production of drugs

Chemical	Substance produced
Acetic anhydride	Heroin, methaqualone
Acetone	Cocaine, heroin, others
Ammonia	Cocaine
Ammonium chloride	Heroin
Ammonium hydroxide	Cocaine, others
Anthranilic acid	Methaqualone
Benzaldehyde	Amfetamines
Benzyl cyanide	Metamfetamine
2-Butanone (MEK)	Cocaine
Chloroform	Cocaine, others
Diethylamine	LSD
Ephedrine	Metamfetamine
Ergometrine	LSD
Ergotamine	LSD
Ethyl ether	Cocaine, heroin others
Hydrochloric acid	Cocaine, heroin others
Isosafrole	Ecstasy, MDA, MDE, etc.
Lysergic acid	LSD
Methylamine	Metamfetamine, ecstasy
3,4-Methylenedioxyphenyl-2-propanone	Ecstasy, MDA, MDE, etc.
Methyl isobutyl ketone (MIBK)	Cocaine
N-acetylanthranilic acid	Methaqualone
Nitroethane	Amfetamines
Phenyl-2-propanone	Amfetamine, metamfetamine
Piperidine	Phencyclidine
Piperonal	Ecstasy, MDE, etc.
Potassium permanganate	Cocaine
Potassium carbonate	Cocaine
Potassium hydroxide	Cocaine
Propionic anhydride	Fentanyl analogues
Pseudoephedrine	Metamfetamine
Pyridine	Heroin
Safrole	Ecstasy, MDA, MDE, etc.
Sodium hydroxide	Cocaine, others
Sodium carbonate/bicarbonate	Cocaine, others
Sulphuric acid	Cocaine, others
Tartaric acid	Heroin

Adapted from the UK Centre for Pharmacy Postgraduate Education distance learning pack 'The treatment of drug dependence'.

some chemicals that may be requested for OTC purchase in order to manufacture drugs of abuse.

Controlling the problem

In terms of abuse potential, OTC medicines offer a number of attractions – they are cheap, easily available and not illegal. Compared with the more widely publicised dangers of illicit drugs, tobacco smoking or alcoholism, OTCs carry an impression of safety because they are 'medicines', which belies their dangers in large doses. Because they are medicines, anyone who abuses them knows exactly what he or she is going to get whenever the product is obtained: the quality assurance procedures that pharmaceutical manufacturers use ensure a reproducible content and potency, and a lack of adulteration. Taken collectively these factors give a feeling of control and a false sense of safety.

From published case reports, factors that seem to increase the likelihood of OTC medicines abuse include mental illnesses (e.g. eating disorders, obsessive–compulsive disorders, schizophrenia), being female, experience of substance misuse, and chronic self-medication.

Despite knowledge of why OTC medicines are abused, which people may be more likely to engage in it, and the dangers associated with abuse, it is not immediately clear what can be done to minimise abuse. However, as stated in the introduction, it affects a minority of OTC medicine purchasers and history reveals that whatever steps are taken to minimise abuse of a substance, the determined individual will find a way around any regulation or control. The additional complicating factor is that any steps taken to prevent OTC medicines being abused need to take account of the fact that the majority of individuals who need, or want, to self-medicate must be able to so without undue inconvenience. With all this in mind, I would make the following observations:

- In an era where high standards of evidence-based practice are applied to medicines available on prescription, the same standards are not always applied to OTC medicines. There are many individual drugs, as well as cocktails of drugs, without proven medicinal benefit. Some of these have been available for many decades with no formal review of their efficacy.
- Printing warnings on medicines stating that the product may be liable to abuse, or can cause dependence, could alert some users to the dangers but may also serve to attract others to 'experiment' with them. It is worth noting that health warnings on cigarettes seem to be a minimal deterrent.
- Restricting all potentially abusable products to 'prescription only' status is unrealistic because most of these products are used to treat minor ailments such as colds, diarrhoea and coughs. The prospect of visiting a family doctor every time a supply of such medicine is required, and paying a charge that far exceeds the cost of the medicine, would meet

resistance from doctors and the public alike. In addition, as Chapter 12 makes clear, prescription-only status is certainly no guarantee against abuse and dependence. Having said this, there is a case for restricting certain products to prescription status if they are particularly liable to abuse and there are non-abusable alternatives available OTC.

- Manufacturers do not always consider abuse potential when marketing new formulations and neither do regulatory authorities.
- For manufacturers there are possible financial barriers to reformulating existing products to make them less liable to abuse. A dialogue with regulatory authorities may be helpful.
- Pharmacists' professional bodies are well placed to offer leadership, guidance and training to their members. Community pharmacists need to train staff in their employment, and standard operating procedures for sales of some medicines liable to abuse may be helpful.
- Research is needed to investigate the scale of the abuse problem, as well as methods of educating the public about it. Further studies could look at the role of treatment and referral guidelines for those affected, and evaluate methods of prevention. In particular, registers for sales of particular products seem a logical way to deter abuse of some medicines. However, research is needed to ascertain how this affects subsequent prevalence and patterns of abuse.
- Patterns of OTC medicine abuse are constantly changing and it would seem a good idea for pharmacies in a given locality to share information about which OTC products are being abused.

References

1. Hughes G F, McElnay J C, Hughes C M, *et al*. Abuse/misuse of non-prescription drugs. *Pharm World Sci* 1999; 21: 251–255.
2. Wazaify M, McElnay J C, Hughes C M. The implementation of a harm minimisation model for the identification and treatment of over-the-counter drug misuse and abuse in community pharmacies. *Int J Pharm Pract* 2002; 10(Suppl): R92.
3. MacFadyen L, Eadie D, McGowan T. Community pharmacists' experience of over-the-counter medicine misuse in Scotland. *J R Soc Promotion Health* 2001; 121: 185–192.
4. Pates R, McBride A J, Li S. Misuse of over-the-counter medicines: a survey of community pharmacies in a South Wales health authority. *Pharm J* 2002; 268: 179–182.
5. Matheson C, Bond C. Misuse of over-the-counter medicines from community pharmacies: a population survey of Scottish pharmacies. *Pharm J* 2002; 269: 66–68.
6. Paxton R, Chapple P. Misuse of over-the-counter medicines: a survey in one English county. *Pharm J* 1996; 256: 313–315.

7. Ball K, Wilde M. OTC medicines misuse in West Cumbria. *Pharm J* 1989; 242: 40.

8. Armstrong D J. The use of over-the-counter preparations by drug users attending an addiction treatment unit. *Br J Addict* 1992; 87: 125–128.

9. Sankey R J, Nunn A J, Sills J A. Visual hallucinations in children receiving decongestants. *BMJ* 1984; 288: 1369.

10. Norvenius G, Widerlov E, Lonnerholm G. Phenylpropanolamine and mental disturbances. *Lancet* 1979; 2: 1367–1368.

11. Bain J, Drennan P C, Miller M G. Visual hallucinations in children receiving decongestants (3 separate letters). *BMJ* 1984; 288: 1688.

12. Leighton K M. Paranoid psychosis after abuse of Actifed. *BMJ* 1982; 284: 789–790.

13. Diaz M A, Wise T N, Semchyshyn G O. Self-medication with pseudo-ephedrine in a chronically depressed patient. *Am J Psychiatry* 1979; 136: 1217–1218.

14. Pugh R, Howie M. Dependence on pseudoephedrine. *Br J Psychiatry* 1986; 149: 798.

15. Loosmore D, Armstrong D. Do-do abuse. *Br J Psychiatry* 1990; 157: 278–281.

16. Lambert M T. Paranoid psychoses after abuse of proprietary cold remedies. *Br J Psychiatry* 1987; 151: 548–550.

17. Sullivan G. Acute psychosis following intravenous abuse of pseudoephedrine: a case report. *J Psychopharmacol* 1996; 10: 324–325.

18. Cockings J G L, Brown M A. Ephedrine abuse causing acute myocardial infarction. *Med J Aust* 1997; 167: 199–200.

19. Martin W R, Sloan J W, Sapira J D, *et al.* Physiologic, subjective and behavioural effects of amphetamine, methamphetamine, ephedrine, phen-metrazine, and methylphenidate in man. *Clin Pharmacol Ther* 1971; 12: 245–258.

20. Herridge C F, A'Brook M F. Ephedrine psychosis. *BMJ* 1968; 1: 160.

21. Roxanas M G, Spalding J. Ephedrine abuse psychosis. *Med J Aust* 1977; 2: 639–640.

22. Whitehouse A M, Duncan J M. Ephedrine psychosis rediscovered. *Br J Psychiatry* 1987; 150: 258–261.

23. Lake C R, Gallant S, Masson E, *et al.* Adverse drug effects attributed to phenylpropanolamine: a review of 142 case reports. *Am J Med* 1990; 89: 195–208.

24. McEwen J. Phenylpropanolamine-associated hypertension after the use of "over the counter" appetite-suppressant products. *Med J Aust* 1983; 2: 71–73.

25. Schlemmer R F. Phenylpropanolamine as an appetite suppressant: a review of its efficacy and safety. *Pharmindex* April 1986, 10–15.

26. Greenway F, Herber D, Raum W, *et al.* Double-blind, randomized, placebo-controlled clinical trials with non-prescription medications for the treatment of obesity. *Obes Res* 1999; 7: 370–378.

27. Tinsley J A, Watkins D D. Over-the-counter stimulants: abuse and addiction. *Mayo Clin Proc* 1998; 73: 977–982.

28. Gruber A J, Pope H G Jr. Ephedrine abuse among 36 female weightlifters. *Am J Addict* 1998; 7: 256–261.

29. Gillies H, Derman W E, Noakes T D, *et al*. Pseudoephedrine is without ergogenic effects during prolonged exercise. *J Appl Physiol* 1996; 81: 2611–2617.

30. Gill N D, Shield A, Blazevich A J, *et al*. Muscular and cardiorespiratory effects of pseudoephedrine in human athletes. *Br J Clin Pharmacol* 2000; 50: 205–213.

31. Swain R A, Harsha D M, Baenziger J, *et al*. Do pseudoephedrine or phenyl-propanolamine improve maximum oxygen uptake and time to exhaustion? *Clin J Sports Med* 1997; 7: 168–173.

32. Blackwood G W. Severe psychological disturbance resulting from abuse of nasal decongestants. *Scott Med J* 1982; 27: 175–176.

33. Shukla P C. Acute ischemia of the hand following intra-arterial oxymeta-zoline injection. *J Emerg Med* 1995; 13: 65–70.

34. Snow S, Logan T P, Hollender M H. Nasal spray 'addiction' and psychosis: a case report. *Br J Psychiatry* 1980; 136: 297–299.

35. Pearson M M, Little R B. The addictive process in unusual addictions: a further elaboration of etiology. *Am J Psychiatry* 1969; 125: 1166–1171.

36. Drug Enforcement Agency News Release: More than 100 arrested in nation-wide methamphetamine investigation. Drug Enforcement Agency Briefs and Background. 10 January 2002. http://www.usdoj.gov/dea/major/me3.html (accessed 28 November 2004).

37. Drug Enforcement Agency News Release. Over 65 arrested in international methamphetamine investigation. Drug Enforcement Agency Briefs and Back-ground. 15 April 2003. http://www.usdoj.gov/dea/pubs/pressrel/pr041503.html (accessed 28 November 2004).

38. Craig D F. Psychosis with Vicks Formula 44-D abuse. *Can Med Assoc J* 1992; 146: 1199–1200.

39. Abed R T, Clark P J. Acute psychotic episode caused by the abuse of Phensedyl. *Br J Psychiatry* 1987; 151: 868.

40. Blau J J. Ephedrine nephrolithiasis associated with chronic ephedrine abuse. *J Urol* 1998; 160: 825.

41. Cornelius J R, Soloff P H, Reynolds C F. Paranoia, homicidal behavior, and seizures associated with phenylpropanolamine. *Am J Psychiatry* 1984; 141: 120–121.

42. Dietz A J Jr. Amphetamine-like reactions to phenylpropanolamine. *JAMA* 1981; 245: 601–602.

43. Pentel P. Toxicity of over-the-counter stimulants. *JAMA* 1984; 252: 1898–1903.

44. Mariani P J. Pseudoephedrine-induced hypertensive emergency. *Am J Emerg Med* 1986; 4: 141–142.

45. Wiesli P, Kupferschmidt H, Koch J. Surreptitious use of phenylpropanolamine parading as pheochromocytoma. *Res Commun Alc Subst Abuse* 1997; 18: 149–156.

46. Bruno A, Nolte K B, Chapin J. Stroke associated with ephedrine use. *Neurology* 1993; 43: 1313–1316.

47. McDowell J R, LeBlanc H J. Phenylpropanolamine and cerebral hemorrhage. *West J Med* 1985; 142: 688–691.

48. Swenson R D, Golper T A, Bennett W M. Acute renal failure and rhabdomyolysis after ingestion of phenylpropanolamine-containing diet pills. *JAMA* 1982; 248: 1216.

49. Hampel G, Horstkotte H, Rumpf W. Myoglobinuric renal failure due to drug-induced rhabdomyolysis. *Hum Toxicol* 1983; 2: 197–203.

50. Szekely J L, Sharpe L G, Jaffe J H. Induction of phencyclidine-like behavior in rats by dextrorphan but not dextromethorphan. *Pharmacol Biochem Behav* 1991; 40: 381–386.

51. Wong B Y, Coulter D A, Choi D W. Dextrorphan and dextromethorphan, common antitussives, are antiepileptic and antagonize N-methyl D-aspartate in brain slices. *Neurosci Lett* 1988; 34: 261–266.

52. Zawertailo L A, Kaplan H L, Busto U E, *et al*. Psychotropic effects of dextromethorphan are altered by the CYP2D6 polymorphism: a pilot study. *J Clin Psychopharmacol* 1998; 18: 332–337.

53. Baumann P, Vlatkovic D, Macciardi F. Intoxication with dextromethorphan in an adolescent with a genetic cytochrome P450 CYP2D6 deficiency. *Therapie* 1997; 52: 607–608.

54. Dodds A, Revai E. Toxic psychosis due to dextromethorphan. *Med J Aust* 1967; 2: 231.

55. Murray S, Brewerton T. Abuse of over-the-counter dextromethorphan by teenagers. *South Med J* 1993; 86: 1151–1153.

56. Schadel M, Sellers E M. Psychosis with Vicks 44-D abuse. *Can Med Assoc J* 1992; 147: 843–844.

57. Price L, Lebel J. Dextromethorphan-induced psychosis. *Am J Psychiatry* 2000; 157: 304.

58. McCarthy J P. Some less familiar drugs of abuse. *Med J Aust* 1971; 2: 1078–1081.

59. Fleming P M. Dependence on dextromethorphan hydrobromide. *BMJ* 1986; 293: 597.

60. Darboe M N, Keenan G R Jr, Richards T K. The abuse of dextromethorphan-based cough syrup: a pilot study of the community of Waynesboro, Pennsylvania. *Adolescence* 1996; 31: 633–644.

61. Wolfe T R, Caravati E M. Massive dextromethorphan ingestion and abuse. *Am J Emerg Med* 1995; 13: 174–176.

62. Polles A, Griffith J L. Dextromethorphan-induced mania. *Psychosomatics* 1996; 37: 71–74.

63. Baker S D, Borys D J. A possible trend suggesting increased abuse from Coricidin exposures reported to the Texas poison network: comparing 1998 to 1999. *Vet Hum Toxicol* 2002; 44: 169–171.

64. Banerji S, Anderson I B. Abuse of Coricidin HBP cough & cold tablets: episodes recorded by a poison center. *Am J Health Syst Pharm* 2001; 58: 1811–1814.

65. Hinsberger A, Sharma V, Mazmanian D. Cognitive deterioration from long-term abuse of dextromethorphan: a case report. *J Psychiatry Neurosci* 1994; 19: 375–377.

66. Walker J, Yatham L N. Benylin (dextromethorphan) abuse and mania. *BMJ* 1993; 306: 896.

67. Orrell M W, Campbell P G. Dependence on dextromethorphan hydrobromide. *BMJ* 1986; 293: 1242–1243.

68. Bornstein S, Czermak M, Postel J. A propos a case of voluntary drug poisoning with dextromethorphan hydrobromide. *Ann Med Psychol* 1968; 1: 447–451.

69. Mendez M F. Mania self-induced with cough syrup. *J Clin Psychiatry* 1992; 53: 173–174.

70. Rammer L, Holmgren P, Sandler H. Fatal intoxication by dextromethorphan: a report of two cases. *Forensic Sci Int* 1988; 37: 233–236.

71. Kathiramalainathan K, Kaplan H L, Romach M K, *et al*. Inhibition of cytochrome P450 2D6 modifies codeine abuse liability. *J Clin Psychopharmacol* 2000; 20: 435–444.

72. Tyndale R F, Droll K P, Sellers E M. Genetically deficient CYP2D6 metabolism provides protection against oral opiate dependence. *Pharmacogenetics* 1997; 7: 375–379.

73. Borrero E. Treatment of 'trash hand' following intra-arterial injection of drugs in addicts – case studies. *Vasc Surg* 1995; 29: 71–75.

74. Jensen S, Hansen A C. Abuse of codeine separated from over-the-counter drugs containing acetylsalicylic acid and codeine. *Int J Legal Med* 1993; 105: 279–281.

75. Elwood W N. Sticky business: patterns of procurement and misuse of prescription cough syrup in Houston. *J Psychoactive Drugs* 2001; 33: 121–133.

76. Krausz M, Verthein U, Degkwitz P, *et al*. Maintenance treatment of opiate addicts with codeine – results of a follow-up study. *Addiction* 1998; 93: 1161–1167.

77. Mattoo S K, Basu D, Sharma A, *et al*. Abuse of codeine-containing cough syrups: a report from India. *Addiction* 1997; 92: 1783–1787.

78. Sakol M S, Stark C S. Codeine abuse. *Lancet* 1989; 334: 1282–1283.

79. Paterson J R, Talwar D K, Watson I D, *et al*. Codeine abuse from co-codaprin. *Lancet* 1990; 335: 224.

80. Fleming G F, McElnay J C, Hughes C M. The separation of codeine from non-prescription analgesic products. *Subst Use Misuse* 2003; 9: 1217–1226.

81. Nathwani B. Abuse potential of Nurofen Plus. *Pharm J* 1998; 261: 489.

82. Bedford K R, Nolan S L, Onrust R, *et al*. The illicit preparation of morphine and heroin from pharmaceutical products containing codeine: 'Homebake' laboratories in New Zealand. *Forensic Sci Int* 1987; 34: 197–204.

83. Ross M W, Stowe A, Loxley W, *et al*. 'Home bake' heroin use by injecting drug users. *Med J Aust* 1992; 157: 283–284.

84. Romach M K, Sproule B A, Sellers E M, *et al*. Long-term codeine use is associated with depressive symptoms. *J Clin Psychopharmacol* 1999; 19: 373–376.

85. Thurston D, Taylor K. Gee's Linctus. *Pharm J* 1984; 233: 63.

86. Kennedy M. Cardiac glycoside toxicity: an unusual manifestation of drug addiction. *Med J Aust* 1981; 2: 686–689.

87. Seow S S W. Abuse of APF Linctus Codeine and cardiac glycoside toxicity. *Med J Aust* 1984; 140: 54.

88. Kilpatrick C, Braund W, Burns R. Myopathy with myasthenic features possibly induced by codeine linctus. *Med J Aust* 1982; 2: 410.

89. Curry K H, Stanhope J M. Codeine linctus and myopathy. *Med J Aust* 1984; 1: 247.

90. Barragry J M, Morris D V. Fatal dependence on kaolin and morphine mixture. *Postgrad Med J* 1980; 56: 180–181.

91. Todd G R G, Blair A L T, McElnay J C, et al. Dependence on kaolin and morphine mixture, hypokalaemia and hypertension. *Ir J Med Sci* 1985; 154: 409–410.

92. Kirkham B, Cowell R, Rees J. Severe hypokalaemia from kaolin and morphine abuse. *Postgrad Med J* 1987; 63: 589–590.

93. Fontebasso M. Diagnosis and treatment of chronic daily headache. *Prescriber* 2004; 15(2): 13–20.

94. Monzon M J, Lainez J M. Chronic daily headache: long-term prognosis following inpatient treatment. *Headache Q* 1998; 9: 326–330.

95. Bahra A, Goadsby P. Chronic overuse of acute antimigraine preparations. *Prescriber* 1999; 10: 109–115.

96. Symon D N K. Twelve cases of analgesic headache. *Arch Dis Child* 1998; 78: 555–556.

97. Madden J S, Wilson C W M. Deliberate aspirin intoxication. *BMJ* 1996; i: 1090.

98. Tiller J, Treasure J. Purging with paracetamol: report of four cases. *BMJ* 1992; 305: 618.

99. Council Statement, Royal Pharmaceutical Society of Great Britain. Sales of preparations containing cyclizine. *Pharm J* 1986; 236: 21.

100. Pearson G, Gilman M, Traynor P. Talking point: the limits of intervention. *Druglink* 1990; 5: 12–13.

101. Bassett K E, Scunk J E, Crouch B I. Cyclizine abuse by teenagers in Utah. *Am J Emerg Med* 1996; 14: 472–474.

102. Gott P H. Cyclizine toxicity. *N Engl J Med* 1968; 279: 596.

103. Gluckman L. Atypical reactions to Marzine. *Aust J Alcohol Drug Depend* 1977; 4: 10–11.

104. Myles J S, Treganza G S. Cyclizine abuse in opiate addicts. *Br J Addict* 1986; 81: 711.

105. Ruben S M, McLean P C, Melville J. Cyclizine abuse among a group of opiate dependents receiving methadone. *Br J Addict* 1989; 84: 929–934.

106. Hughes A, Coote J. Cyclizine dependence. *Pharm J* 1986; 236: 130.

107. Cox D, Ahmed Z, McBride A J. Diphenhydramine dependence. *Addiction* 2001; 96: 516–517.

108. Feldman M D, Behar M. A case of massive diphenhydramine abuse and withdrawal from use of the drug. *JAMA* 1986; 255: 3119–3120.

109. Bartlik B, Galanter M, Angrist B. Dimenhydrinate addiction in a schizophrenic woman. *J Clin Psychiatry* 1989; 50: 476.

110. Young G B, Boyd D, Kreeft J. Dimenhydrinate: evidence for dependence and tolerance. *Can Med Assoc J* 1988; 138: 437–438.

111. Craig D F, Mellor C S. Dimenhydrinate dependence and withdrawal. *Can Med Assoc J* 1990; 142: 970–973.

112. Isabelle C, Warner A. Long-term heavy use of diphenhydramine without anti-cholinergic delirium. *Am J Health Syst Pharm* 1999; 56: 555–557.

113. Malcolm R, Miller W C. Dimenhydrinate (Dramamine) abuse: hallucinogenic experiences with a proprietary antihistamine. *Am J Psychiatry* 1972; 128: 1012–1013.

114. Brown J H, Sigmundson H K. Delirium from misuse of dimenhydrinate. *Can Med Assoc J* 1969; 101: 49–50.

115. Rowe C, Verjee Z, Koren G. Adolescent dimenhydrinate abuse: resurgence of an old problem. *J Adolesc Health* 1997; 21: 47–49.

116. Gardner D M, Kutcher S. Dimenhydrinate abuse among adolescents. *Can J Psychiatry* 1993; 38: 113–116.

117. de Nesnera A P. Diphenhydramine dependence: a need for awareness. *J Clin Psychiatry* 1996; 57: 136–137.

118. MacRury S, Neilson R, Goodwin K. Benylin dependence, metabolic acidosis and hyperglycaemia. *Postgrad Med J* 1987; 63: 587–588.

119. Roberts K, Gruer L, Gilhooly T. Misuse of diphenhydramine soft gel capsules (Sleepia): a cautionary tale from Glasgow. *Addiction* 1999; 94: 1575–1578.

120. Woodhead M. Drug users injecting antihistamines. *Aust Doct* August 2003, 5.

121. Dinndorf P A, McCabe M A, Frierdich S. Risk of abuse of diphenhydramine in children and adolescents with chronic illnesses. *J Pediatrics* 1998; 133: 293–295.

122. Neims D M, McGill J, Giles T R, *et al*. Incidence of laxative abuse in community and bulimic populations: a descriptive review. *Int J Eat Disord* 1995; 17: 211–218.

123. Weltzin T E, Bulik C M, McConaha C W, *et al*. Laxative withdrawal and anxiety in bulimia nervosa. *Int J Eat Disord* 1995; 17: 141–146.

124. Colton P, Woodside D B, Kaplan A S. Laxative withdrawal in eating disorders: treatment protocol and 3 to 20 month follow-up. *Int J Eat Disord* 1999; 25: 311–317.

125. Kofoed L L. OTC drug overuse in the elderly: what to watch for. *Geriatrics* 1985; 40: 55–60.

126. Baker E H, Sandle G I. Complications of laxative abuse. *Ann Rev Med* 1996; 47: 127–134.

127. Bytzer P, Stokholm M, Andersen I, *et al*. Prevalence of surreptitious laxative abuse in patients with diarrhoea of uncertain origin: a cost benefit analysis of a screening technique. Gut 1989; 30: 1379–1384.

128. Duncan A, Morris A J, Cameron A, *et al*. Laxative induced diarrhoea – a neglected diagnosis. *J R Soc Med* 1992; 85: 203–205.

129. Forbes D A, O'Loughlin E V, Scott R B, *et al*. Laxative abuse and secretory diarrhoea. *Arch Dis Child* 1985; 60: 58–60.

130. Wald A. Is chronic use of stimulant laxatives harmful to the colon? *J Clin Gastroenterol* 2003; 36: 386–389.

131. Leather J. Blotto and minty: Anchorage has a problem with chronic inebriates and mouthwash isn't helping any. *Anchorage Press* 22–28 August 2002.

132. Abel D. Homeless cited in mouthwash thefts: high alcohol content spurs street popularity. *Boston Globe* 1 May 2003.

133. Köppel C, Tenczer J, Schirop T, *et al*. Camphor poisoning: abuse of camphor as a stimulant. *Arch Toxicol* 1982; 51: 101–106.
134. Huntimer C M, Bean D W. Delirium after ingestion of mentholatum. *Am J Psychiatry* 2000; 157: 483–484.
135. Luke E. Addiction to mentholated cigarettes. *Lancet* 1962; i: 110.

14

Caffeine

As far as she could recall no one had ever, given the choice, said 'No, I will not touch horrible coffee anymore! It's a long black ground-acorn substitute for me, with extra floating gritty bits.'
Terry Pratchett, 'Monstrous Regiment'

History

Caffeine is an important constituent of several plants that are widely consumed. The most popular of these are listed in Table 14.1, together with their caffeine content. Other plant sources of caffeine are discussed in Chapter 17.

The tea plant is native to South-East Asia. It has been consumed in China as a hot infusion for many centuries. The Chinese character for tea is pronounced 'tay' or 'cha' depending upon the dialect. Tea was introduced into Europe in the early 1600s and in Britain was originally termed 'tay'; the modern pronunciation 'tea' originated in the 18th century.

The coffee plant is native to Ethiopia and local legend relates that the earliest human use was by a holy man who prepared an infusion of the seeds in water so that he might stay awake at night to pray. The plant was first cultivated by man in the vicinity of Mocha in Yemen, the plants having been originally taken from Kefa in Ethiopia. Until the end of the 17th century, this region supplied most of the world's coffee. From the mid-17th century onwards, coffee and tea consumption increased rapidly once Europeans acquired a taste for these beverages, and coffee houses in London, for example, became important centres for political, literary and business dealings. Cultivation of both plants consequently spread to meet the demand. European nations, especially the British and Dutch, encouraged their colonies to grow the plants.

Chocolate is a relatively minor source of caffeine. It is prepared from the seeds of the cacao tree (*Theobroma cacao*), which is native to South America. A drink prepared from the seeds by the Aztecs was 'chocalatl' (bitter), and was described as the food of the gods.

Table 14.1 Major dietary sources of caffeine

Foodstuff	Plant (parts used commercially)	Plant caffeine content	Caffeine dose per typical cup
Tea	*Thea sinensis* (dried leaves)	1–5%	10–100 mg (average 40 mg)
Coffee	*Coffea arabica,* etc. (beans)	0.75–2.5%	30–150 mg (average 60–80 mg)
'Decaffeinated' coffee	*Coffea arabica,* etc. (beans)		2–4 mg
Cocoa	*Theobroma cacao* (seeds)	0.03–1.7%	2–50 mg (average 5 mg)
Chocolate	*Theobroma cacao* (seeds)		2–63 mg per 50 g
Cola drinks	*Cola acuminata* (nuts)	1.5–2%	25–100 mg*

*Cola drinks contain added synthetic caffeine.

Effects sought

Caffeine is taken primarily for its stimulant effect on the central nervous system (CNS). It is the most widely used psychotropic substance in the world. Caffeine produces increased alertness, decreased fatigue, clear-headedness, intellectual stamina and enhanced physical endurance. In those who regular consume caffeine, administration gives rise to a contentment, possibly related to the avoidance of withdrawal symptoms but also influenced by the social ease associated with the drinking of caffeinated drinks and the personal expectation of CNS stimulation. Research supports the importance of negative reinforcement as a drive towards the daily consumption of caffeinated drinks.[1,2] Those habituated to caffeine show a strong preference for caffeinated drinks as opposed to caffeine-free varieties, even when the caffeine content is not known to the consumer.[1] The effect is particularly apparent in the morning, because enforced overnight caffeine abstinence produces dysphoria, which is alleviated by ingestion of caffeine.[2] It has been further proposed that a liking for the taste and smell of caffeinated beverages is driven by Pavlovian-like conditioning: taste and smell alerting the brain that a stimulating caffeine 'reward' is about to arrive.[1] As with other psychotropic substances, many of the effects are at least partly determined by the expectation of the user.

Interestingly, studies suggest that coffee protects against the development of diabetes mellitus. A dose-related protective effect has been observed with coffee and decaffeinated coffee, but not with tea.[3,4]

Administration

Caffeine intake has been arbitrarily classified according to the following values for daily consumption:

- low: 0–250 mg per day
- moderate: 250–750 mg per day
- high: in excess of 750 mg per day.

Note that this is not a universally accepted definition and many authors of research papers use their own definitions for low, medium and high intake.

The amount of caffeine consumed by the average person is difficult to estimate because of the various forms of each beverage and the different methods of preparing them. For example, percolated coffee usually contains more caffeine than instant varieties. If the coffee grounds are boiled during preparation – a method popular in many Scandinavian countries – the caffeine content can be as high as 500 mg per cup. Similarly, tea brewed directly from the crushed leaf releases more caffeine into the infusate than tea bags. The various strains of coffee and tea plants also differ in their caffeine content.

Plain chocolate contains more caffeine than milk chocolate. Chocolate also contains large amounts of theobromine, another methylxanthine with approximately 10% of the pharmacological activity of caffeine. Products flavoured with chocolate contain only small amounts of caffeine (e.g. chocolate ice cream typically has 2–5 mg of caffeine per 50 g).

A variety of other preparations also contain caffeine. These include over-the-counter (OTC) analgesic medicines and stimulants (see Chapter 13) and herbal products such as guarana (see Chapter 17).

Pharmacokinetics and pharmacology

Caffeine is a member of the group of compounds known as methylxanthines, which also includes the asthma drug, theophylline. Many of the effects of methylxanthines are thought to be mediated via competitive antagonism of adenosine. Adenosine is a neurotransmitter with largely inhibitory actions in the CNS. Benzodiazepines are thought to act in part as adenosine agonists and it is therefore not surprising that methylxanthines and benzodiazepines have opposing CNS actions.

In vitro, methylxanthines inhibit phosphodiesterase, the enzyme that causes breakdown of cyclic AMP. This group of drugs also has effects on the intracellular movement of calcium ions. However, neither of these actions is likely to occur to a significant extent in humans, except at very high doses. Caffeine can also increase the concentration of circulating catecholamines, but the mechanism of this and its importance to methylxanthine pharmacology is uncertain.

The average half-life of caffeine in adults is 5 hours but with considerable variation between individuals (range 2–12 hours). The main metabolite is paraxanthine, which is inactive, but small amounts of theobromine and theophylline are also produced. Each of these metabolites is subject to further enzymatic degradation before elimination. Following oral administration, caffeine is almost 100% bio-available and reaches peak plasma concentration 15–45 minutes after ingestion. Like theophylline, the clearance of caffeine is accelerated by drugs that induce the cytochrome P450 isoenzyme CYP1A2. Thus, for example, tobacco smoking will increase caffeine clearance, but clearance is appreciably slowed in women taking oestrogen-containing oral contraceptives or HRT (hormone replacement therapy).[5,6]

Adverse effects

On being told that coffee was a slow-acting poison, an aged Voltaire is said to have remarked: 'I think it must be so, for I have been drinking it for 65 years and I am not dead yet.' There is no proven association between caffeine intake and any fatal illness at normal levels of consumption. However, caffeine is pharmacologically active and can produce a range of effects in man. It is difficult to specify the dose of caffeine required to produce particular effects because the amount that individuals ingest is rarely known. In addition, the sensitivity to methylxanthines and the pharmacokinetic profile varies markedly between individuals; dose-related effects are also affected by tolerance, which can develop quickly.

Caffeine-related adverse effects may be wrongly attributed to other causes through ignorance. Recurrent headaches, persistent anxiety, inability to concentrate, muscular tremor/tension and chronic insomnia are probably the commonest of these reactions. The psychostimulant action of caffeine upon the CNS is dose-related, but in individuals who do not regularly consume it, even quite small amounts can cause irritability, insomnia and nervousness. The escalation of stimulant effects with increasing dose is illustrated in Table 14.2.

Severe psychiatric upset and convulsions are the ultimate, if rarely observed, sequelae of high-dose usage. Some of the other pharmacological effects of caffeine are also shown in Table 14.2. At regular daily doses above 0.5–1 g, a condition known as 'caffeinism' may develop. This frequently has a presentation akin to anxiety neurosis because the CNS effects predominate. Other possible symptoms are given in the table.

High, regular caffeine intake can exacerbate the symptoms of pre-existing **psychiatric illnesses** such as anxiety, depression and schizophrenia.[7–11] The stimulant effect of caffeine may encourage patients to consume large quantities in order to overcome the sedative effects of psychiatric medication. If this resulted simply in the reversal of unacceptable sedation then it would be helpful, but caffeine can also antagonise the therapeutic actions of benzodiazepines and phenothiazines. High-caffeine consumers who are taking these medications require larger doses of drug to control their symptoms. In the case of benzodiazepines, this is probably due to the opposing pharmacological action of caffeine on adenosine. Superimposing the adverse psychiatric effects of high intake of caffeine on top of an existing

Table 14.2 Side-effects of caffeine

Low to moderate intake of caffeine
- Diuresis
- Increased gastric acid secretion
- Fine tremor
- Increased skeletal muscle stamina
- Mild anxiety, insomnia

High intake of caffeine
- Chronic insomnia
- Persistent anxiety, restlessness, tension, agitation, excitement, panic attacks, inability to concentrate
- Confusion, disorientation, paranoia, delirium
- Tremors, muscle twitching, muscle tension, convulsions
- Vertigo, dizziness, tinnitus, auditory and visual disturbance
- Facial flushing, increased body temperature, raised blood pressure
- Tachycardia, palpitations, arrhythmias
- Nausea, vomiting, abdominal discomfort
- Headaches
- Tachypnoea

Lethal acute adult dose: 5–10 g caffeine

psychiatric disorder may change the clinical presentation. The new predominating symptoms may not be ameliorated by existing medication.

A high caffeine intake is also undoubtedly a reason behind some prescriptions for hypnotics and anxiolytics. Persistent caffeine stimulation encourages those adversely affected to take CNS depressant medication in an attempt to restore the normal sleep/wake cycle of the body. In the elderly, in whom the sleep/wake cycle is naturally subject to increased disruption, caffeine may have more obvious sleep-disturbing properties. Unfortunately, many elderly patients find it difficult to believe that tea and coffee, which most have been drinking for several decades, could be part of the cause of their insomnia.

Many patients with a high caffeine intake may also take considerable quantities of a very common CNS depressant – alcohol. The role of caffeinism in fuelling alcoholism has not been adequately researched. Caffeine is also suspected of involvement in the aetiology of some cases of the restless legs syndrome.

Caffeine has been investigated as a potential causative agent of several **cancers**. It can cause mutagenesis in bacteria, but studies in laboratory animals reveal no evidence of carcinogenicity. Despite initial concerns, epidemiological studies have not proved a link between caffeine consumption and any cancer in humans. Specifically, investigations have not revealed an association between caffeine intake and human cancer of the breast, pancreas, bladder, ovary or colon. However, such studies are complicated by the widescale use of caffeine and the difficulty of excluding all other confounding variables.

Similar arguments apply to studies of the relationship between caffeine intake and **coronary heart disease**. Small amounts of daily coffee do not seem to be associated with an increased risk, but as the daily intake increases the likelihood of an association also increases. The overall risk associated with coffee drinking is probably small.[12,13] However, high-dose methylxanthines do stimulate the myocardium so that it would seem wise for those with existing cardiovascular disease to avoid excessive intake. Large amounts of boiled unfiltered fresh coffee have been known for some time to raise plasma cholesterol.[14] More recently it has been demonstrated that as little as five or six cups of cafetière coffee per day can increase total plasma cholesterol levels by 6–10% (low-density lipoprotein cholesterol by 9–14%).[15] This has been suggested to increase the risk of coronary heart disease by 12–20%. The effect is thought to be caused by two diterpenes in coffee – cafertol and kahweol – and is reversible upon cessation of cafetière coffee intake.

Plasma cholesterol levels are not raised after drinking equivalent amounts of filter coffee because the diterpenes are retained on the paper filter. The same study showed that cafetière coffee raises serum alanine aminotransferase (which is a signal for liver damage) in all patients, but that this only exceeded the upper limit of normal in 36%. The clinical relevance of these findings to liver function is not known at present.

Caffeine encourages urinary excretion of calcium but a link between caffeine intake and osteoporosis has not been demonstrated.

Caffeinated drinks may have **gastrointestinal** side-effects. Caffeine can stimulate the production of gastric acid, so potentially worsening the symptoms of acid-related gastrointestinal disease in susceptible individuals. Decaffeinated coffee is at least as detrimental in this respect as caffeine-containing varieties, suggesting that caffeine is not the sole culprit and that patients with acid-related gastrointestinal disease will not benefit by swapping from caffeinated to decaffeinated coffees.[16,17] Some other effects produced by caffeine-containing beverages are not caused by the caffeine itself. For example, the high tannin content of tea can cause constipation whereas the essential oils in coffee may give rise to gastrointestinal upset and diarrhoea. Table 14.3 lists some of the known ingredients of coffee and tea.

Table 14.3 Chemicals found in tea and coffee plants

Tea leaves	Coffee beans
Tannin (10–24%)	Fixed coffee oil (15%) including linoleic and oleic acids
Caffeine (1–5%)	Various proteins (11%)
Various proteins	Sucrose and other sugars (8%)
Theobromine, theophylline	Chlorogenic/caffeic acids (6%)
Volatile oils	Caffeine (0.75–2.5%)
Over 20 amino acids	Trigonelline
About 30 polyphenolic compounds (e.g. theaflavine, thearubigins)	Volatile oils
12 sugars	Oxalic and tannic acids
6 organic acids (e.g. oxalic)	Minerals (e.g. magnesium, potassium)
Various B-group vitamins	Various B-group vitamins (especially nicotinic acid)
Minerals (e.g. manganese, fluoride)	

Caffeine dependence and withdrawal

It should be noted that the DSM-IV (*Diagnostic and Statistical Manual of Mental Disorders* – Fourth Edition) definition of dependence suggests that physical, emotional or behavioural impairment should occur. How often regular daily intake of caffeine constitutes dependence is not clear, but it does happen.[18,19] Dependence on caffeine is most easily observed in those who experience tolerance, side-effects from taking too much (perhaps with unsuccessful attempts to cut down), and who develop a withdrawal reaction when attempting to decrease use. However, these collective effects are not seen in most regular users of caffeine. It is true that withdrawal reactions are widely reported, but withdrawal by itself is not dependence (see Chapter 1). Tolerance to the stimulant effect of caffeine also develops to some extent but, unlike many psychoactive substances, there generally seems to be no particular desire to increase the amount of caffeine consumed with time. Most consumers continue to drink caffeinated beverages at roughly the same intake for their lifetime, experience no substantial side-effects from it and no withdrawal because they make no attempt to reduce their intake. Moreover, regular use of caffeine does not cause the majority of users distress, lead them to abandon important responsibilities, or even demand a great deal of their time. Consequently the majority of those who drink caffeinated beverages on a daily basis are not characterised as dependent.

There is a psychological component to regular use, whether this ever becomes dependency or not. This is best characterised by the rituals, habits and beliefs associated with ingestion. For example, many people always take caffeine at certain times of the day (e.g. afternoon tea, coffee with breakfast) and there is a strong desire to continue taking caffeinated substances to maintain/achieve a sense of well-being. Extra drinks may be consumed in the belief that they will help an individual to cope with a particularly difficult experience. Caffeinated drinks form an important part of many social occasions and are part of the cultural background to many societies. 'Tea time' and 'coffee breaks' are terms used to describe points in the day when caffeine may be taken, but these terms are used even by those that do not take caffeine at these times.

Caffeine withdrawal[18-23] is typified by symptoms such as:

- headache
- irritability, restlessness
- dysphoria, anxiety, depression, feeling antisocial
- lethargy, fatigue, sleepiness, yawning
- poor concentration.

Less-common features of withdrawal include flu-like symptoms, muscular tension and pains, sweating, rhinorrhoea, dizziness and nausea. Some sufferers experience craving for caffeine. Headache is the most common feature of withdrawal. Symptoms usually start within 24 hours of abstinence, peak during the next 1 or 2 days and last up to a week. In those who consume moderate amounts of caffeine each day, dysphoric symptoms can be observed every morning, after only overnight abstinence.[2] Withdrawal reactions are seen only after chronic administration, but is not limited to those with a high caffeine intake. Most users are aware, even if only subconsciously, that the symptoms of withdrawal can be rapidly reversed by ingesting more caffeine. Negative reinforcement may therefore play a part in ensuring continued dependence.

Headaches that occur in many patients following surgery under general anaesthetic have been attributed to caffeine withdrawal caused

Table 14.4 Steps to help reduce caffeine intake

- Educate the subject regarding the potential effects of caffeine and discuss how health may be improved by stopping or reducing caffeine intake. The individual should understand the nature (symptoms) and time course of withdrawal.
- It is important to identify all the current means of caffeine intake and the patterns of use (frequency, quantities). Ensure that one form of caffeine intake is not inadvertently swapped for another. Check for medication or herbal products that may contain caffeine, as well as tea, coffee and cola drinks.
- Withdrawal is probably easier if it is not abrupt. Drinking tea or coffee that is gradually made weaker than usual may help. The frequency of ingestion and perhaps the volume of beverage can also be progressively reduced.
- Substitution of caffeinated drinks wholly or partly with decaffeinated varieties may help, especially as these have a similar taste and presentation to caffeinated varieties. Again, this may need to be a gradual changeover.
- In order not to disrupt the psychological aspects of the daily routine and to keep social rituals alive, the subject should be encouraged to drink something at the time of the day when caffeine was normally taken, e.g. non-caffeine-containing hot drinks, herbal teas (but check that these do not contain caffeine). A visit to a health food store is instructive in identifying alternatives.
- Short-term, non-caffeine-containing analgesics may be helpful to treat withdrawal headache.
- If caffeine intake is to be reduced rather than stopped completely, the subject may find it helpful to limit consumption to certain fixed times of the day, e.g. one coffee with breakfast and one after lunch.

by forced abstinence. Table 14.4 (page 285) gives suggestions for making caffeine withdrawal less unpleasant.

Interaction with medicines

In some situations it has been the practice to mix psychiatric medication into caffeinated drinks to encourage patients to take it. This practice could be considered unethical if undertaken without the patient knowing that the drink contained medication. However, in the case of phenothiazine neuroleptics there are additional reasons for avoiding this practice. Caffeine-containing drinks may cause phenothiazines to precipitate when the two are mixed.[24] This may be caused by the tannic acid content.[25] Tea may be more potent than coffee in causing precipitation, although the effect is not related to the caffeine content of these beverages. Stomach acid reverses the precipitation *in vitro*[25] but in some animal studies the absorption of phenothiazines has still been impaired.[24] The practice of mixing phenothiazines with tea or coffee should not be encouraged because:

- If only a proportion of the drink is consumed it is impossible to ascertain how much medication has been consumed. The precipitate is unpalatable and may discourage a patient from finishing a drink.
- The precipitate might settle in the cup, or stick to the sides of it, so that the drug is not ingested even if a substantial proportion of the drink is consumed.
- In patients taking antacids or drugs that reduce acid secretion from the stomach, the reversal of precipitation in the gut may not occur.
- Precipitation in a drink and its potential reversal in the stomach introduces unnecessary uncertainty into drug therapy. The extent of precipitation, the degree of reversal (and therefore response to therapy) may vary according to the physiology of the individual, the drug and beverage involved, and concomitant drug therapy. The response to phenothiazines could vary from day to day in the same patient because of this practice.

Some medicines may increase the plasma levels of caffeine largely by inhibiting its metabolism via cytochrome P450 isoenzyme CYP1A2.[26] These medicines can include ethinylestradiol and other oestrogens, fluvoxamine, verapamil, fluconazole, methoxsalen, mexiletine, theophylline and some quinolone antibiotics. Caffeine may also increase the plasma levels of some medicines metabolised via CYP1A2 and examples include clozapine and theophylline.[26]

Pregnancy and breastfeeding

Pregnancy

Studies involving several thousand women have shown that caffeine is unlikely to cause congenital anomalies or other problems at normal intake. There is less information on high caffeine consumption. Human studies suggest that higher doses might be associated with spontaneous abortion or reduced birth weight but this has not been proven. A single large prospective study suggested that regular intake of more than eight cups of coffee per day increased the risk of stillbirth, an effect that has also been demonstrated in monkeys,[27] but this study requires confirmation.

Reversible cardiac arrhythmias have been described in the human fetus and newborn after exposure to high caffeine doses.[28] In 1988, eight newborns with apparent caffeine withdrawal symptoms were described. Their mothers had consumed very large amounts of caffeine (average 863 mg per day). Symptoms included jitteriness and vomiting.[29]

The evidence for adverse effects from caffeine in human pregnancy is not compelling, but reducing caffeine intake during pregnancy would seem a sensible precaution, especially in those who usually consume large amounts.

Breastfeeding

Caffeine passes into breast milk but does not concentrate there. It is commonly taken by breastfeeding women and there are no apparent serious adverse effects upon the nursing infant at normal levels of intake. Caffeine is used therapeutically at a dose of up to 10 mg/kg per day (of base) to treat neonatal apnoea. This is a considerably higher dose than could be achieved via exposure to breast milk containing caffeine and it is not associated with significant side-effects. However, a change in infant behaviour during maternal high-dose caffeine administration should prompt a reduction in consumption.

References

1.   Rogers P J, Richardson N J, Elliman N A. Overnight caffeine abstinence and negative reinforcement of preference for caffeine containing drinks. *Psychopharmacology* 1995; 120: 457–462.

2.   Richardson N J, Rogers P J, Elliman N A, *et al*. Mood and performance effects of caffeine in relation to acute and chronic caffeine deprivation. *Pharmacol Biochem Behav* 1995; 52: 313–320.

3.   Salazar-Martinez E, Willett W C, Ascherio A, *et al*. Coffee consumption and risk for type 2 diabetes mellitus. *Ann Intern Med* 2004; 140: 1–8.

4.   Tuomilehto J, Hu G, Bidel S, *et al*. Coffee consumption and risk of type 2 diabetes mellitus among middle-aged Finnish men and women. *JAMA* 2004; 291: 1213–1219.

5.   Balogh A, Klinger G, Henschel L, *et al*. Influence of ethinylestradial containing combination oral contraceptives with gestodene or levonorgestrel on caffeine elimination. *Eur J Clin Pharmacol* 1995; 48: 161–166.

6.   Pollock B G, Wylie M, Stack J A, *et al*. Inhibition of caffeine metabolism by estrogen replacement therapy in postmenopausal women. *J Clin Pharmacol* 1999; 39: 936–940.

7.   Smith G A. Caffeine reduction as an adjunct to anxiety management. *Br J Clin Psychol* 1988; 27: 265–266.

8.   Greden J F, Fontaine P, Lubetsky M, *et al*. Anxiety and depression associated with caffeinism among psychiatric inpatients. *Am J Psychiatry* 1978; 135: 963–966.

9.   Shisslak C M, Beutler L E, Scheiber S, *et al*. Patterns of caffeine use and prescribed medications in psychiatric inpatients. *Psychol Rep* 1985; 57: 39–42.

10. De Freitas B, Schwarts G. Effects of caffeine in chronic psychiatric patients. *Am J Psychiatry* 1979; 136: 1337–1338.

11. Mikkelsen E J. Caffeine and schizophrenia. *J Clin Psychiatry* 1978; 39: 732–736.

12. Stensvold I, Tverdal A, Jacobsen B K. Cohort study of coffee intake and death from coronary heart disease over 12 years. *BMJ* 1996; 312: 544–545.

13. Marchioli R, Di Mascho R, Marfisi R M, *et al*. Coffee intake and death from coronary heart disease. *BMJ* 1996; 312: 1539.

14. Thelle D S. Coffee, cholesterol and coronary heart disease. *BMJ* 1991; 302: 804.

15. Urgert R, Meyboom S, Kuilman M, *et al*. Comparison of effect of cafetière and filtered coffee on serum concentrations of liver aminotransferases and lipids: six month randomised controlled trial. *BMJ* 1996; 313: 1362–1366.

16. Cohen S, Booth G H. Gastric acid secretion and lower esophageal sphincter pressure in response to coffee and caffeine. *N Engl J Med* 1975; 293: 897–899.

17. Feldman E J, Isenberg J I, Grossman M I. Gastric acid and gastrin response to decaffeinated coffee and peptone meal. *JAMA* 1981; 246: 248–250.

18. Strain E C, Mumford G K, Silverman K, *et al*. Caffeine dependence syndrome – evidence from case histories and experimental evaluations. *JAMA* 1994; 272: 1043–1048.

19. Strain E C, Griffiths R R. Caffeine dependence: fact or fiction? *J R Soc Med* 1995; 88: 437–440.

20. Silverman K, Evans S M, Strain E C, *et al*. Withdrawal syndrome after the double-blind cessation of caffeine consumption. *N Engl J Med* 1992; 327: 1109–1114.

21. Hughes J R. Clinical importance of caffeine withdrawal. *N Engl J Med* 1992; 327: 1160–1161.
22. Smith R. Caffeine withdrawal headache. *J Clin Pharm Ther* 1987; 12: 53–57.
23. van Dusseldorp M, Katan M B. Headache caused by caffeine withdrawal among moderate coffee drinkers switched from ordinary to decaffeinated coffee: a 12 week double blind trial. *BMJ* 1990; 300: 1558–1559.
24. Cheeseman H J, Neal M J. Interactions of chlorpromazine with tea and coffee. *Br J Clin Pharmacol* 1981; 12: 165–169.
25. Curry M L, Curry S H, Marroum P J. Interaction of phenothiazine and related drugs and caffeinated beverages. *Ann Pharmacother* 1991; 25: 437–438.
26. Carrillo J A, Benitez J. Clinically significant pharmacokinetic interactions between dietary caffeine and medications. *Clin Pharmacokinet* 2000; 39: 127–153.
27. Wisborg K, Kesmodel U, Bech B H, *et al.* Maternal consumption of coffee during pregnancy and stillbirth and infant death in first year of life: prospective study. *BMJ* 2003; 326: 420–423.
28. Oei S, Vosters R P L, van der Hagen N L J. Fetal arrhythmia caused by excessive intake of caffeine by pregnant women. *BMJ* 1989; 298: 568.
29. McGowan J D, Altman R E, Kanto W P. Neonatal withdrawal symptoms after chronic maternal ingestion of caffeine. *South Med J* 1988; 81: 1092.

15

Tobacco

*A custom loathsome to the Eye, hateful to the Nose, harmful to
the Braine, dangerous to the Lungs, and in the black, stinking fume
thereof, nearest resembling the horrible Stygian smoke of the pit
that is bottomless.*
King James I, 'Counterblaste to Tobacco', 1604

History

Tobacco is the dried leaf of *Nicotiana tobaccum*, one of a number of
Nicotiana species containing similar alkaloids and that can be smoked.
Nicotine is found in small quantities in several other solanaceous plants
(e.g. aubergine, tomatoes), but the amounts are generally too small to
have pharmacologically significant effects after human ingestion.
However, there are a large number of compounds in *Nicotiana* leaves
other than nicotine, and tobacco smoke contains over 3000 different
chemicals.

    Nicotiana plants are members of the Solanaceae or potato family
and are indigenous to the Americas. When Columbus landed there in
1492 he observed the natives smoking rolls of dried *Nicotiana* leaves
that were known as 'tobacos'. The plant and related species were widely
known to the North American Indians and the Aztecs, who had probably already been using them for over a thousand years by the time that
Columbus arrived. Once brought back to Europe, the popularity of
tobacco smoking spread rapidly in the 16th century. Sir Walter Raleigh
was a famous advocate of pipe smoking in Elizabethan England, a practice that found less favour under the Stuart King, James I. Jean Nicot is
reputed to have introduced tobacco to France in 1560, his name being
commemorated in the genus *Nicotiana* and the principle alkaloid, nicotine (which was isolated in 1828). The essayist Sir Francis Bacon seems
to have been the first to describe the addictive powers of tobacco when
in 1610 he recorded how difficult it was to stop. Smoking of tobacco
was initially via pipes, but in the 18th century the taking of snuff
became popular. Both of these methods were largely superseded by

cigars, which became the most popular method of taking tobacco in the 19th century. Cigarettes were introduced in the mid-19th century, but did not enter mass production until the late 1900s. From this point onwards cigarettes rapidly became the predominant method by which to smoke tobacco.

The number of smokers worldwide is estimated at 1.3 billion, although the prevalence of smoking in the Western world has been slowly declining. For example, in Great Britain in 1948, 52% of the population aged over 16 years smoked (65% of men and 41% of women). The 2002/3 figures for Britain showed this had fallen to 26% of the population (27% of men and 25% of women).[1] Prevalence rates in Britain are highest in the 20- to 24-year-old age group, where 37% of men and 38% of women smoke, and lowest in those aged over 60, where 17% men and 14% women smoke. An interesting newer trend is that in those aged 16–19, more women smoke than men (29% vs 22%). This is the only age group in Britain for which female smokers out-number male. There have been similar reductions in smoking prevalence in many other Western countries. However, despite some success in reversing the tobacco epidemic in the developed world, it is unpleasant to learn that the number of tobacco smokers continues to increase rapidly in less-developed continents such as Asia, Africa and South America. In many of the countries affected there are insufficient resources to meet even basic healthcare needs, let alone the conse-quences of widespread population self-poisoning. The World Health Organization (WHO) estimated that nearly 5 million people died worldwide in 2000 as a consequence of smoking tobacco.[2] About 80% of these were men. It has been estimated that if current trends continue, 70% of the projected 10 million global deaths from tobacco in 2025 will occur in developing countries.[3] In the light of statistics such as these, and the very well-known adverse health consequences for indi-viduals that smoke, it is remarkable that tobacco continues to be used. It is a sad tribute to the power of dependence. Unlike most other drugs of abuse, tobacco is a legal substance in every country in the world.

There is a significant international tobacco lobby, supported of course by millions of dependent individuals, and this will always make it very difficult to tackle this epidemic more rigorously. More cynically, tobacco and tobacco-related products generate vast sums for govern-ments each year in taxes – in the UK, for example, tobacco duty revenue was £8.1 billion in 2002.[1] When asked to ban smoking in France, Napoleon was candid: 'This vice brings in one hundred million francs in taxes every year. I will certainly forbid it at once – as soon as you can name a virtue that brings in as much revenue.'

Effects sought

Individuals typically begin smoking tobacco when young, commonly in the early to mid teenage years. As with other abused substances, the reasons for starting are multifactorial: a combination of factors such as peer pressure, teenage rebellion and the desire to experiment. Additionally, as with under-age drinking of alcohol (see Chapter 16), advertising can play an important part in recruiting new users – both explicit commercial advertisements and the use of tobacco by significant role models in films and on television. A systematic review of available studies into this aspect of recruitment has concluded that: 'tobacco advertising and promotion increases the likelihood that adolescents will start to smoke'.[4] The importance of all these factors cannot be over-stated – few people enjoy their first cigarette – and yet in England in 2002, 10% of children aged 11–15 smoked cigarettes regularly,[1] and in the USA in 2003, 28% of 12-year-olds and 54% of 16-year-olds had smoked tobacco at least once.[5] So preventing young people from taking their first few cigarettes is a highly significant intervention. Children and young adolescents who smoke tend to come from environments where smoking is already accepted behaviour (e.g. at home), from relatively deprived areas, to be under-achievers at school, and to have low self-esteem.[6] By the age of 20, 80% of smokers regret ever having started.[6]

Smokers claim that smoking alleviates anxiety and stress, and promotes relaxation. In fact nicotine is a stimulant and at least initially it has general mood-elevating properties, and causes arousal, increased concentration, and loss of appetite. Nicotine can reach the brain within 7 seconds of inhaling cigarette smoke and rapid-onset, short-lasting peaks of mild mood stimulation are believed to be important aspects of positive reinforcement. However, nicotine does not produce the intense euphoria of drugs such as cocaine. The initial effect is a mild 'buzz' or headiness to which the chronic smoker soon becomes largely tolerant. Negative reinforcement results from the desire to avoid nicotine withdrawal symptoms (which include anxiety), and this effect soon predominates as the principal reason for continuing to smoke. Anxiety also tends to stimulate habitual behaviour per se (e.g. biting nails, drumming fingers), and smoking is clearly a habitual pursuit.

Administration

Tobacco is smoked in cigarettes, which may be purchased ready-made or rolled by the smoker using tobacco and cigarette paper. Ready-made cigarettes usually have a filter that removes varying proportions of the constituents of the smoke before it enters the smoker's lungs. Tobacco may also be smoked in a pipe or as cigars. Tobacco smoke contains over 3000 chemicals, including many known to be carcinogenic, such as various nitrosamines and polycyclic aromatic hydrocarbons.

Nicotine is a liquid that normally boils at about 250°C. The end of a burning cigarette is at least 800°C and such temperatures are high enough to volatilise nicotine so that it can be inhaled. Occasionally tobacco is chewed; those who use this route tend to keep a 'quid' of tobacco in the side of the mouth, thus enabling buccal absorption. This allows a gentle peak plasma level of nicotine to develop. Nicotine is absorbed if swallowed but at least three-quarters of the dose is destroyed by the liver before reaching the systemic circulation. Snuff is a form of tobacco inhaled directly into the nose from the hand. It was much more popular in the 18th and 19th centuries than it is today.

Pharmacokinetics and pharmacology

Nicotine is metabolised mainly in the liver. Although several metabolic pathways are involved, the most important is the conversion of nicotine to the inactive cotinine by the cytochrome P450 isoenzyme 2A6. Nicotine has an average half-life of around 2 hours. Cotinine's longer half-life of 20 hours makes it a useful marker for exposure to tobacco.

Nicotine is an agonist at the so-called nicotinic receptors for acetylcholine. Most of its actions are confined to the central nervous system (CNS) at the doses achieved through smoking. Much larger amounts are needed to affect the nicotinic receptors on skeletal muscle. The mechanism of the psychotropic effects of nicotine is not known. The drug binds to nicotinic receptors in central ganglia of the autonomic nervous system where it can be an agonist or antagonist, depending upon the dose. Nicotine also triggers the release of many CNS neurotransmitters.

Adverse effects

About 350 years after a pronouncement from King James I about the evils of tobacco – an extract from which is reproduced at the beginning of this chapter – the true harmful effects of smoking began to be realised, in particular the effects of smoking on lung function and the development of lung cancer. As already mentioned, the WHO estimated that nearly 5 million people died worldwide as a result of tobacco smoking in 2000. Half of all smokers die prematurely as a result of smoking and lose on average 8 years of life. In developed countries this makes stopping the most significant health intervention in smokers. The majority of deaths are from lung cancer and coronary heart disease. Table 15.1 lists some of the other diseases known to be caused by smoking. Stopping at any age has both immediate and long-term health benefits, but the benefits are less in old age than in the young. Those who stop before the age of 35 have only a marginally decreased life expectancy compared to those who have never smoked.

Besides the serious health consequences, the tobacco smoker frequently suffers from a range of other more minor ailments, including decreased exercise tolerance, reduced appetite, weight loss, halitosis and an increased susceptibility to coughs and colds.

Non-smokers who are exposed to significant amounts of tobacco smoke may cough, become pale and feel nauseous. Other common complaints amongst passive smokers include dizziness, feeling faint,

Table 15.1 Mortality and morbidity linked to tobacco smoking[7]

Cancers caused by smoking
- Cancer of lung, mouth, pharynx and larynx
- Cancer of oesophagus, stomach, bladder, kidney and pancreas

Cancers less strongly linked to smoking
- Cancer of liver, cervix, nose and lip
- Adult myeloid leukaemia

Other diseases linked to smoking
- Chronic obstructive airways disease, pneumonia
- Ischaemic heart disease, myocardial infarction, pulmonary heart disease, aortic aneurysm
- Peripheral vascular disease
- Cerebrovascular disease
- Peptic ulcer, Crohn's disease, hernia, periodontal disease
- Osteoporosis, hip fracture
- Impotence, male infertility
- Cataracts, blindness (macular degeneration)
- Cot deaths for babies exposed to passive smoking
- Fires are an important cause of accidental death or injury that may result from careless smoking

tremor, headache, palpitations, loss of appetite and exacerbation of existing asthma. Passive smoking also increases the risk of developing lung cancer.

Intriguingly, epidemiological data suggest that some diseases seem to be less common in smokers. These may include cancer of the endometrium, hyperemesis gravidarum, ulcerative colitis, recurrent aphthous ulcers and Parkinson's disease.[8]

Dependence

Most smokers become dependent upon tobacco to some extent; they also exhibit tolerance. It is well established that nicotine is the substance in tobacco that causes physical dependence. Symptoms of withdrawal are not apparent in all smokers, but for the majority who do experience them they are the biggest barrier to quitting. Symptoms begin within 24 hours of cessation and can include:

- craving for nicotine
- restlessness, anxiety, irritability, emotional lability, frustration, anger
- depression
- inability to concentrate, drowsiness
- insomnia
- increased appetite, weight gain
- headaches.

These symptoms are at their most intense for the first week, but many of them subside over the ensuing 3 weeks or so.[6] However, craving for nicotine and increased appetite can last for months. Most smokers need several attempts at cessation before they are successful and most relapses occur early because of the unpleasant nature of withdrawal.

Non-pharmacological treatment

Various pharmacological methods have been used to help smokers stop, but non-pharmacological methods are also important. Simply attempting to stop with personal 'willpower' is effective in about 3% of attempts. These attempts are probably more effective if smokers plan a method for stopping: setting a definite date to stop, deciding on a technique for stopping (abrupt cessation or cutting down slowly), identifying a reason for stopping, enlisting help from friends and family, and specifying a reward if the attempt is successful.

Brief advice from a healthcare professional on smoking cessation increases the success rate by about 2%. Other non-pharmacological methods include self-help materials, and group and individual counselling or behavioural therapy. Behavioural and counselling therapies are more effective if conducted by fully trained professionals outside of a clinical setting. About 8% of patients motivated to attend such sessions do quit as a result.[9]

It is important to note that these non-pharmacological methods also boost the response to drug therapy. It is vital that patients understand that while medication can help them to quit they are not miracle cures for tobacco dependence – with any intervention the patient must still be motivated to stop.

Nicotine replacement therapy

This is a technique for replacing nicotine from tobacco with synthetic nicotine, and then withdrawing it from the patient – usually in a stepwise fashion – until the patient is no longer receiving any. Usually a course lasting 6–8 weeks is given.

The main advantage of nicotine replacement therapy (NRT) is that it replaces the principal dependence-producing agent in tobacco with a clean pharmaceutical source. The patient is thus no longer exposed to all the other chemicals in tobacco smoke that are responsible for the majority of serious side-effects. NRT also helps to prevent withdrawal symptoms by a method that removes the patient from the rituals, and environmental and social cues associated with smoking cigarettes. For successful withdrawal from tobacco, patients must learn to cope with triggers that might otherwise encourage recidivism, and NRT may help by initially maintaining dependency in the absence of the usual cues for lighting a cigarette.

NRT utilises various forms of drug delivery, including transdermal patches, nicotine-impregnated chewing gum, nasal sprays, lozenges and inhalers. All treatments significantly increase the success rate for attempts to stop smoking to about 17% at 1 year (compared to 10% for those on placebo).[10,11]

The rate of success with NRT is probably limited because replacing 'smoked' nicotine with 'therapeutic' nicotine is not an end in itself – just a different source of the problem. NRT does not completely prevent withdrawal and patients still have to cope with it to a greater or lesser extent. Also, none of the formulations reproduce identically the very rapid attainment of high nicotine levels that smokers come to expect from cigarettes.

There seems insufficient evidence to ascertain whether any one form of NRT is significantly more effective than another,[10,11] and there may be an advantage in encouraging patients themselves to choose between them in an informed way, and thus feel in greater control of the process. Patients may prefer one formulation over another after considering factors such as dosing schedule, ease of use, likely side-effects, and cost. For example, compared to other formulations, transdermal nicotine has the advantage of once-daily application, but it does not reproduce the frequently recurring high peaks in plasma nicotine levels that occur in smokers, and the dose cannot be suddenly increased acutely to help with craving. Patches can also cause local irritation at the site of administration. The gum formulation can cause a range of local side-effects such as mouth ulcers, salivation problems and sore throat as a consequence of the irritant properties of nicotine, and some users find the taste unpleasant. Similar side-effects have been reported with nicotine sublingual tablets. Furthermore, the gum requires a chewing technique that may not be easy to master. For those using nasal sprays, the irritant nature of nicotine can produce sneezing, runny nose, watery eyes and sore throat. Oral inhalers can also cause throat and mouth irritation. Because sprays provide more immediate psychoactive effects than any other form of NRT they may theoretically be more open to abuse.

Bupropion

This was originally marketed as an antidepressant, but it helps patients to stop smoking whether they are depressed or not. The mode of action is not clear. Treatment needs to start 1–2 weeks before the anticipated date for stopping smoking, and if initially successful it may continue for about 8 weeks. Bupropion significantly increases the success rate for attempts to stop smoking to about 19% at 1 year (compared to 9% for those on placebo).[10] At doses up to 300 mg daily, it has been associated with convulsions in 0.1% of recipients, and those at risk of seizures should not receive it.[12] The manufacturer gives a detailed warning about this and various other aspects of use of this medicine.[12]

Lobeline

In some countries over-the-counter (OTC) oral preparations are available that contain the nicotine-related alkaloid lobeline. These products have not been adequately tested in clinical trials.[13] The lack of data on effectiveness of lobeline led the Food and Drug Administration (FDA) in the USA to order the withdrawal of such products from the market.

Silver acetate

Silver acetate reacts with the constituents of cigarette smoke to produce an unpleasant taste in the mouth. Products utilising this effect include chewing gums and mouthwashes. Existing trials show little evidence of benefit.[14] The FDA has also removed them from sale in the USA.

Other drugs

Various anxiolytics have been used in an attempt to help smokers to stop, but results have been disappointing. They may be more useful in patients with overt anxiety. Clonidine has been used successfully, but its side-effects limit its usefulness in practice.[15] Larger clinical trials involving naltrexone are needed to assess any role that it may have.

Interaction with medicines

Polycyclic hydrocarbons in tobacco seem to induce the metabolism of some drugs. The classic example of a drug affected by this interaction is theophylline. Smokers exhibit a shorter theophylline half-life than non-smokers and may need bigger doses. A similar effect has been noted with, for example, propranolol, chlorpromazine, olanzapine, haloperidol, dextropropoxyphene and related drugs. It has also been noted that tobacco smokers with diabetes seem to require bigger doses of insulin for reasons that are not understood.

Women taking the combined oral contraceptive pill are at increased risk of thromboembolic disease. Smoking tobacco seems to further increase this risk.

Pregnancy and breastfeeding

Pregnancy

Tobacco smoking is associated with reduced oxygen supply and blood flow to the fetus. It has been well established that smoking in pregnancy increases the risks of the following effects: intra-uterine growth retardation, low birth weight, prematurity, ectopic pregnancy, spontaneous abortion, placental abruption, premature rupture of the membranes and increased perinatal mortality (including sudden infant death syndrome). These effects are probably more likely in women who are heavy smokers. Tobacco smoking has not been proven to cause specific congenital abnormalities, but studies have suggested a link between maternal smoking during pregnancy and childhood obesity[16] or asthma,[17] and a possible association with oral clefts. Abnormal behaviour and impairment of cognition may persist into childhood but these effects are often mild and it is difficult to be certain that they are not due to other factors that have not been separated from the effects of tobacco smoking. However, several studies suggest an association between exposure to tobacco in the womb and teenage or adult conduct disorders. The effects of reduced growth are usually overcome in early infancy.

Breastfeeding

Nicotine can be concentrated in milk and its metabolites are found in the urine of babies who ingest it. Nicotine has been suggested to cause infantile colic,[18,19] yet exposure to tobacco in pregnancy may also increase the risk of infantile colic post-partum.[20] The baby is exposed to nicotine partly via breast milk and partly via passive inhalation of smoke while the mother or other people smoke near to the infant. Passive smoking is associated with increased respiratory tract infections and sudden infant death syndrome. Nursing mothers who smoke may find that they stop breastfeeding sooner than non-smokers,[19] and they may also be less inclined to initiate breastfeeding.[21] Smokers who breastfeed may expose their babies to significantly higher amounts of cadmium than mothers who do not smoke.[22]

Mothers should not smoke just before feeding, to reduce infant exposure to peak milk levels of nicotine; they should also avoid smoking near the baby and should try to reduce consumption if possible.

References

1. Office of National Statistics. Smoking: rates highest in early 20s. Available at http://www.statistics.gov.uk/cci/nugget.asp?id=921 (published 29 July 2004; accessed 28 November 2004).
2. Anonymous. World deaths in 2000 attributable to selected leading risk factors. World Health Organization, 2002 (ref WHR 2002).
3. Mackay J, Crofton J. Tobacco and the developing world. Br Med Bull 1996 52: 206–221.
4. Lovato C, Linn G, Stead L F, *et al.* Impact of tobacco advertising and promotion on increasing adolescent smoking behaviours (Cochrane review). In:

The Cochrane Library, Issue 1, 2004. Chichester, UK: John Wiley & Sons Ltd.

5. Johnston L D, O'Malley P M, Bachman J G, *et al*. *Ecstasy Use Falls for Second Year in a Row, Overall Teen Drug Use Drops*. National press release, University of Michigan News and Information Services, Ann Arbor, 19 December 2003.

6. Jarvis M J. ABC of smoking cessation: why people smoke. *BMJ* 2004; 328: 277–279.

7. Wald N J, Hackshaw A J. Cigarette smoking: an epidemiological overview. *Br Med Bull* 1996; 52: 3–11.

8. Baron J A. Beneficial effects of nicotine and cigarette smoking: the real, the possible and the spurious. *Br Med Bull* 1996; 52: 58–73.

9. Coleman T. ABC of smoking cessation: use of simple advice and behavioural support. *BMJ* 2004; 328: 397–399.

10. *Guidance on the use of nicotine replacement therapy (NRT) and bupropion for smoking cessation*. Technology Appraisal No. 39. London: National Institute for Clinical Excellence, March 2002.

11. Silagy C, Lancaster T, Stead T, *et al*. Nicotine replacement therapy for smoking cessation (Cochrane review). In: *The Cochrane Library*, Issue 1, 2004. Chichester, UK: John Wiley & Sons Ltd.

12. Summary of Product Characteristics for Zyban. GlaxoSmithKline UK. Last updated 25 September 2003. http://www.emc.medicines.org.uk (accessed 28 November 2004).

13. Stead L F, Hughes J R. Lobeline for smoking cessation (Cochrane review). In: *The Cochrane Library*, Issue 1, 2004. Chichester, UK: John Wiley & Sons Ltd.

14. Lancaster T, Stead L F. Silver acetate for smoking cessation (Cochrane review). In: *The Cochrane Library*, Issue 1, 2004. Chichester, UK: John Wiley & Sons Ltd.

15. Gourlay S G, Stead L F, Benowitz N L. Clonidine for smoking cessation (Cochrane review). In: *The Cochrane Library*, Issue 1, 2004. Chichester, UK: John Wiley & Sons Ltd.

16. von Kries R, Toschke A M, Koletzko B, *et al*. Maternal smoking during pregnancy and childhood obesity. *Am J Epidemiol* 2002; 156: 954–961.

17. Jaakkola J J K, Gissler M. Maternal smoking in pregnancy, fetal development, and childhood asthma. *Am J Public Health* 2004; 94: 136–140.

18. Said G, Patois E, Lellouch J. Infantile colic and parental smoking. *BMJ* 1984; 289: 660.

19. Matheson I, Rivrud G N. The effect of smoking on lactation and infantile colic. *JAMA* 1989; 261: 42–43.

20. Sondergaard H, Henriksen T B, Obel C, *et al*. Smoking during pregnancy and infantile colic. *Pediatrics* 2001; 108: 342–346.

21. Leung G M, Ho L-M, Lam T-H. Maternal, paternal and environmental tobacco smoking and breast feeding. *Paediatr Perinat Epidemiol* 2002; 16: 236–245.

22. Milnerowicz H, Chmarek M. Effect of smoking on concentrations of cadmium, copper, iron and zinc in early transitional human milk. *Acta Toxicologica* 2003; 11: 85–91.

16

Alcohol

Caesar was the only sober man who ever tried to wreck the
Constitution.
Cato the Younger (95–46 BC)

History

Ethyl alcohol, ethanol or more simply 'alcohol' is very widely available, and compared with most other substances of abuse it has a simple chemical structure. It is produced by the action of yeast on sugars found in fruit and other plant material, and has been available to humans for several thousand years. It is easy to assume that alcohol was one of the first intoxicants used by early peoples because the manufacturing process is so straightforward. However, most of the fruits used to produce alcohol today have been artificially selected for their high sugar content so that the manufacture of fruit wines is a relatively simple process, but this was not so in prehistoric times when sugar-rich plants and sugars themselves were comparatively rare.[1] Therefore other plant-derived psychotropic substances that could simply be eaten without preparation almost certainly pre-date alcohol. The first cultures to produce alcohol are thought to have been based in the eastern Mediterranean and Mesopotamia. During the 4th millennium BC they probably fermented dates. The warm climate and the high sugar content of the dates were ideal for the purpose.[1] As the process spread, a whole range of naturally occurring substances were used to produce alcoholic drinks. Some of these are listed in Table 16.1.

The introduction of distillation enabled early civilisations to make more-concentrated alcoholic drinks. This process was probably discovered independently by several ancient societies. Concentrating the active constituent in this way enabled the alcohol to act as a preservative and beverages could be stored for longer. In Britain, the strength of alcohol-containing drinks was traditionally measured in terms of 'percentage proof'; 100 per cent proof is equal to 57.1% ethanol by volume. However, it is now standard practice to state alcohol content in terms

Table 16.1 Natural products used to produce alcoholic beverages

Source	Alcoholic beverage
Grapes	Wine (from which sherry, port and brandy are derived), grappa (Italy)
Barley	Beer (hops are added as a preservative and for flavour)
	Whisky (Irish varieties may also include fermented oats)
Rye	Rye whisky
Maize	Bourbon whisky
Rice	Saké (Japan)
Sugar cane or molasses	Rum
Apples	Cider, calvados
Pears	Perry
Plums	Slivovitz (E Europe)
Agave cactus	Tequila and Pulque (Mexico)
Palm sap	Toddy (Sri Lanka), palm wine (W Africa)
Cereal, potatoes or sugar beet	Vodka, poteen (Ireland), raki (Turkey), kvass (Russia and Eastern Europe)
Figs	Boukha (Tunisia)
Dates	Mahia (Morocco), thibarine (Tunisia)
Mare's milk	Koumish or milchsnapps
Honey	Mead

of percentage by volume, and to refer to the content of individual drinks in terms of 'units' (see Table 16.2).

In many Islamic countries the consumption of alcohol is illegal because it is condemned in the Qur'an and other Muslim texts. Elsewhere, alcohol is very widely accepted, even being used as a central part of the Christian religious ceremony known as the Communion or Mass. It is also commonly used in a celebratory context in association with major events in people's lives – weddings, birthdays and special celebrations. A vast and profitable industry exists to supply the public with this inebriant, which can have very pleasurable effects but which can also kill. It is not surprising that many people feel that society has a rather hypocritical attitude to psychotropic substances: condemning illicit substances on the one hand while condoning the wide-scale use of alcohol on the other.

Table 16.2 Alcohol content of different drinks as expressed in the UK[3]

Alcoholic beverage	Alcohol content (% v/v)
Beers and lagers	2.5–5.5
Cider	3.5–5
Wine	9.5–15
Sherry, port	16–23
Spirits, liqueurs	35–55

Examples of applying the alcohol unit concept to specific drinks:
One pint (568 mL) of ordinary strength lager, beer or cider (3.5%) = 2 units
One pint (568 mL) of strong lager (5.2%) = 3 units
A glass (175 mL) of red or white wine (11.5%) = 2 units
A club measure (25 mL) of spirits (40%) = 1 unit
One bottle (275 mL) of an alcopop (5%) = 1.5 units

A comparison of alcohol consumption per capita of population (all ages) in several countries in 2000 has been published.[2] This expressed consumption in terms of litres of pure alcohol. Alcohol consumption was highest in France with 10.5 litres per capita. For other countries the approximate figures were the UK 8, Australia 7.8, and USA 6.5. In the UK in 2002/3 the amount of alcohol consumed per person aged over 16 was 11.5 litres.[3] In 2002, total UK expenditure on alcohol by consumers was £38.4 billion.[3] In all studies, the amount of alcohol consumed is greatest amongst men, and greatest of all in men aged 20–29.

In 2001 the Australian government estimated that 10% of the population aged over 14 consumed alcohol at a level considered 'risky' or 'high risk' for long-term alcohol-related harm.[4] A UK household survey in 2001 showed that 27% of men and 15% of women drank more than the recommended weekly amounts of alcohol on average – more than 21 and 14 units respectively.[3] These figures have remained reasonably constant since 1992. A separate survey in Great Britain in 2000 suggested that 7% of the adult population were dependent upon alcohol.[3] In the USA, there were an estimated 11 million alcoholics in 1995 – some 4–5% of the population.[5]

There has been increasing concern that teenagers may be encouraged to consume large amounts of alcohol by the marketing of concentrated alcoholic beverages in forms similar to soft drinks, such as lemonades and other sweet, fruit-flavoured drinks. These are sometimes called alcopops. There is also concern about the effects of alcohol advertising on adolescents – both explicit advertising and indirect via films, television and music.[6] In the USA, 46% of 12-year-olds surveyed in 2003 reported that they had ever consumed alcohol, and 20% had been drunk at least once.[7] For 16-year-olds, 77% had ever consumed alcohol, and 58% had been drunk at least once. In England in 2002, 24% of 11- to 15-year-olds in a national survey said they had consumed alcohol in the past week – but this was 5% of 11-year-olds and 47% of 15-year-olds.[3] However, this figure does not illustrate sufficiently the prevalence of under-age drinking in the UK: a survey of 758 schoolchildren aged 12–15 in Dundee, Scotland, in 1996 concluded that over half of them had been drunk at least once.[8] Another study of 7722 pupils aged 15 and 16 from across the UK published in 1996 revealed that 94% of participants had already consumed alcohol and 78% of these had become drunk at least once.[9]

Effects sought

Alcohol is a central nervous system (CNS) depressant that encourages disinhibition because the highest levels of brain function are most susceptible to it. Depression of the cerebral cortex causes reduced inhibition, merriment, loquacity, risk-taking behaviour and impaired judgement. As with nearly all psychoactive substances, the precise effects vary according to the dose, the mood of the user, and the environment. Blood alcohol concentrations of 0.2–0.7 g/L are required for these effects to occur.

It has been shown that a moderate daily intake of alcohol (up to 3 drinks per day) can reduce overall mortality, and that in people consuming these amounts there is a reduced incidence of coronary heart disease, diabetes and ischaemic stroke.[10-15] Not all studies individually support this finding, but the larger studies and meta-analyses do support it. Cardiovascular deaths in hypertensive men are also significantly reduced by regular alcohol consumption.[16] Another study has suggested that people with higher cholesterol levels may benefit more from alcohol.[17] There is insufficient evidence to be certain whether particular types of alcoholic drink confer greater protection.

Administration

Alcohol is taken orally, primarily in the form of a drink. The alcohol content of drinks varies considerably so, as a means of enabling people to compare the intoxicating potential of different drinks, the idea of an alcohol 'unit' was created. A unit of alcohol is equivalent to 10 mL (8 g) of pure alcohol. This concept has proved popular, but it may be promoted differently in different countries. In the UK, the government has offered guidance on the typical number of units per alcoholic drink (see Table 16.2), and has also stated that the recommended maximum weekly intake for men is 21 units and for women 14 units, divided equally over the course of the week.[3] Recommendations on intake vary in other countries. As well as focusing on suitable daily and weekly intakes, the social and health consequences of binge drinking should be stressed as acute episodes of intoxication are linked to a variety of adverse social, criminal and health consequences. Frequent episodes of binge drinking may also be a prelude to alcoholism.

In addition to use as a beverage, alcoholic drinks are used in cooking as flavourings. Alcohol is also employed as a solvent, cleaner and fuel in products such as liquid metal polishes, aftershaves, mouthwashes and methylated spirits. Unfortunately, these products are sometimes consumed by alcoholics as a cheap or more readily available source of concentrated alcohol.

Pharmacokinetics and pharmacology

Alcohol has a variety of actions on the brain.[18] Although it has a relatively non-specific mode of action it does affect particular neurotransmitter systems and is not simply a general CNS depressant as was once thought. However, there is no ethanol 'receptor': alcohol interacts with other CNS receptors by altering their configuration, thus affecting the binding of endogenous chemicals. Alcohol seems to augment the actions of the inhibitory neurotransmitter gamma-aminobutyric (GABA) and to antagonise certain effects of the excitatory glutamate. This is probably the mechanism of many of the CNS depressant actions of alcohol. The effects on GABA, plus an ability to trigger the release of neurotransmitters such as exogenous opioids and dopamine, may explain the pleasurable feelings evoked by alcohol and its reinforcing potential. Stimulation of $5HT_3$ receptors may be part of the reason for alcohol causing nausea and vomiting.

Alcohol is absorbed passively from the gastrointestinal tract – a process that begins as soon as alcohol enters the mouth. It is absorbed from the stomach but passes across the mucosa of the small intestine much more rapidly because of the larger surface area. Food in the stomach will therefore decrease the rate of absorption by delaying the passage of alcohol into the small intestine. The alcohol will continue to be absorbed from the stomach but at a slower rate. Peak concentrations are achieved in blood 20–60 minutes after ingestion, depending on the amount of alcohol ingested, its concentration and whether there is food in the stomach.

Alcohol is deactivated mainly via metabolism in the liver, although about 5% is lost in the breath, urine and sweat. The majority of alcohol ingested is metabolised by alcohol dehydrogenase to acetaldehyde. However, the cytochrome P450 isoenzyme 2E1 also facilitates the conversion as does, to a small extent, the enzyme catalase. Acetaldehyde is further degraded to acetic acid, mainly by aldehyde dehydrogenase in the liver. Acetic acid is then either converted to carbon dioxide and water in peripheral tissues and excreted or – because acetic acid is formed by a variety of means in the body – incorporated into the metabolic pathways of carbohydrate or lipid.

Alcohol dehydrogenase is only available in small amounts in infants under 5, hence their comparatively increased sensitivity to alcohol. One form of aldehyde dehydrogenase is commonly deficient in a high proportion of Oriental races; affected individuals often dislike alcohol ingestion because of the build-up of acetaldehyde, which causes flushing and nausea.

The half-life is dose-dependent because the amount of alcohol ingested is usually too great for enzyme systems to handle (i.e. zero-order kinetics). The conversion of alcohol to acetaldehyde is the limiting step. The rate of human elimination of ethanol varies from 80 to 150 mg/kg per hour; the average clearance is 100 mg/kg per hour.

Adverse effects

The adverse effects of alcohol on society are difficult to measure. The World Health Organization (WHO) estimates that in 2000, 1.8 million people died worldwide as a result of the effects of alcohol.[19] Over 90% of these deaths were in men. In economic terms, the drug has significant impact upon health and industry expenditures, and the costs of crime must also be met. Taking account of these factors, in the USA an estimate of the economic costs of alcohol abuse for 1998 was $184.6 billion for the whole country.[20] It was estimated that in 2003, alcohol abuse in the UK cost up to £20 billion.[3] (Interestingly, total UK tax revenue from alcoholic drinks in the same period was £11.7 billion.)

A detailed list of potential adverse effects is given in Table 16.3. Some of these are discussed in more detail below.

Acute effects

Acute intake of alcohol can produce a wide range of effects in the **central nervous system**. Intoxication is an important factor in many

Table 16.3 Adverse effects of alcohol

Acute effects
- Intoxication leading to accidents, emotional lability, aggression, risk-taking behaviour and criminal acts
- Incoordination, ataxia, slurred speech
- Dulled mentation, reduced audiovisual acuity, drowsiness, loss of consciousness, respiratory depression, death
- Flushing, hypothermia
- Diuresis, dehydration
- Gastritis, nausea, vomiting, oesophageal reflux, haematemesis
- Sleep apnoea, inhalation of vomit
- Hypoglycaemia
- Raised blood pressure, arrhythmias

Effects of chronic heavy ingestion
- Oral, pharyngeal and laryngeal cancers
- Reflux oesophagitis, Mallory–Weiss tears (rupture of oesophageal mucosa), oesophageal cancer, oesophageal varices
- Gastritis, impaired healing of upper gastrointestinal ulcers, diarrhoea
- Fatty liver, liver cirrhosis, alcoholic hepatitis, liver cancer
- Pancreatitis, pancreatic cancer
- Malnutrition, weight loss, dehydration
- Alcoholic cardiomyopathy, tachyarrhythmias (especially atrial fibrillation), sudden death
- Hypertension
- Hypomagnesaemia, hypocalcaemia, hypophosphataemia, hypokalaemia
- Hyperuricaemia, metabolic acidosis
- Gynaecomastia, decreased libido, impotence, decreased male fertility, menstrual irregularities
- Increased risk of breast cancer
- Myopathy, muscle weakness, muscle pain, rhabdomyolysis
- Peripheral neuropathy, sensory and motor polyneuritis
- Wernicke's encephalopathy, Korsakoff's psychosis, stroke, CNS infection, tobacco–alcohol amblyopia, cerebellar degeneration, central pontine myelinolysis
- Depression, paranoia, anxiety
- Memory loss, blackouts

accidents involving both the affected individual (drowning, falling, suffocation) and other people (road traffic accidents). In Great Britain it is estimated that in 2002, there were 20,140 casualties in traffic accidents where alcohol levels in the blood were above legal limits.[3] This was about 6% of all traffic accident casualties. It is also a significant factor in a high proportion of violent crimes and acts of aggression. The changes produced by disinhibition can result in fights and other forms of antisocial behaviour, unprotected sex, and the desire to use other substances of abuse. The effects of alcohol may result in serious disruption to important relationships.

As the concentration of alcohol in the bloodstream increases to about 1–1.5 g/L, basic brain functions become affected (loss of taste, reduced audiovisual acuity, slurred speech, awkward gait). The ultimate sequelae of CNS depression – loss of consciousness, respiratory depression and death – are seen at blood alcohol concentrations greater than 3–4 g/L.

One or two units of alcohol will encourage **sleep** through simple CNS depression, but larger doses tend to cause poor sleep because the somatic sympathetic nervous system is activated by alcohol, and its stimulating effects dominate once the effects of ethanol wear off. Sleep in the early morning is therefore often restless and punctuated by vivid dreams. Alcohol may cause or exacerbate snoring and obstructive sleep apnoea, which also gives rise to poor quality sleep in those affected.

Acute physical adverse effects of alcohol are well known. **Flushing** occurs because alcohol depresses the vasomotor centre in the medulla, resulting in dilation of blood vessels in the skin. Alcohol can sometimes cause hypothermia in cold weather when cutaneous vasodilation is coupled with inhibition of the thermoregulatory centre in the hypothalamus. **Diuresis** is a consequence of the inhibition of antidiuretic hormone production from the pituitary and, especially in hot environments, it can give rise to dehydration.

Gastrointestinal effects are common. Gastritis, vomiting and oesophageal reflux can result from acute intake of large amounts of alcohol because alcohol inhibits gastric emptying, as well as irritating the gastric mucosa. Gastric irritation is a direct action of alcohol, as well as a consequence of the stimulation of the production of gastric secretions. Haematemesis may occur in severe cases. When unconsciousness occurs, death may arise from inhalation of vomit.

Cardiac arrhythmias, especially atrial fibrillation, are established effects of acute heavy alcohol consumption in non-alcoholics, which often resolve spontaneously and do not recur if future alcohol intake is moderated.[21,22]

Alcohol hangover

This is a term used to describe the unpleasant aftermath of an acute excess of alcohol. It typically ensues a few hours after the last drink, but not all those who drink alcohol experience it. Symptoms may include:

- headache
- nausea, vomiting, stomach cramps, diarrhoea, loss of appetite
- tiredness, fatigue
- tremor
- anxiety, remorse
- overall poor sense of well-being.

During a hangover the levels of various hormones in the body are altered – in particular the levels of anti-diuretic hormone, aldosterone and renin are all raised. Alcohol also alters the mode of cytokine production, such that thromboxane-B_2 levels in plasma are increased.

It is not known what causes the hangover, and it may be due to a variety of factors. However, on balance, perhaps 'congeners' are the most likely causative agents of alcohol hangover.[23,24] Congeners are the other organic compounds found in alcoholic drinks besides ethanol, and include substances such as methanol and aldehydes. Drinks with a high congener content (e.g. red wine, brandy and whisky) tend to cause worse and more frequent hangovers than low congener drinks (e.g. vodka, gin). This has been demonstrated in experiments where volunteers were given equivalent amounts of alcohol as high-congener and low-congener drinks, and the incidence and severity of hangovers compared.

Effects of chronic high-dose use

Regular intake of large amounts of alcohol can lead to dependence, also known as alcoholism. Physical dependence is evidenced by tolerance to the effects of alcohol and an unpleasant withdrawal reaction when administration ceases (see below). Alcoholics may put considerable effort into maintaining a high alcohol intake in order to stave off withdrawal, often despite adverse social and medical consequences. The social consequences may include disrupted relationships, unemployment, poverty, acts of violence, criminality and loneliness. Alcoholism can give rise to a range of serious adverse medical effects, some of which can be fatal. Women and individuals under 50 years of age seem to be the groups most at risk of dying early (from any cause) as a result of prolonged heavy intake. Some of these effects are described below.

The **liver** is notoriously susceptible to alcohol-induced damage. Abuse of alcohol for a few days causes a fatty liver in most people, but this is an asymptomatic condition that is reversible after a short period of abstinence. The more serious forms of liver disease that occur in alcoholics include hepatitis and cirrhosis, which may develop sequentially, simultaneously, or either may occur in isolation.[25] Hepatotoxicity may be associated with a wide range of symptoms depending on the duration and severity of liver damage, including oesophageal varices, gastrointestinal bleeding, jaundice, ascites, hepatic encephalopathy and increased susceptibility to infection. Patients who continue to drink alcohol after recovering from hepatitis have a 7-year survival rate of 50%, whereas those who manage to stop have an 80% survival rate.[25] Cirrhosis can cause permanent damage to the liver if the characteristic fibrotic changes are extensive; its prognosis is difficult to estimate but is generally worse if major complications exist such as ascites. Liver transplant is sometimes an option for patients with alcoholic liver disease who have a low risk of resuming alcohol intake afterwards. Liver cancer is more common in alcoholics, as are cancers of the mouth, oesophagus and stomach. Long-term alcohol intake can also cause pancreatitis.

The **cardiovascular** consequences of alcoholism include hypertension, which is commonly seen in alcoholics, and may contribute to the evolution of other cardiovascular problems. Cardiomyopathy is a recognised consequence of long-term heavy drinking, which is probably reversible in the early stages if alcohol consumption is abandoned.[26] It is sometimes called alcoholic heart muscle disease. Tachyarrhythmias, especially atrial fibrillation,[22] are also associated with alcoholism, as is sudden death (perhaps due to ventricular fibrillation). Electrolyte disturbances may play a part in some cases of cardiac toxicity: for example hypomagnesaemia is a well-known problem caused by chronic alcohol excess.

Neurological disorders are common in alcoholics.[27] Some of these arise as a result of poor diet. Malnutrition results when alcoholics come to depend upon alcohol as a source of energy to the exclusion of food: 1 g of alcohol supplies about 7 calories. Water-soluble vitamins are markedly susceptible to depletion because they are not stored in the body and depend upon dietary intake to maintain their role. Vitamin B_1 (thiamine) deficiency is a particular problem because its absence can cause the death of certain neurones. Alcoholics have a reduced dietary intake of this vitamin, but oral absorption of thiamine can also be reduced in alcoholism, as can its metabolic activation. Vitamin B_1 deficiency is the primary cause of Wernicke's encephalopathy. This is characterised by symptoms such as confusion, unsteadiness, double vision, memory impairment, hypothermia with hypotension, or decreased level of consciousness. Patients with any signs, or potential signs, of this condition must be treated with high-dose parenteral thiamine immediately, as the condition is reversible if treated early.[28] The active transport mechanism by which thiamine enters the brain is slow and easily saturable; high parenteral doses ensure that thiamine crosses the blood–brain barrier more rapidly and in greater amounts by establishing a favourable concentration gradient for passive diffusion.[29]

Ideally, thiamine should be given to all alcoholics admitted to hospital because most are likely to be deficient to some extent, even if this is not clinically apparent. Low-dose oral thiamine, or compound vitamin B tablets, are of no value in treating suspected Wernicke's encephalopathy because the thiamine content is too low. However, some practitioners may use high-dose oral thiamine during detoxification in patients without Wernicke's symptoms in an attempt to correct any deficiency in a non-invasive manner. Similarly, low-dose daily 'maintenance' doses of oral thiamine or compound vitamin B tablets may be prescribed for alcoholics after detoxification in an attempt to correct the reduced dietary intake of B group vitamins on an ongoing basis. It is not known whether these prophylactic oral measures are effective – compliance is likely to be a significant problem in those given maintenance doses who return to drinking.

Korsakoff's syndrome is another serious brain disorder that has also been linked to thiamine deficiency. Unlike Wernicke's, to which it may be a sequel, it does not appear to be reversible. The patient characteristically has a gross failure of recent memory and may cope with this inability to remember by confabulation. Other symptoms can include psychosis, delirium and painful extremities.

Sensory and motor neuropathies occur commonly in alcoholics, particularly in the lower limbs. They can result from thiamine deficiency, but also from a direct toxic effect of alcohol or its metabolites. Non-alcoholic patients with thiamine deficit neuropathy have been compared with alcoholic patients who have neuropathy but no thiamine deficiency.[30] This suggests that alcohol itself causes a slowly progressing, sensory-dominant neuropathy with superficial pain or painful burning sensations. Thiamine deficiency seems to cause a motor-dominant neuropathy that is acutely progressive. In practice, alcoholics understandably seem to show a mixture of these two presentations.

Cerebellar malfunction manifests primarily as ataxia and dysarthria, and is potentially also linked to thiamine deficiency. Central pontine myelinolysis is characterised by demyelination of neurones at the base of the pons. This can result in paralysis. The condition is probably caused by iatrogenic over-rapid correction of hyponatraemia, but the exact mechanism is not known.[27]

The mechanism of the ischaemic or haemorrhagic strokes that occur in those ingesting large amounts of alcohol chronically is probably multifactorial, involving alcohol effects on blood coagulability, blood pressure, emboli arising due to cardiac toxicity, and reductions in cerebral blood flow.[14]

The long-term **endocrine** effects of alcohol are largely confined to carbohydrate metabolism and reproductive function. Chronic heavy consumption of alcohol is associated with an increased risk of developing diabetes.[15] It may also cause gynaecomastia, decreased libido, impotence and infertility in men, largely because of inhibition of hormone production at both pituitary level and testis. In women, alcohol may be the cause of absent or irregular menstruation.

Alcohol withdrawal

In the alcoholic, acute withdrawal usually begin within 12 hours of the last intake of alcohol and lasts for up to a week. Symptoms are summarised in Table 16.4. It should be noted that a minority of heavy regular consumers of alcohol do not experience withdrawal symptoms at all.

Table 16.4 Symptoms of alcohol withdrawal

Common features
- Hand tremor
- Sweating, flushing
- Anxiety, agitation, confusion, disorientation
- Minor transient hallucinations which the patient knows are due to withdrawal
- Tachycardia
- Nausea, vomiting, anorexia, diarrhoea
- Insomnia
- Convulsions

Less-common features
- Arrhythmias, hypertension
- Paraesthesiae
- Hepatic dysfunction
- Suicidal ideation

Delirium tremens
- Severe hallucinations often evoking extreme fear (mainly visual but may be tactile or auditory)
- Delirium, violent behaviour, severe depression
- Hyperpyrexia, dehydration, electrolyte abnormalities
- Convulsions

Acute withdrawal can progress to delirium tremens in about 5% of cases. If this happens there is a deterioration in the patient's level of consciousness and cognition, and frightening hallucinations are common. Delirium tremens may be fatal.

Many alcoholics have intermittent periods of reduced alcohol intake when symptoms of withdrawal may occur, but this usually encourages a return to old habits (negative reinforcement). Full-scale 'detoxification' usually requires admission to a psychiatric hospital, specialised alcohol detoxification unit or a general medical ward. In the UK, chlordiazepoxide is generally used during withdrawal to ease the patient's symptoms. In other countries, diazepam and clomethiazole are also used. Drug users rate the euphoria from diazepam much more highly than that from chlordiazepoxide, and this may be because diazepam has a faster onset of action.[31] Because chlordiazepoxide may be less liable to abuse than diazepam it should be the preferred drug; it also has a longer half-life than clomethiazole. These drugs alleviate many of the symptoms of alcohol withdrawal, but it is important to realise that their function is to make withdrawal more bearable – they do not prevent it.

There are two approaches to prescribing sedatives for alcohol withdrawal. The first uses a fixed dose reduction schedule starting with high doses on the first day of withdrawal – for example 60 mg or more of chlordiazepoxide in divided doses – and this dose is then reduced every day in a predetermined way. The second method is to allow patients to receive a dose of sedative 'as required', whenever an evaluation of their symptoms exceeds a predetermined score on a rating scale. The second method is as effective as the first, although more labour intensive, but it allows individualisation of therapy, usage of less drug, and a shorter period of medication.[32,33] Whichever method is used, lower doses should generally be used in the elderly, and in patients with severe liver impairment where hepatic encephalopathy is a potential adverse effect of administering sedative drugs. The amount of drug used should become less each day and then must be stopped completely.

Clomethiazole has gained some notoriety in the UK as a drug on which alcoholics can become dependent, and which can have dangerous CNS depressant actions if taken with alcohol.[34,35] It also has a shorter half-life than the benzodiazepines chlordiazepoxide or diazepam. This has led to UK recommendations that clomethiazole be avoided as an aid to alcohol withdrawal.[34,28] However, many of the problems associated with clomethiazole may have been caused by prescribing inappropriately long courses of treatment, inadequate patient supervision, failure to review treatment regularly and, worst of all, prescribing 'maintenance' doses that serve no purpose but do encourage dependence and dangerous additive effects with alcohol if drinking is resumed. Although these problems have been particularly associated with clomethiazole, benzodiazepines can also have additive CNS depressant effects with alcohol and can cause dependence if prescribed inappropriately. Consequently, courses of sedative drugs prescribed for alcohol withdrawal should not be extended because of the risk of adding sedative dependence to the patient's existing problems. Similarly, inpatients should not be allowed to take supplies of medication home with them when they leave hospital – not only because of the risk of dependence but because in the (common) event of recidivism, the effects of alcohol and sedatives are additive. Alcoholics might also sell sedative drugs on the black market.

Carbamazepine has been used to treat acute alcohol withdrawal and limited evidence suggests that it has some potential advantages over the sedatives discussed above in terms of tolerability and speed of response.[36] Clonidine relieves some of the withdrawal symptoms mediated by the sympathetic nervous system (e.g. tremors, palpitations) but has no anxiolytic, sedative or anticonvulsant actions. It is therefore not widely used. Intravenous alcohol has sometimes been used in intensive care units to treat alcohol withdrawal. However, the evidence to support this practice is weak – being mainly derived from small open studies – and there are significant concerns about dosing, monitoring and safety.[37]

The anticonvulsant action of benzodiazepines or clomethiazole is often sufficient to prevent withdrawal seizures, but if convulsions do occur, diazepam rectal solution or lorazepam injection can be given. Recurrent fitting can be controlled with a regular anticonvulsant (e.g. carbamazepine) but alcoholics may not comply.

Haloperidol is sometimes advocated for the alleviation of distressing hallucinations or aggressive behaviour.[38] However, neuroleptic agents with anti-dopamine actions in the CNS may exacerbate delirium. Furthermore, most antipsychotic drugs tend to lower the seizure threshold and can cause liver damage, hepatic encephalopathy or interfere with temperature regulation. Neuroleptics such as haloperidol must therefore be used with extreme caution. It is rare to encounter a situation where the simple sedative actions of benzodiazepines are insufficient, and many detoxification units never use neuroleptics.[39]

During the process of acute withdrawal many alcoholics will require rehydration and correction of electrolyte abnormalities, according to their individual circumstances.

Maintaining abstinence

After passing through the period of acute withdrawal, the patient requires other forms of support to maintain abstinence. Especially during the first 6 months of abstinence there may be craving for alcohol, often associated with depression. Aspects of lifestyle that help to fuel dependence need to be addressed, e.g. unemployment, homelessness and problems with relationships. Some alcoholics also suffer from specific psychiatric disorders such as depression, schizophrenia or anxiety, which may require treatment. Various forms of counselling and support are available but the self-help methods offered by Alcoholics Anonymous remain popular. However, some drug therapies are available that may also help.

Acamprosate is used to maintain abstinence in alcoholics following withdrawal. In alcohol-dependent laboratory animals it reduces the voluntary ingestion of alcohol in a dose-related manner. A derivative of the amino acid taurine, acamprosate potentiates the actions of the inhibitory neurotransmitter GABA in the CNS and antagonises the excitatory transmitter glutamate, i.e. it has a similar action to alcohol. Glutamate receptors have been observed to proliferate in the brains of alcoholics, suggesting that overactivity of excitatory neurosystems in the brain upon withdrawal of alcohol may be at least partly responsible for craving. If chronic alcohol consumption disrupts the balance between excitatory and inhibitory neurotransmission in the CNS, acamprosate may act by helping to restore it and thus reduce craving. Acamprosate does seem to increase the likelihood of maintaining abstinence in alcoholics after withdrawal reasonably consistently, and several studies have assessed effectiveness over the course of a year.[40] However, the magnitude of response varies quite considerably between trials. Acamprosate does not treat withdrawal, prevent alcohol intoxication, interact with it or lessen any of the harmful effects of alcohol. It also does not produce intoxication or dependence, and is generally well tolerated.

Naltrexone is an opioid antagonist and, as has already been noted, alcohol seems to increase the release of endogenous opioids. Like acamprosate, laboratory work has shown that alcohol-dependent animals will choose to take alcohol less often when administered naltrexone. A Cochrane review of published studies suggested short-term effectiveness, but noted the limited number of clinical trials and that the beneficial effects of naltrexone may not last long after the cessation of treatment.[41] As with acamprosate there is variability between clinical trials in terms of the magnitude of response observed.

Selective serotonin reuptake inhibitors (SSRIs) such as citalopram and fluoxetine have been shown in limited studies to reduce the desire to consume alcohol. In animal research, the boosting of central serotonin levels seems to reduce the voluntary consumption of alcohol. In humans, only small-scale, short-term studies are available, and these have shown that although SSRIs may significantly reduce craving for alcohol, this does not always correspond to a marked decrease in intake. The response to treatment is highly variable.[42] Larger and longer-term studies are needed.

Disulfiram is occasionally used to try to control alcohol intake. It usually produces unpleasant symptoms if the recipient imbibes alcohol during the course of treatment. Drugs of this kind are termed antidipsotropics. Disulfiram irreversibly inhibits the enzyme aldehyde dehydrogenase, and this results in greatly increased plasma levels of acetaldehyde if alcohol is ingested. Symptoms of acetaldehyde accumulation include facial flushing, pulsing headache, nausea, dizziness, weakness, orthostatic hypotension and palpitations. Some of these effects can last for several days. The inhibiting effect on the enzyme is permanent and one dose of disulfiram can continue to be effective for up to 2 weeks. However, the benefits of disulfiram are limited – not all alcoholics will accept this treatment and even those that appear to accept it may not comply. In addition, some alcoholics do not experience the so-called 'disulfiram reaction' with alcohol or may experience symptoms that can be tolerated; for others the reaction may cause a wide range of serious adverse effects (e.g. arrhythmias, heart failure, hepatotoxicity).

Interactions with medicines

The interactions between alcohol and medicines have been reviewed in detail elsewhere.[43,44] However, some example interactions are:

1. **Additive side-effects.** When alcohol is consumed by patients taking medicines with CNS depressant actions, there tends to be an additive effect producing sedation, incoordination, etc. Medicines that may interact in this way include amitriptyline, benzodiazepines and opioids. The combination can be unexpectedly potent in some people.

   Alcohol may increase the gastrointestinal bleeding associated with aspirin and non-steroidal anti-inflammatory drugs, and chronic consumption may potentiate the hepatotoxicity of medicines such as paracetamol and isoniazid.

2.   **Metabolism of medicines.** Intake of moderate amounts of alcohol does not seem to affect the metabolism of warfarin. However, chronic heavy alcohol intake may accelerate its metabolism.

3.   **Disulfiram reaction.** When taken with alcohol some medicines may produce an unpleasant reaction characterised by gastrointestinal upset, facial flushing and other features. Medicines that can be affected include metronidazole, procarbazine and cefamandole.

Pregnancy and breastfeeding

Pregnancy

The effects of alcohol in pregnancy are probably dose-dependent so continued heavy drinking is more likely to affect the fetus, and the worst adverse effects are seen in alcoholics. In terms of damage to the fetus, it is particularly difficult to separate the contribution made directly by high levels of ethanol from other aspects of the alcoholic's lifestyle. For example, alcoholics often have a very poor diet and are more likely to smoke. Despite this it is generally believed that alcohol is teratogenic. Fetal alcohol syndrome (FAS) has been identified in babies born to alcoholics and those who regularly drink heavily, although many of these women are delivered of apparently healthy babies. FAS has the following characteristics:

*   intra-uterine growth retardation (including reduced weight at birth and decreased head circumference);
*   characteristic facial changes;
*   neurological defects (eg reduced mental ability and brain anomalies).

There may also be a link with other congenital abnormalities (e.g. heart damage, genitourinary defects) but the evidence to support an association is more limited. In addition, FAS is associated with delayed mental development, retardation, low IQ and various behavioural problems later in life. Reduced growth rate and small size can also continue into childhood, although facial changes may diminish with time. FAS has been associated with 'heavy drinking' but the precise definition of this in terms of the quantity of alcohol required is unclear. FAS probably represents the worst end of a spectrum of dose-related damage that alcohol can cause to the fetus. Babies born to women who drink smaller amounts of ethanol than consumed by an alcoholic can still show evidence of harm such as minor anomalies, growth deficiency and behavioural problems. Moderate to heavy alcohol use in pregnancy may also be associated with an increased risk of spontaneous abortion.

Some neonates appear to be delivered with CNS depression caused by alcohol and experience withdrawal reactions. Symptoms include tremors, irritability, apnoea, restlessness, hypertonia and agitation. These usually appear within a few hours of birth and resolve within a few days.

There is no particular evidence that an occasional single drink is associated with an adverse effect on pregnancy outcome but a 'safe' level of drinking in pregnancy has not been established. It is also not clear whether alcohol can cause damage at any stage of pregnancy or whether there are periods of lesser risk.

Breastfeeding

Alcohol passes into breast milk, although acetaldehyde, the major pharmacologically active metabolite, does not. Very large maternal doses caused a reversible 'Cushing's syndrome-like' effect in one breastfed infant[45] and 'drunkenness' in another baby.[46] However, these are isolated reports. A more ubiquitous property of alcohol is its ability to inhibit milk ejection in a dose-dependent way by blocking the release of oxytocin from the pituitary in response to suckling.[47] A high intake of alcohol can inhibit milk flow completely. When breastfeeding occurs immediately after consuming an alcoholic drink, the infant is found to consume only about three-quarters of the amount of milk that it would do otherwise.[47] The precise reasons for this are unclear but it may be that alcohol imparts a disagreeable taste to the milk.

One study has suggested that regular alcohol intake can adversely affect motor development at 1 year.[48] One drink a day had only slight effects, occasional drinking had no effect. The impairment was more marked if more than six drinks a day were taken during nursing. No adverse mental effects were reported.

Notwithstanding these effects, it is generally considered acceptable to consume small amounts of alcohol while breastfeeding. However, it is easy to avoid breastfeeding for 1 or 2 hours after a single alcoholic drink – thus reducing infant exposure – and this should be recommended.

References

1.   Rudgley R. *The Alchemy of Culture: Intoxicants in Society*. London: British Museum Press, 1993, 30–33.

2.   Australian Institute of Criminology. Total alcohol consumption by country 2000. In: *Alcohol and Illicit Drugs in Australia*. Canberra: Australian Government, 2003.

3.   *Statistics on alcohol: England, 2003*. Statistical Bulletin 2003/20. London: National Statistics Office and Department of Health. 30 October 2003. http://www.publications.doh.gov.uk/public/sb0320.pdf (accessed 28 November 2004).

4.   *Statistics on Drug Use in Australia 2002. Drug Statistics Series No. 12*. Cat no. PHE 43. Canberra: Australian Institute of Health and Welfare, February 2003.

5.   Williams G D, Stinson F S, Parker D A, *et al*. J. Epidemiologic Bulletin No. 15: Demographic trends, alcohol abuse and alcoholism, 1985–1995. *Alcohol Health Res World* 1987; 11: 80–83, 91.

6.   Strasburger V C. Alcohol advertising and adolescents. *Pediatr Clin North Am* 2002; 49: 353–376.

7.   Johnston L D, O'Malley P M, Bachman J G, *et al. Ecstasy Use Falls for Second Year in a Row, Overall Teen Drug Use Drops*. National press release, University of Michigan News and Information Services, Ann Arbor, 19 December 2003.

8.   McKeganey N, Forsyth A, Barnard M, *et al*. Designer drinks and drunkenness amongst a sample of Scottish schoolchildren. *BMJ* 1996; 313: 401.

9.   Miller P McC, Plant M. Drinking, smoking and illicit drug use among 15 and 16 year olds in the United Kingdom. *BMJ* 1996; 313: 394–397.

10. Rimm E B, Klatsky A, Grobbee D, *et al*. Review of moderate alcohol consumption and reduced risk of coronary heart disease: is the effect due to beer, wine or spirits? *BMJ* 1996; 312: 731–736.

11. Di Castelnuovo A, Rotondo S, Iacovelli L, *et al*. Meta-analysis of wine and beer consumption in relation to vascular risk. *Circulation* 2002; 105: 2836–2844.

12. Rimm E B, Stampfer M J. Wine, beer, and spirits: are they really horses of a different colour? *Circulation* 2002; 105: 2806–2807.

13. Mukamal K J, Conigrave K M, Mittleman M A, *et al*. Roles of drinking pattern and type of alcohol consumed in coronary heart disease in men. *N Engl J Med* 2003; 348: 109–118.

14. Reynolds K, Lewis L B, Nolen J D L, *et al*. Alcohol consumption and risk of stroke: a meta-analysis. *JAMA* 2003; 289: 579–588.

15. Howard A A, Arnsten J H, Gourevitch M N. Effect of alcohol consumption on diabetes mellitus: a systematic review. *Ann Intern Med* 2004; 140: 211–219.

16. Malinski M K, Sesso H D, Lopez-Jimenez F, *et al*. Alcohol consumption and cardiovascular disease mortality in hypertensive men. *Arch Intern Med* 2004; 164: 623–628.

17. Hein H O, Suadicani P, Gyntelberg F. Alcohol consumption, serum low density lipoprotein cholesterol concentration, and risk of ischaemic heart disease: six year follow up in the Copenhagen study. *BMJ* 1996; 312: 736–741.

18. Nutt D J, Peters T J. Alcohol: the drug. *Br Med Bull* 1994; 50: 5–17.

19. Anonymous. World deaths in 2000 attributable to selected leading risk factors. World Health Organization, 2002 (ref WHR 2002).

20. Harwood H. Updating Estimates of the Economic Costs of Alcohol Abuse in the United States: Estimates, Update, Methods and Data. Report prepared by The Lewin Group for the National Institute on Alcohol Abuse and Alcoholism, 2000.

21. Thornton J R. Atrial fibrillation in healthy non-alcoholic people after an alcoholic binge. *Lancet* 1984; ii: 1013–1014.

22. Koskinen P, Kupari M. Alcohol and cardiac arrhythmias. *BMJ* 1992; 304: 1394–1395.

23. Wiese J G, Shlipak M G, Browner W S. The alcohol hangover. *Ann Intern Med* 2000; 132: 897–902.

24. Calder I. Hangovers: not the ethanol – perhaps the methanol. *BMJ* 1997; 314: 2–3.

25. Menon K V N, Gores G J, Shah V H. Pathogenesis, diagnosis, and treatment of alcoholic liver disease. *Mayo Clin Proc* 2001; 76: 1021–1029.

26. Preedy V R, Atkinson L M, Richardson P J, *et al*. Mechanisms of ethanol-induced cardiac damage. *Br Heart J* 1993; 69: 197–200.

27. Charness M E, Simon R P, Greenberg D A. Ethanol and the nervous system. *N Engl J Med* 1989; 321: 442–454.

28. Thomson A D, Cook C C H, Touquet R, *et al*. The Royal College of Physicians report on alcohol: guidelines for managing Wernicke's encephalopathy in the accident and emergency department. *Alcohol Alcohol* 2002; 37: 513–521.

29. Cook C C H, Hallwood P M, Thomson A D. B vitamin deficiency and neuropsychiatric syndromes in alcohol misuse. *Alcohol Alcohol* 1998; 33: 317–336.

30. Koike H, Iijima M, Sugiura M, *et al*. Alcoholic neuropathy is clinicopathologically distinct from thiamine-deficiency neuropathy. *Ann Neurol* 2003; 54: 19–29.

31. Griffiths R R, Wolf B. Relative abuse liability of different benzodiazepines in drug abusers. *J Clin Psychopharmacol* 1990; 10: 237–243.

32. Daeppen J-B, Gache P, Landry U, *et al*. Symptom-triggered vs fixed-schedule doses of benzodiazepine for alcohol withdrawal. *Arch Intern Med* 2002; 162: 1117–1121.

33. Saitz R, Mayo-Smith M F, Roberts M S, *et al*. Individualized treatment for alcohol withdrawal. *JAMA* 1994; 272: 519–523.

34. McInnes G T. Chlormethiazole and alcohol: a lethal cocktail. *BMJ* 1987; 294: 592.

35. Gregg E, Akhter I. Chlormethiazole abuse. *Br J Psychiatry* 1979; 134: 627–629.

36. Kosten T R, O'Connor P G. Management of drug and alcohol withdrawal. *N Engl J Med* 2003; 348: 1786–1795.

37. Hodges B M. Critical care therapeutics: pharmacotherapy for alcohol withdrawal. *Hosp Pharm* 2003; 38: 420–425.

38. Anonymous. Alcohol problems in the general hospital. *Drug Ther Bull* 1991; 29: 69–71.

39. Gillman M A, Lichtigfeld F J. The drug management of severe alcohol withdrawal syndrome. *Postgrad Med J* 1990; 66: 1005–1009.

40. Overman G P, Teter C J, Guthrie S K. Acamprosate for the adjunctive treatment of alcohol dependence. *Ann Pharmacother* 2003; 37: 1090–1099.

41. Srisurapanont M, Jarusuraisin N. Opioid antagonists for alcohol dependence (Cochrane review). In: *The Cochrane Library*, Issue 1, 2004. Chichester, UK: John Wiley & Sons Ltd.

42. Naranjo C A, Knoke D M. The role of selective serotonin reuptake inhibitors in reducing alcohol consumption. *J Clin Psychiatry* 2001; 62(Suppl. 20): 18–25.

43. Stockley I H (ed). *Stockley's Drug Interactions*, 6th edn. London: Pharmaceutical Press, 2002.

44. Fraser A G. Pharmacokinetic interactions between alcohol and other drugs. *Clin Pharmacokinet* 1997; 33: 79–90.

45. Binkiewicz A, Robinson M J, Senior B. Pseudo-Cushing syndrome caused by alcohol in breast milk. *J Pediatr* 1978; 93: 965–967.

46. Bisdom W. Alcohol and nicotine poisoning in nurslings. *JAMA* 1937; 109: 178.

47. Cobo E. Effect of different doses of ethanol on the milk ejecting reflex in lactating women. *Am J Obstet Gynecol* 1973; 115: 817–821.

48. Little R E, Anderson K W, Ervin C H, *et al*. Maternal alcohol use during breast feeding and infant mental and motor development at one year. *N Engl J Med* 1989; 321: 425–430.

17

Plants and fungi

Within the infant rind of this small flower,
Poison hath residence, and medicine power.
Romeo and Juliet, William Shakespeare

Deliberate self-intoxication with plants or fungi is an ancient human practice. Mescaline-containing cacti have been used by the people of Central America for at least 10,000 years, as have hallucinogenic mushrooms in Africa. Cannabis was probably known to the Chinese in 4000 BC as well as to the ancient Egyptians. Tobacco, tea, coffee and cannabis are conspicuous examples of psychotropic plant materials that are still widely used as crude plant products – these have been the subject of earlier chapters in this book – but many street drugs have strong links with the plant kingdom. Cocaine is derived directly from a plant (*Erythroxylum coca*), and opioids are all ultimately analogues of the morphine found in the opium poppy, *Papaver somniferum*. LSD (lysergide) is a modified form of the psychotropically inactive lysergic acid found in the rye fungus or ergot (*Claviceps purpurea*). However, there are many other LSD-like compounds found in nature that are psychoactive. Several examples of amfetamine-like substances have also been isolated from plants.

In the past, taking plants for their mind-altering effects was largely confined to the region where the plant was indigenous, and even within that region to the season during which the plant was available. However, the Internet enables rapid communication with the rest of the world about any novel product with psychotropic effects, and this applies no less to plants. Modern horticultural, storage and distribution techniques may enable seasonal plants to be available all year round.

As with herbal medicines, those selling or advocating the use of plants or fungi for their psychotropic effects are keen to stress that their wares are 'natural' or 'organic' and so somehow safer than synthetic alternatives. This is not necessarily true, as the details below make clear, and besides it should be clear that what is being promoted is a psycho-tropic drug effect no matter where the causative agent originates. When using plant material there are also the dangers of incorrect identification, deliberate adulteration and inability to estimate the correct dose due to the natural variation in psychoactive constituents. All of these are especially important considerations for novices, and inexperienced users may be poisoned or may inadvertently take an overdose. Another attraction for users is that possession of a wide variety of psychoactive plant materials is not illegal in most countries. Of course plants that are grown personally or harvested from nature are also free.

Healthcare professionals may be required to treat patients who are intoxicated after consuming plants or fungi – patients may have taken an overdose or be suffering from side-effects. The main potential problems for the professional are an inability to identify the plant, a lack of familiarity with its effects, and limited evidence to guide treatment.

Some of the plants that are taken throughout the world today for their psychoactive effects are considered below, and their similarities with more well-known drugs highlighted. Although discussed individually, it is quite common for mixtures of some plants to be sold in tablet or capsule form with names such as 'Herbal High'.

Ayahuasca[1-3]

This is native to the Amazon basin of South America and in a local native language means 'vine of the souls', reflecting a long history of use in association with religious ritual. It is also widely known by the Portuguese transliteration 'hoasca', and various local names such as 'yage'. It is increasingly popular in the West, and is widely promoted on the Internet.

Ayahuasca is a generic name for a mixture of at least two plants. The first is a large woody vine or liana, *Banisteriopsis caapi*, which contains beta-carboline alkaloids, principally harmine. These alkaloids are known to inhibit monoamine oxidase A (MAO-A), an enzyme that in the human body is responsible for the inactivation of various amines including neurotransmitters such as serotonin, dopamine and noradrenaline (norepinephrine). The second constituent is a plant that contains *N,N*-dimethyltryptamine (DMT) or closely related compounds. The identity of the second plant is variable, but is commonly *Psychotria viridis*.

DMT is hallucinogenic if administered parenterally or intranasally, but if taken orally it is not active as it is destroyed by MAO-A in the human gut wall and liver. However, the beta-carbolines in *Banisteriopsis caapi* prevent this deactivation and allow DMT into the circulation, and from there it enters the brain. The psychotropic effects produced by ayahuasca are thus mainly due to DMT.

Effects and administration

Ayahuasca is traditionally taken orally as a drink. The effects attributed to this combination of plants are complex. It seems to promote dream-like hallucinations, perceptual distortions, happiness and emotional insight, and it is taken to promote spiritual revelation, contentment, improved cognition, a greater understanding of self, and even to treat psychiatric disorders and substance misuse.

The acute effects begin within an hour of ingestion, peak at about 2 hours, and abate within 4 hours.

Adverse effects

Nausea and vomiting are seen frequently, and dysphoric reactions can occur. Small increases in blood pressure have also been observed.

Given the ability of ayahuasca to inhibit monoamine oxidase, it is important to realise that this product might interact with various foods and medicines in the same way that monoamine oxidase inhibitor (MAOI) antidepressants may interact. The same cautions that apply to MAOIs should therefore be exercised when selecting conventional medicines for known ayahuasca users. A reaction similar to the serotonin syndrome has been described in an individual who took ayahuasca while being treated with fluoxetine.[4]

Betel

The chewing of betel is widespread in India, southern China, South-East Asia and the South Pacific. It is the fourth most commonly used drug in the world after tobacco, alcohol and caffeine.[5]

Effects and administration

Traditionally, users prepare a 'quid' for chewing that contains three key ingredients: the 'nut' of the betel or areca palm (seed of *Areca catechu*),

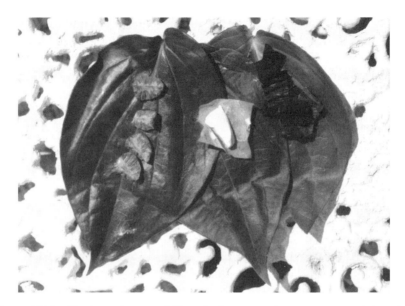

Figure 17.1 The large leaves of *Piper betle* are used to wrap around the other ingredients to make a betel 'quid'. These ingredients include the seed of *Areca catechu* or betel 'nut' (left), slaked lime (middle), and dried tobacco leaves (right).

betel pepper leaf (from *Piper betle*) and slaked lime (Figure 17.1). Sometimes tobacco or other ingredients are added as well. More recently areca nut has been refined, packaged commercially, and sold worldwide in various attractive oral presentations, which may be sweetened and may also contain tobacco.[5] This product is known generically as 'pan masala' and its advent has enabled easier global transportation.

Betel chewing is reported to relax the user, improve concentration and lift mood but it also has stimulant properties, creating a feeling of alertness, decreased fatigue and reduced appetite. In adverse climatic conditions it may enable individuals to work for longer periods. It also causes a mild state of intoxication and euphoria, and a sensation of warmth. The precise mode of action is not known for certain, and areca nut contains many alkaloids that could contribute to its pharmaco-logical effects. Some of the psychotropic properties may be mediated via the inhibitory neurotransmitter gamma-aminobutyric acid (GABA) in the brain. Arecoline, a cholinergic agonist, is the main alkaloid con-stituent of *Areca catechu* but it is not itself psychoactive. However, chewing with lime results in arecoline hydrolysis to arecaidine and this product is a powerful inhibitor of GABA uptake.[6] The alkaline environment produced by the lime also facilitates absorption from the mouth. In addition, some preparations of betel nut have been shown to elevate plasma levels of adrenaline and noradrenaline by mechanisms that are unknown.[7] This weak adrenergic effect may contribute to some of its observed actions. To complicate matters further, betel pepper leaves are also thought to contain psychoactive ingredients.

Adverse effects

Chewing betel releases a red dye into the mouth that stains the oral mucosa dark red. Teeth may also be stained brown. Although the rate of periodontal disease is increased in betel nut users, the incidence of dental caries is reduced.[8] The hypersalivation and constant moistness of the lips produced by chronic use of betel causes 'betel chewer's per-leche', characterised by fissures at the angles of the mouth.[8]

Other adverse effects from chewing betel include hot facial flushing, sweating, tachycardia, mouth ulcers, giddiness, abdominal pains and diarrhoea.[8,9] The cholinergic properties of arecoline are probably the cause of many of the side-effects of betel, and chronic users can become tolerant to many of them. The cholinergic actions of the preparation may also explain a reduced effectiveness of the antimuscarinic drug procyclidine in protecting against phenothiazine-induced extrapyramidal symptoms in two patients who chewed betel.[10] In addition, betel nut chewing has been associated with bronchospasm and acute exacerbation of asthma, which might similarly be a result of arecoline's cholinergic effects.[8,11] A variety of other serious side-effects have been occasionally reported, including psychosis, cardiac arrhythmias and cholinergic crisis.[8]

An examination of epidemiological studies by the International Agency for Research on Cancer on behalf of the World Health Organization (WHO) in 2003 concluded that betel chewing causes oral cancer, even when it is used without tobacco.[12]

Withdrawal symptoms have been described in some users after enforced cessation of a long-term habit. Lack of concentration, memory lapses, tiredness and despondency were described in one user upon withdrawal.[13] Anxiety, fidgeting, despondency and paranoia developed in a second patient.[13] Although there is a paucity of published material, a review from the National Addiction Centre in London concluded that betel chewing was associated with a dependence syndrome, with a mild stimulant-like withdrawal reaction.[5]

Caffeine-containing plants

Several plants contain caffeine as the principal pharmacologically active constituent, and some are listed in Table 17.1. Caffeine itself is discussed in more detail in Chapter 14.

Effects and administration

Guarana is a popular product, sold in health food shops and pharmacies, which contains larger amounts of caffeine than any of the other plants listed. It has attracted attention perhaps because of its tropical origins in the Amazon basin and its exotic-sounding name. Some who use amfetamine and ecstasy claim that it helps them to cope with the depressant and fatiguing aftermath of a 'trip'. This is not surprising because both amfetamines and caffeine are central nervous system (CNS) stimulants, and it is common for those taking illicit stimulants to experience tiredness and lethargy as the effects wear off. Other than the effects attributable to caffeine, claims that guarana has any special psychoactive or energy-boosting properties are unfounded.[14,15] However, it is known that guarana may have a more prolonged stimulant effect than other caffeine-containing plants because the caffeine is extensively bound to tannins, which only release the alkaloid slowly in the human gut.[16] The high tannin content can give rise to constipation if guarana is taken regularly.

The chewing of cola (kola) nuts is popular in West Africa.[17] Sometimes flavourings are added before chewing to ameliorate the bitter taste. Towards the end of the 19th century, an extract of cola was mixed with an extract of the coca plant to form the drink Coca-Cola. It thus originally contained a mixture of caffeine and cocaine. The modern formula does not utilise drugs extracted from plants: synthetic caffeine is used and cocaine is no longer included!

Adverse effects

See Chapter 13 (caffeine).

Table 17.1 Plants containing caffeine

Coffee	*Coffea arabica* (and other species)
Tea	*Thea sinensis*
Cola	*Cola acuminata* and *C. nitada*
Maté	*Ilex paraguensis*
Guarana	*Paullinia cupana*

Ephedra

Although *Ephedra sinica* is the plant most closely associated with the generic name of herbal ephedra, there are about 40 species of *Ephedra*, amongst which are *E. equisetana*, *E. major* and *E. distachya*. Most of these species contain ephedrine and related alkaloids, which can exceed 2% of the plant weight. Up to 90% of this alkaloid content can be ephedrine itself.[18] In traditional Chinese medicine, ephedra is known as 'ma huang' and it is used as an anti-inflammatory.

Effects and administration

Ephedrine is a sympathomimetic with properties similar to, although milder than, amfetamine, and both ephedrine and ephedra are taken orally for their psychotropic or stimulant effects. Over-the-counter (OTC) products containing ephedrine and related compounds are also known to be subject to abuse (see Chapter 13). Herbal ephedra has been marketed as a legal alternative to illicit stimulants, under trade names such as 'herbal ecstasy', 'cloud 9' and 'Xphoria'. In the late 1990s, the plant was associated with a number of patient deaths in the USA, leading at least some states to prohibit its sale when advertised as an alternative to illicit substances for producing psychotropic effects. In December 2003, the US Food and Drug Administration (FDA) announced its intention to prohibit the sale of dietary supplements containing ephedra because they 'present an unreasonable risk of illness or injury and should not be consumed'.[19] Furthermore the FDA stated:

> The totality of the available data showed little evidence of ephedra's effectiveness except for short-term weight loss, while confirming that the substance raises blood pressure and otherwise stresses the circulatory system. These reactions have been conclusively linked to significant adverse health outcomes, including heart ailments and strokes.[19]

In the UK, the government stated in 1997 that the marketing of herbal products like ephedra as alternatives to illicit substances was illegal.[20]

Adverse effects

More details of the potential side-effects of ephedrine are given in Chapter 12. Notably, ephedrine-containing medicines have caused severe psychiatric disturbances such as psychosis and mania, and circulatory problems (see Chapter 13), and similar effects have been attributed to ephedra ingestion.[19,21,22]

Ginseng

A variety of plants are referred to as 'ginseng'. Usually the species taken is *Panax ginseng* (Korean, Chinese or Asian ginseng).

Effects and administration

Ginseng is known to produce CNS stimulation. In 1979 a study was made of 133 chronic ginseng users.[23] All users reported stimulation as an effect of ginseng and many described feelings of well-being or increased cognitive ability; euphoria was mentioned by 18 users. The CNS arousal produced by ginseng is probably effected by glycoside constituents, which vary according to the species. Although most took ginseng orally, nine had experimented with intranasal administration and four had tried injection.

Ginseng is also claimed to have a stimulant effect upon athletic performance but this has not been substantiated.[24]

Adverse effects

In the study of 133 chronic ginseng users cited above, the 'ginseng abuse syndrome' was described in 14 users of oral *Panax ginseng*.[23] This was characterised as 'hypertension together with nervousness, sleeplessness, skin eruptions and morning diarrhoea'. Oedema, agitation, confusion and tremor were side-effects noted in some individuals, but these did not form part of the syndrome identified. Some used up to 15 g of powdered ginseng root per day and it was noted that all sufferers also took caffeinated drinks, but details of the quantities consumed were not given.

Kava

Kava is a traditional beverage in the South Pacific islands[25] and is derived from the macerated root and stem of a shrub, *Piper methysticum*. It is also known as 'kava-kava', 'kawa', 'ava' and 'awa'.

Effects and administration

Kava has mild intoxicating and relaxant properties that are similar to those of alcohol and, like alcohol in the West, it has an important social and cultural role amongst the inhabitants of the islands of Oceania. The principal active ingredients seem to be a group of compounds called kava-lactones and plant extracts containing them may be effective clinically in relieving anxiety.[26]

Adverse effects

Between 2000 and 2003 the European Union, Canada and Australia removed licensed kava products from sale following reports of idiosyncratic liver toxicity associated with the drug.[27] In 2002, the Medicines Control Agency in the UK analysed the 70 known worldwide cases of liver toxicity: four patients died and seven required a liver transplant.[27] This has led to medicinal products containing kava being withdrawn from the market in Europe and Canada and the marketing of any new products is prohibited.

The spread of chronic heavy kava abuse among the Aborigines of northern Australia in the 1980s caused much concern, not least because of the detrimental effects that it is known to have on general health – being associated with malnutrition, weight loss, hepatic dysfunction and dyspnoea for example.[28–30] A wide variety of laboratory blood and urine tests can become abnormal in chronic heavy users. Chronic heavy use also produces a characteristic dry scaly skin, puffy face, increased photosensitivity and reddened eyes.[25,26,29] All of these side-effects gradually improve once kava is discontinued, or the dose reduced, and a healthy diet initiated.

Psychotic-type reactions and cases of acute dyskinesia (e.g. choreoathetosis) have been described infrequently.[30]

Khat

Khat is known by a variety of other names including 'qat', 'chat' or 'miraa'. It is the common name for *Catha edulis*, an evergreen shrub with a native range extending from North and East Africa (Ethiopia, Kenya, Somalia) through Yemen to Afghanistan. The leaves of the plant are used for their psychotropic effects. They have a characteristic shape and the two principal active constituents are cathine ([+]-norpseudo-ephedrine) and cathinone, which have structures and psychostimulant effects similar to amfetamines[31,32] (Figure 17.2). Cathinone is the keto-analogue of cathine and is the constituent primarily responsible for the psychoactive effects sought by users.

Khat should not be confused with methcathinone, commonly called 'cat'. Although structurally very similar to cathinone, methcathinone is a

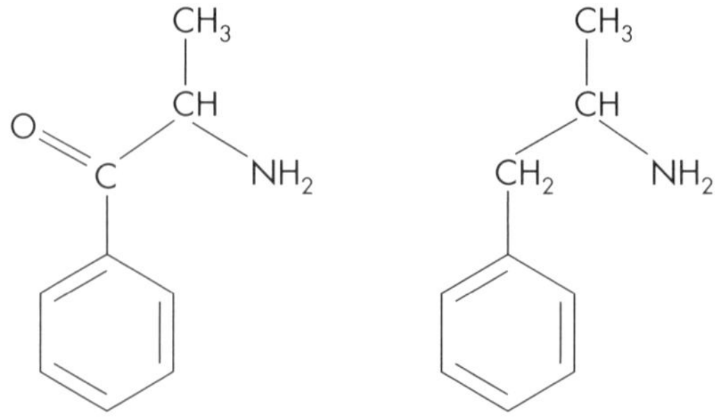

Figure 17.2 Cathinone, from khat, is related to amfetamine.

synthetic substance made from OTC sympathomimetics such as pseudo-ephedrine. It is sold as an alternative to illicit amphetamines.

Effects and administration

In many of the countries of origin, khat is the main social drug used – tobacco and alcohol being less freely available or culturally acceptable.[31,33] For example, khat may be considered a permissible alternative to alcohol for Muslims. The plant has an important cultural and social significance in many of these communities, and its use frequently continues when immigrant communities become established in a new country. The leaves are usually chewed – being retained in the mouth for some time to allow periodic re-chewing. Sometimes the leaves are smoked, sprinkled on food or prepared as an infusion. Khat reduces tiredness and hunger, and causes heightened alertness, sociability, talkativeness and creativity, as well as a mild euphoria and occasionally hallucinations.

Cathinone is very labile and the amount contained in leaves diminishes rapidly after collection, so for maximum effect leaves must be consumed while fresh, and certainly within 2–3 days of harvesting. Refrigeration or freezing is sometimes used to retard loss of potency. In the past this rapid denaturing has limited the spread of khat use, but during the 1980s exportation of leaves by air began and this has enabled immigrants in the UK, much of Europe and the USA to continue their traditional habit. Importation and possession of khat is illegal in some Western countries (e.g. USA, France, Sweden) but legal in others (e.g. the UK). In the UK in 2001, it was estimated that over a tonne of leaves was imported into the country every day,[31,34] whereas in the same year in the USA the total quantity seized at ports of entry was only 37 tonnes.[35]

Adverse effects

Reported side-effects are similar to amfetamines and include sympatho-mimetic-like reactions, anorexia, insomnia, hyperthermia, dry mouth and hypertension.[31–33,36] Tolerance may develop to many of these side-effects. Less commonly, 'bad trips', mania, psychosis[36–38] and arrhythmias have been described. The development of lethargy, tiredness or depression after use is well known.

There may be a link between chronic khat chewing and certain oral cancers.[39] In addition, khat tends to stain teeth brown and cause constipation, stomatitis and gastritis because of the tannins it contains. One small study has also suggested that chronic use can decrease semen volume, the proportion of normal sperm, sperm count and motility.[40]

Chronic use may be associated with dependence and mild withdrawal symptoms after discontinuation such as lethargy, depression, tremor and disrupted sleep.[31–33,36,41] However, dependence is likely to affect only a small minority of the population that consume khat.[31] The lack of tolerance to the psychotropic effects of khat with prolonged use may be due to the physical limits on the amount that may be chewed, and the fact that the drug is taken by mouth.

Morning glory

The species of morning glory with hallucinogenic potential is *Ipomoea tricolor*, also known as *I. violacea*, which is native to Central and South America. The European morning glory (*I. purpurea*) does not contain psychoactive alkaloids.[42] However, the seeds of *I. tricolor* can be purchased on the Internet or from gardening shops. The principal active constituent is D-lysergic acid amide (ergine), which is closely related in structure and actions to LSD (lysergide). *Rivea corymbosa* is a related plant with similar effects to *I. tricolor*. Both are known as 'ololiuqui' in Mexico where use for psychotropic effects dates back to at least the time of the Aztecs.

Effects and administration

At least 200 seeds are needed to produce a 'trip'. The seeds are ground up and then eaten or prepared into an infusion. The subjective effects are similar to those of LSD with perceptual changes, hallucinations and mood changes.[43–45]

Adverse effects

Side-effects include gastrointestinal upset, muscle tension, drowsiness and peripheral numbness. One patient had a persisting repetition of his psychedelic experience over a period of weeks, which was so distressing that he committed suicide.[44] One case of persistent drug-induced psychosis was described amongst a series of three patients who took morning glory seeds.[45] Another patient in this series injected a seed extract and suffered from a severe shock-like reaction; the same patient later experienced flashbacks.[45]

Mushrooms

Across the world there are many fungi that contain psychoactive compounds. Collectively, they are often referred to as 'magic mushrooms'. The extent of abuse is very difficult to quantify but a survey of over 7000 school pupils aged 11–15 in England in 2003 revealed that 2% had used magic mushrooms in the past year.[46] A study of 3075 university students in the UK in 1996 found that 16% had used hallucinogenic mushrooms on at least one occasion.[47] Only 0.4% of the 3075 students used them regularly (at least once a week).

As already stated, incorrect identification of plants or fungi may lead to accidental poisoning. This is of particular concern when novices harvest wild mushrooms, because correct identification is not easy and superficially similar or closely related species can have very different, and potentially dangerous, pharmacological actions. Furthermore, those purchasing mushrooms on the black market may be sold inactive harmless forms or varieties that have been injected with LSD, phencyclidine or other psychoactive substances. Several studies have shown that only a small percentage of mushrooms offered for sale are true hallucinogenic species.

The limited seasonal availability of mushrooms, and the fact that unpleasant 'trips' seem to be quite common, means that chronic use or dependence is unlikely to be common.

Psilocybin-containing species

There are over 180 species of fungi from around the world that contain the alkaloids psilocybin and psilocin. These compounds were identified as the psychoactive constituents by Albert Hofmann in 1958, who was also the first to describe the mind-altering effects of LSD. Psilocybin-

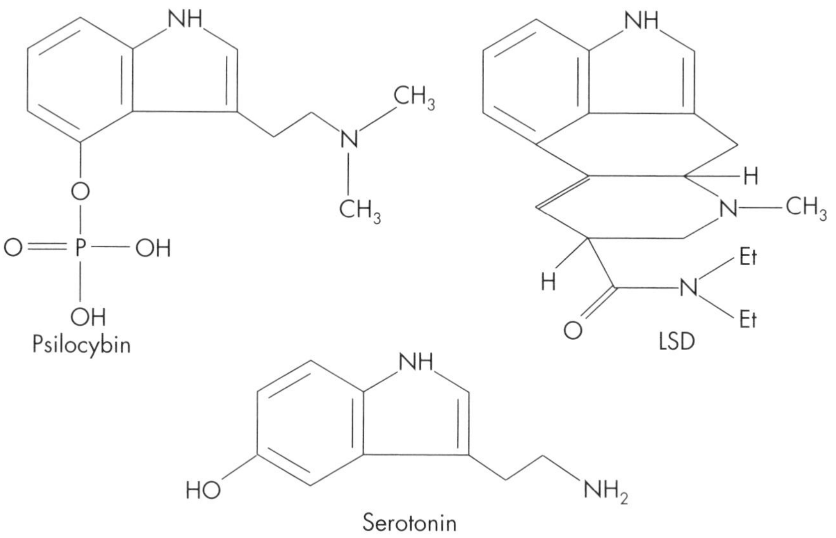

Figure 17.3   Similarity of psilocybin structure to serotonin and LSD.

containing fungal species can be found amongst genera such as *Psilocybe*, *Panaeolus*, *Gymnopilus*, *Conocybe* and *Copelandia*. Both psilocybin and psilocin have an indole-based structure reminiscent of the neurotransmitter serotonin and LSD (see Figure 17.3). However, psilocybin is now known to be a pro-drug that is very rapidly converted to psilocin after ingestion, and it is psilocin that is biologically active.[48] Psilocin has only 0.5–1% of the psychotropic activity of LSD. The clinical and pharmacological effects of the alkaloids, and the mushrooms themselves, have not been investigated systematically and data on their biological effects are derived from a limited number of small observational studies and case reports.

Fungal species containing psilocybin and psilocin are found in Central America and were used by the Aztecs as part of their religious rites. The main species abused in Britain and northern Europe is *Psilocybe semilanceata*; it is also found in the USA. In Britain and the USA it is commonly known as 'liberty cap', although this term has been applied to other *Psilocybe* species. Its psychotropic effects have been comparatively well studied.[49–55] It is commonly found in damp areas of open places such as parks, fields and meadows. It grows from late summer to the end of autumn and the yellow to buff-coloured mushrooms are up to 10 cm high, with a characteristic nipple at the apex of the mushroom (Figure 17.4). Intoxication with the species *Psilocybe*

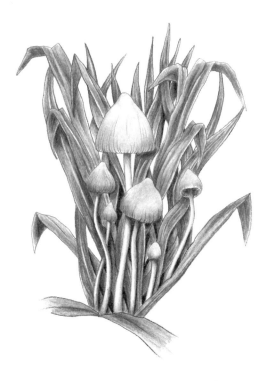

Figure 17.4 The small, unobtrusive mushrooms of liberty cap (*Psilocybc semilanceata*) belie its potential for intense pyschoactive effects (Photo courtesy of Multimedia Research Partners Ltd).

cubensis has also been described in the medical literature. This species is native to the USA and Australia.[43,56,57]

Many users know that fresh mushrooms containing psilocybin develop a dark blue colouration within an hour of being bruised or cut. This is said to be a positive test for psilocybin and it is commonly used to distinguish 'magic mushrooms' from other varieties, but it is not completely reliable.[58]

Effects and administration

The fresh mushrooms may be eaten raw or cooked. They may be dried or frozen for later use, or made into a drink by infusing in hot water. Intravenous injection of prepared fungal extracts has been reported but is probably extremely rare.[59] The amount ingested plays a major role in determining the effects produced. The exact number of mushrooms required depends upon the species, the psilocybin/psilocin content, and the tolerance or expectation of the user. For *Psilocybe semilanceata* a small number of mushrooms (two to four) may be enough to promote relaxation and/or mild euphoria but some 20–100 are usually required to produce a full psychedelic experience.

The psychotropic effects are variable.[43,49–53,55,56] The experience begins with feelings of relaxation, and is commonly followed by euphoria. Perceptual distortions seem to be an almost universal occurrence – they are mainly visual and may include aberrant perception of colours, distortions of the passage of time, and sometimes synaesthesia. Frank hallucinations are less frequently reported. In many respects, the effects of psilocybin/psilocin intoxication are very similar to those of LSD, although LSD tends to cause more profound mental changes and may be less likely to cause euphoria.

If an infusion is consumed, the effects can begin within a few minutes of ingestion but if the mushrooms themselves are eaten, at least half an hour is required. The onset of effects can sometimes be delayed by a few hours if the mushrooms are not broken up into small enough pieces and if they are eaten with a meal. The usual duration of the most intense phase of the psychedelic experience is less than 4 hours from the time of onset, but the whole experience is typically complete within 12 hours of ingestion.

Adverse effects[43, 49–53,55–57]

The desired experience may be heralded or accompanied by sympathomimetic effects such as flushing, tachycardia and dry mouth. On examination, dilated pupils are common and there may be some blurring of vision. Raised blood pressure and hyperreflexia may also be seen.

As with all psychoactive drugs of abuse, a bad 'trip' may occur at any time and may include panic reactions, severe agitation, frightening illusions or hallucinations, and other dysphoric reactions. These unpleasant psychotropic effects are the commonest reason for recreational use of magic mushrooms to come to the attention of healthcare professionals. The frequency of unpleasant reactions is suggested by a unique published account revealing that of 100 young people who ingested *Psilocybe semilanceata* one evening in Wales, 19 sought medical assistance because of psychotropic effects that caused concern.[52]

Large doses may cause a reaction that appears similar to acute psychosis. This may resolve over a period of a few days.[53] One case report describes a patient with persistent daily panic attacks that developed

2 weeks after a dysphoric reaction to *Psilocybe semilanceata* mushrooms.[54] Two similar cases are briefly described in a study of 27 mushroom exposures.[49] Given that psilocin intoxication is similar to that produced by LSD, it is not surprising that more traditional 'flashbacks' have also been reported.[50,56]

Other common side-effects are nausea and vomiting, abdominal cramps, disturbed behaviour, and paraesthesia. Ataxia, convulsions and urinary incontinence have been reported rarely.

In an analysis of 318 cases of *Psilocybe semilanceata* intoxication reported from the UK in 1983, no deaths were reported even though one patient reportedly consumed 200 mushrooms.[50]

After the acute psychotropic effects have worn off, users may have a strong desire to sleep. Sometimes depression and lethargy persisting for several days between doses is reported by regular users.[57]

Intravenous use has resulted in cyanosis, recurrent vomiting, acute muscle pain, and severe 'flu-like symptoms such as myalgia, hyperpyrexia, rigors and headache.[59]

Amanita species[43,60]

The most well known of these is *Amanita muscaria*, also known as fly agaric. It is native to the USA, UK, northern Europe and northern Asia and has long been employed by humans for its psychedelic effects. There is a particularly well-established history of use in Siberia, which seems to date back millennia. Rock paintings in the Sahara of a mushroom that is probably *A. muscaria* may be as much as 11,000 years old.

The mushrooms have a very distinctive appearance. The cap is round and red with small white flecks on the upper surface, and a white underside – the typical 'toadstool' of childhood fiction (Figure 17.5). There are a number of other *Amanita* species that have psychedelic effects, but there are also highly poisonous species, so correct identification is vital. *Amanita muscaria* mushrooms are usually found in autumn in woods or other areas under the shelter of trees. They generally occur singly but sometimes in small groups.

Amanita muscaria has two principal psychoactive constituents: ibotenic acid and muscimol (Figure 17.6). In contrast to psilocin, which interacts with the central serotonergic system, the active constituents of *A. muscaria* seem to have more depressant actions on the CNS. Its two main psychotropic constituents both affect CNS neurotransmitters: ibotenic acid has a similar structure to glutamate, and muscimol resembles GABA (gamma-aminobutyric acid). However, unlike glutamate

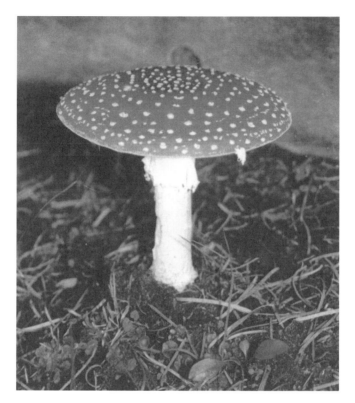

Figure 17.5 *Amanita muscaria* or fly agaric.

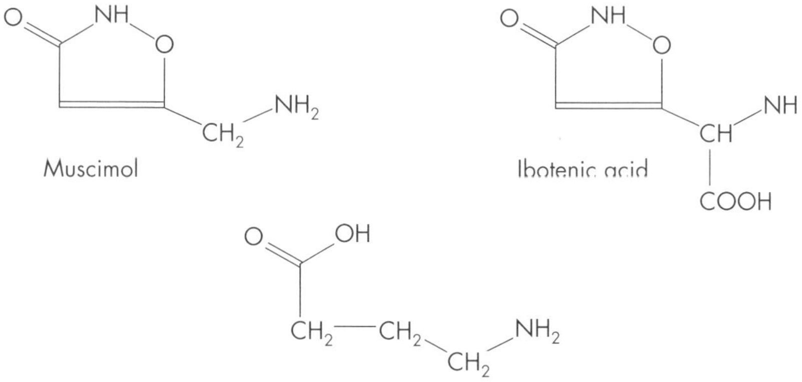

Muscimol

Ibotenic acid

Gamma-aminobutyric acid (GABA)

Figure 17.6 Ibotenic acid is converted to muscimol, which may exert psychotropic effects via GABA.

and GABA, muscimol and ibotenic acid cross the blood–brain barrier. Ibotenic acid is rapidly converted to muscimol *in vivo* and this latter is believed to be the main compound responsible for the mushroom's psychotropic effects via GABA. GABA is an inhibitory neurotransmitter that tends to reduce the activity of neurones in the brain – hence *A. muscaria*'s CNS depressant effects.

Effects and administration

The quantity of active ingredients in *A. muscaria* is particularly subject to variation according to environmental conditions at the time of growth; in addition it declines with increased duration of storage. The mushrooms also vary greatly in size. Consequently the dose required can only be determined by experience. Mushrooms are usually taken orally, but may sometimes be dried for smoking.

A 'trip' typically starts within 30–120 minutes of ingestion. It begins with feelings of drowsiness but may then progress to confusion, perceptual distortions, slurred speech, incoordination and sometimes euphoria.

Adverse effects

Side-effects include headaches, vomiting, dizziness, muscle spasms and convulsions. Often the experience is completed by a deep sleep, which may include vivid dreams.

Nutmeg

The hard kernel contained within the fruit of the tree *Myristica fragrans* is commonly called nutmeg (Figure 17.7). Nutmeg contains a variety of compounds that may contribute to its psychotropic effects, but the main aromatic ether it contains is called myristicin, and this is generally believed to be the principal psychoactive constituent. Myristicin is structurally related to amfetamine derivatives such as ecstasy. Human metabolism may actually introduce the side chain amino group necessary for true amfetamine status (see Figure 17.8). After administration it takes some hours for psychotropic actions to develop, lending support to the idea that metabolic conversion is needed to produce psychotropic effects. The effects usually begin within 6 hours.

Other plants, such as parsley and carrots, contain myristicin, but not in high enough concentration to have significant pharmacological action.

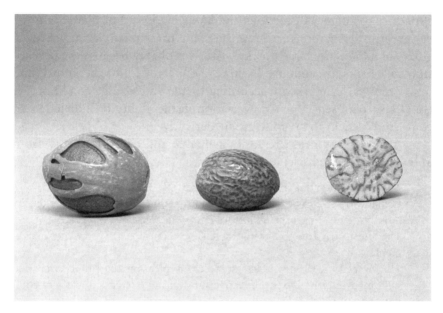

Figure 17.7 Nutmeg. The central kernel is nutmeg and the surrounding red arillus is mace (Photo courtesy of Multimedia Research Partners Ltd).

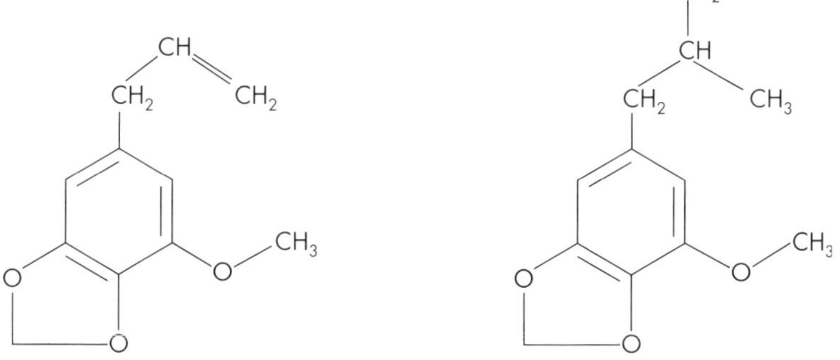

Myristicin

MMDA

Figure 17.8 Myristicin may be converted to methoxymethylenedioxyamfetamine (MMDA) *in vivo*.

Effects and administration[43,61-67]

Nutmeg is ground to a fine powder before use. It is then usually ingested mixed with a drink, although it can be smoked, inhaled nasally or vaporised. By mouth, as little as one nutmeg may be enough to provoke euphoria, perceptual distortions and hallucinations, but there is a great variation in the response to nutmeg: some users report no psychedelic effects at all, despite large doses.[66] This is probably because the psychotropic elements are contained within the volatile oil of the kernel, and oil content varies markedly according to age and storage conditions. It could also represent a genetic variation in the ability of individuals to convert myristicin to an amfetamine derivative.

Although nutmegs are easily available and cheap, abuse is probably uncommon because:

- The abuse potential is not widely known.
- Preparation is cumbersome and administration is awkward: if taken by mouth the taste of large quantities is very unpleasant.
- The effects are slow to onset – there is no intense 'high' or rush of excitement.
- The overall experience is less subjectively pleasant than that associated with many alternative psychoactive substances. Side-effects are very common and not well tolerated (see below).

For these reasons, nutmeg abuse is often a single experimental experience, or occurs amongst knowledgeable individuals in situations where access to alternative psychoactive drugs is limited.

Adverse effects[43,61-68]

Reports of nutmeg intoxication commonly describe severe headaches, tingling and numbness of the extremities, and nausea or vomiting. This may be accompanied by antimuscarinic-like reactions including dry mouth, flushing, tachycardia, palpitations and sweating. Unpleasant psychotomimetic effects are also common such as agitation, frightening hallucinations, depersonalisation, and a sense of impending doom. Other frequently cited acute effects include dizziness, drowsiness and confusion. Muscle twitching and restlessness is sometimes described. Usually the actions of nutmeg last for up to 24 hours but occasionally longer and, as with synthetic amfetamine derivatives, the user often feels very tired or weak afterwards.

Serious side-effects have been occasionally reported and several cases of nutmeg abuse requiring medical attention have been described. Most of these have arisen because of unpleasant psychotropic effects coupled with persistent physical symptoms such as headache or vomiting. Severe reactions in cases of poisoning have included hypotension and shock.[69] A case of chronic psychosis linked to long-term nutmeg administration has also been documented.[68] Interestingly, the patient's condition was complicated by polydipsia, and hyponatraemia secondary to water overload; these symptoms have also been described in ecstasy users (see Chapter 8).

Peyote cactus

The Peyote cactus, *Lophophora williamsii*, is found in the wild in Mexico and Texas. The heads of the cactus are eaten whole or are made into an infusion. The plant has been used for its psychotropic effects for at least 10,000 years by New World peoples such as the Aztecs. The psychoactive component mescaline is chemically related to the amfetamines and may produce hallucinations, out-of-body experiences and synaesthesia.

Potato family

The plants of the potato family (Solanaceae) are economically and pharmacologically very important. The tobacco plant (*Nicotiana tabacum*) is the most widely used recreationally today, but historically the solanaceous plants were important psychotropic substances in Europe. The four main plants involved were mandrax (*Mandragora officinarum*), henbane (*Hysocyamus niger*), deadly nightshade (*Atropa belladonna*) and the thorn apple (*Datura stramonium*).

All of these species contain the antimuscarinic compounds hyoscine (scopolamine), hyoscyamine and atropine.

Effects and administration

Antimuscarinic drugs are known to have the potential for abuse and prescription medicines are sometimes taken for this purpose even today (see Chapter 12). The use of the plants above – the so-called 'hexing herbs' – has been associated with witchcraft. Mixtures of them were formed into an ointment and topical application is known to produce a range of effects including sensations of flying through the air and illusions of human transformation into animals – typical features of witch folklore. Witches sometimes carried sticks to facilitate ointment application to the anus or genitals, where absorption occurred more rapidly. In order to avoid suspicion these may have been disguised as broomsticks or other apparently innocent items.[70–72]

Modern day abuse of *Datura* is not infrequently reported in the USA, where it grows wild and is commonly known as Jimson weed.[43,73,74] Users are typically adolescent males who seek hallucinogenic effects, usually by drinking an aqueous infusion of the plant material or eating the seeds. The roots, seeds and leaves are all used but the seeds contain the most atropine. Occasionally the leaves are prepared as a 'reefer' and smoked. After oral administration, pharmacological effects begin within about an hour but may persist for 48 hours or longer, because antimuscarinic drugs inhibit the motility of the gastrointestinal tract and thereby reduce their own rate of absorption.

Adverse effects

The symptoms of antimuscarinic toxicity and intoxication are aptly described by the following lines:

Hot as a hare,	(hyperthermia)
Blind as a bat,	(dilated pupils, blurred vision)
Dry as a bone,	(dry mouth, dry eyes, reduced sweating)
Red as a beet,	(flushing)
Mad as a hatter.	(disorientation, incoherency, hallucinations, agitation)
The bowel and bladder lose their tone,	(constipation and urinary retention)
And the heart runs on alone.	(tachycardia)

Other effects may include sedation, headache, nausea, vomiting, hyper-reflexia, combative behaviour, seizures and coma. Several deaths have been reported. In 1993, the American Association of Poison Control Centers Toxic Exposure Surveillance System was notified of 318 cases of *Datura stramonium* toxicity.[74] More recently, abuse of the related species *Datura inoxia* has been reported. This also contains antimuscarinics.[75]

Salvia divinorum

Salvia divinorum is a large herb, a member of the mint family and native to South and Central America. It has been used by the Mazatec Indians of Mexico for its psychotropic effects for centuries. The main psychoactive constituent is a diterpene, known as salvinorin A.

Effects and administration

The plant material has an unpleasant bitter taste but to experience psychoactive effects it can be eaten fresh, chewed as a 'quid', drunk as an infusion, or dried and then smoked. Psychotropic effects last for a few hours depending upon dose. The effects reported by users are mainly 'mystical' experiences such as visions, or more frank hallucinations. Synaesthesia has also been reported, and the plant's effects have been variously compared to ketamine, psilocin, LSD or mescaline.[76,77]

Adverse effects

Information on side-effects is minimal, but might include slurred speech, dizziness, and a chill.[77]

Yohimbe

This is the name of a West African tree *Pausinystalia yohimbe* (or *Corynanthe yohimbe*). The bark and roots contain an alkaloid called yohimbine and both the alkaloid and the plant itself have been widely used as an aphrodisiac or as a treatment for impotence.

However, anecdotally the plant is also used as an ecstasy-like drug because it produces hallucinations and stimulant-like effects.[78] It has also been used to assist athletic training as an alternative to anabolic steroids. Unfortunately these effects have not been systematically studied in humans. Side-effects of yohimbine include raised blood pressure.

References

1. Riba J, Rodriguez-Fornells A, Urbano G, *et al.* Subjective effects and tolerability of the South American psychoactive beverage ayahuasca in healthy volunteers. *Psychopharmacology* 2001; 154: 85–95.
2. Grob C S, McKenna D J, Callaway J C, *et al.* Human psychopharmacology of hoasca, a plant hallucinogen used in ritual context in Brazil. *J Nerv Ment Dis* 1996; 184: 86–94.
3. Ott J. Pharmahuasca: human pharmacology of DMT plus harmine. *J Psychoactive Drugs* 1999; 31: 171–177.
4. Callaway J C, Grob C S. Ayahuasca preparations and serotonin reuptake inhibitors: a potential combination form severe adverse interactions. *J Psychoactive Drugs* 1998; 30: 367–369.
5. Winstock A. Areca nut – abuse liability, dependence and public health. *Addict Biol* 2002; 7: 133–138.

6. Johnston G A R, Krogsgaard-Larsen P, Stephenson A. Betel nut constituents as inhibitors of gamma-aminobutyric acid uptake. *Nature* 1975; 258: 627–628.
7. Chu N-S. Sympathetic response to betel chewing. *J Psychoactive Drugs* 1995; 27: 183–186.
8. Nelson B S, Heischober B. Betel nut: a common drug used by naturalized citizens from India, Far East Asia, and the South Pacific Islands. *Ann Emerg Med* 1999; 34: 238–243.
9. Arjungi V K N. Areca nut: a review. *Arzneim Forsch* 1976; 26: 951–956.
10. Deahl M P. Psychostimulant properties of betel nuts. *BMJ* 1987; 294: 849.
11. Taylor R F H, Al-Jarad N, John L M E, *et al*. Betel-nut chewing and asthma. *Lancet* 1992; 339: 1134–1136.
12. Anonymous. Betel-quid and areca-nut chewing and some areca-nut related nitrosamines. International Agency for Research on Cancer Monographs on the Evaluation of Carcinogenic Risk to Humans, Vol 85, 11–18 June 2003.
13. Wiesner D M. Betel nut withdrawal. *Med J Aust* 1987; 146: 453.
14. Briggs C. Guarana. *Can Pharm J* 1992; May: 222–224.
15. Houghton P. Guarana. *Pharm J* 1995; 254: 435–436.
16. Aktuell. Guarana – der 'neue' Muntermacher. *Dtsch Apotheker Zeit* 1993; 133: 218.
17. Rudgley R. *The Alchemy of Culture*. London: British Museum Press, 1993, 116–118.
18. World Health Organization. Herba ephedrae. *WHO Monographs on Selected Medicinal Plants*, Vol. 1. Geneva: WHO, 1996: 145–153.
19. US Food and Drug Administration. *Consumer Alert: FDA Plans Regulation Prohibiting Sale of Ephedra-Containing Dietary Supplements and Advises Consumers to Stop Using These Products*. FDA reference number PO3-106, 30 December 2003. http://www.fda.gov/oc/initiatives/ephedra/december 2003/advisory.html (accessed 28 November 2004).
20. Anonymous. Sales of "herbal high" drugs are to be halted. *Pharm J* 1997; 259: 316.
21. Capwell R R. Ephedrine induced mania from an herbal diet supplement. *Am J Psychiatry* 1995; 152: 647.
22. Doyle H, Kargin M. Herbal stimulant containing ephedrine has also caused psychosis. *BMJ* 1996; 313: 756.
23. Siegel R K. Ginseng abuse syndrome – problems with the panacea. *JAMA* 1979; 241: 1614–1615.
24. Bahrke M S, Morgan W P. Evaluation of the ergogenic properties of ginseng. *Sports Med* 1994; 18: 229–248.
25. Singh Y N. Kava: an overview. *J Ethnopharmacol* 1992; 37: 13–45.
26. Anonymous. Is kava calming? *Drug Ther Perspect* 1999; 13: 15–16.
27. Medicines Control Agency. *MCA Investigation of Kava-Kava Leads to Ban Following Voluntary Withdrawal*. Press statement number 2002/0528. London: MCA, 20 December 2002.
28. Cawte J. Macabre effects of a 'cult' for kava. *Med J Aust* 1998; 148: 545–546.
29. Mathews J D, Riley M D, Fejo L, *et al*. Effects of the heavy usage of kava on physical health: summary of a pilot survey in an Aboriginal community. *Med J Aust* 1998; 148: 548–555.

30. Cairney S, Maruff P, Clough A R. The neurobehavioural effects of kava. *Aust N Z J Psychiatry* 2002; 36: 657–662.

31. Griffiths P. *Qat Use in London: A Study of Qat Use Among a Sample of Somalis Living in London*. Drugs Prevention Initiative Paper No. 26. London: Home Office, Central Drugs Prevention Unit, 1998.

32. Kalix P. Khat: a plant with amphetamine effects. *J Subst Abuse Treat* 1988; 5: 163–169.

33. Kalix P. Khat: scientific knowledge and policy issues. *Br J Addict* 1987; 82: 47–53.

34. BBC News Online. Fears rise over khat leaf. http://news.bbc.co.uk/2/hi/health/1425780.stm (6 July 2001; accessed 28 November 2004).

35. US Drug Enforcement Authority. Drug Intelligence Brief. *Khat*. http://www.usdoj.gov/dea/pubs/intel/02032/02032.html (June 2002; accessed 28 November 2004).

36. Pantelis C, Hindler C G, Taylor J C. Use and abuse of khat (*Catha edulis*): a review of the distribution, pharmacology, side effects and a description of psychosis attributed to khat chewing. *J Psychol Med* 1989; 19: 657–688.

37. Critchlow S, Seifert R. Khat-induced paranoid psychosis. *Br J Psychiatry* 1987; 150: 247–249.

38. Jager A D, Siveling L. Natural history of khat psychosis. *Aust N Z J Psychiatry* 1994; 28: 331–332.

39. Soufi H E, Kameswaran M, Malatani T. Khat and oral cancer. *J Laryngol Otol* 1991; 105: 643–645.

40. El-Shoura S M, Abdel Aziz M, Ali M E, *et al*. Deleterious effects of khat addiction on semen parameters and sperm ultrastructure. *Hum Reprod* 1995; 10: 2295–2300.

41. Giannini A J, Miller N S, Turner C E. Treatment of khat addiction. *J Subst Abuse Treat* 1992; 9: 379–382.

42. Capper K R. Lysergic acid derivatives in morning glory seeds. In: Wilson C W M, ed. *The Pharmacological and Epidemiological Aspects of Adolescent Drug Dependence*. New York: Pergamon Press, 1968, 75–81.

43. Spoerke D G, Hall A H. Plants and mushrooms of abuse. *Emerg Med Clin North Am* 1990; 8: 579–593.

44. Cohen S. Suicide following morning glory seed ingestion. *Am J Psychiatry* 1964; 120: 1024–1025.

45. Fink P J, Goldman M J, Lyons I L. Morning glory seed psychosis. *Arch Gen Psychiatry* 1966; 15: 209–213.

46. National Centre for Social Research/National Foundation for Educational Research. *Drug Use, Smoking and Drinking among Young People in England in 2003: headline figures*. London: Department of Health, 2004.

47. Webb F, Ashton C H, Kelly P, *et al*. Alcohol and drug use in UK university students. *Lancet* 1996; 348: 922–925.

48. Hasler F, Bourquin D, Brenneisen R, *et al*. Determination of psilocin and 4-hydroxyindole-3-acetic acid in plasma by HPLC-ECD and pharmacokinetic profiles of oral and intravenous psilocybin in man. *Pharm Acta Helvetica* 1997; 72: 175–184.

49. Peden N R, Bissett A F, Macaulay K E C, *et al*. Clinical toxicology of 'magic mushroom' ingestion. *Postgrad Med J* 1981; 57: 543–545.

50.   Francis J, Murray V S G. Review of enquiries made to the NPIS concerning *Psilocybe* mushroom ingestion 1978–1981. *Hum Toxicol* 1983; 2: 349–352.

51.   Mills P R, Lesinkas D, Watkinson G. The danger of hallucinogenic mushrooms. *Scott Med J* 1979; 24: 316–317.

52.   Harris A D, Evans V. Sequelae of a 'magic mushroom' banquet. *Postgrad Med J* 1981; 57: 571–572.

53.   Hyde C, Glancy G, Omerod P, *et al*. Abuse of indigenous psilocybin mushrooms: a new fashion and some psychiatric complications. *Br J Psychiatry* 1978; 132: 602–604.

54.   Benjamin C. Persistent psychiatric symptoms after eating psilocybin mushrooms. *BMJ* 1979; 1: 1319–1320.

55.   Peden N R, Pringle S D. Hallucinogenic fungi. *Lancet* 1982; 1: 396–397.

56.   Schwartz R R, Smith D E. Hallucinogenic mushrooms. *Clin Pediatr* 1988; 27: 70–73.

57.   McCarthy J P. Some less familiar drugs of abuse. *Med J Aust* 1971; 2: 1078–1081.

58.   Benedict R G, Tyler V E, Watling R. Blueing in Conocybe, Psilocybe and Stropharia species and the detection of psilocybin. *Lloydia* 1967; 30: 150–152.

59.   Curry S C, Rose M C. Intravenous mushroom poisoning. *Ann Emerg Med* 1985; 14: 900–902.

60.   Michelot D, Melendez-Howell L M. Amanita muscaria: chemistry, biology, toxicology, and ethnomycology. *Mycol Res* 2003; 107: 131–146.

61.   Faguet R A, Rowland K F. 'Spice cabinet' intoxication. *Am J Psychiatry* 1978; 135: 860–861.

62.   Panayotopoulos D J, Chisholm D D. Hallucinogenic effect of nutmeg. *BMJ* 1970; 1: 754.

63.   Sjoholm A, Lindberg A, Personne M. Acute nutmeg intoxication. *J Intern Med* 1998; 243: 329–331.

64.   Venables G S, Evered D, Hall R. Nutmeg poisoning. *BMJ* 1976; 1: 96.

65.   Payne R B. Nutmeg intoxication. *N Engl J Med* 1963; 269: 36–8.

66.   Weil A T. Nutmeg as a psychoactive drug. *J Psychedelic Drugs* 1971; 3: 72–80.

67.   Quin G I, Fanning N F, Plunkett P K. Nutmeg intoxication. *J Accid Emerg Med* 1998; 15: 287–288.

68.   Brenner N, Frank O S, Knight E. Chronic nutmeg psychosis. *J R Soc Med* 1993; 86: 179–180.

69.   Green R C Jr. Nutmeg poisoning. *JAMA* 1959; 171: 1342–1344.

70.   Richardson P M. *Encyclopedia of Psychoactive Drugs: Flowering Plants – Magic in Bloom* (British edition). London: Burke Publishing Co., 1988.

71.   Rudgley R. *The Alchemy of Culture: Intoxicants in Society*. London: British Museum Press, 1993, 90–99.

72.   Harner M J, ed. *Hallucinogens and Shamaninsm*. London: Oxford University Press, 1973, 126–150.

73.   Shervette R E, Schydlower M, Lampe R M, *et al*. Jimson 'loco' weed abuse in adolescents. *Pediatrics* 1979; 63: 520–523.

74.   Centers for Disease Control and Prevention. Jimson weed poisoning – Texas, New York and California 1994. *MMWR* 1995; 44: 41–44.

75. Centers for Disease Control and Prevention. Suspected moonflower intoxication – Ohio 2002. *MMWR* 2003; 52: 788–791.

76. US Drug Enforcement Administration. Salvia divinorum, ska Maria Pastora, salvia (salvinorin A, divinorin A). *Drugs and Chemicals of Concern*, September 2002. http://www.deadiversion.usdoj.gov/drugs_concern/salvia_d/summary.htm (accessed 28 November 2004).

77. Valdes L J III. Salvia divinorum and the unique diterpene hallucinogen salvinorin (divinorin) A. *J Psychoactive Drugs* 1994; 26: 277–283.

78. 'Legal Highs' Drug Information. DrugScope, 2002. Accessed via http://www.drugscope.org.uk, Jan 2004.

18

Alkyl nitrites

Poppers make you feel really heady when you're dancing but you have to keep sniffing it every few minutes because it doesn't last long. Sometimes it makes you feel a bit dizzy.

Comment from user, 1996

History

Three alkyl nitrites are commonly abused: amyl nitrite, butyl nitrite and isobutyl nitrite. Amyl nitrite was used from 1867 until the earlier part of the 20th century as a treatment for angina attacks. It was supplied in small glass 'capsules' (or vitrellae) that were broken open during an attack of angina and the contents inhaled. The nitrites are essentially vasodilators, being converted to the endogenous mediator nitric oxide *in vivo*.

The popping sound made when vitrellae were broken has given rise to the most popular street name for alkyl nitrites – 'poppers'. The name has persisted despite the fact that this particular preparation has not been available at street level for many years. Sometimes alkyl nitrites are also known as 'snappers', 'rush' or 'amyl'.

The legal controls on alkyl nitrites vary widely around the world. They are often sold under the guise of 'room odourisers', with warnings that they should not be inhaled, and no overt claims are made concerning medicinal or intoxicating properties. In this way laws aimed at circumventing their use because they are medicines or intoxicating substances can sometimes be bypassed. In practice, whatever restrictions are imposed, alkyl nitrites are easily available to most people in the Western world. In some countries, propyl nitrites have been abused because they are not covered by limited existing legal controls.

Alkyl nitrites are very popular in some communities (e.g. gay men). Studies in Australia in the late 1990s suggested that between a third and a half of gay men had used nitrites in the past 6 months.[1] In the general population, usage levels are much lower. A survey of schoolchildren aged 11–15 in England in 2002 revealed that 4% of them had used alkyl nitrites in the past year, and the same incidence was seen in 16- to 24-year-olds from both England and Wales.[2] This compares with 1.2% for the general adult population under 60.[3] However, when asked about lifetime use of alkyl nitrites, 15% of 16- to 24-year-olds had used them at least once.[2] In the USA, the proportion of 16-year-olds at high school who had ever abused nitrites was 1.6% in 2003.[4]

Administration

The alkyl nitrites are volatile, yellowish clear liquids with a distinctive smell, often likened to 'old socks'. The liquid is irritant and may burn the skin if spilled. It is also inflammable and so care should be taken to avoid contact with fire (e.g. lighted cigarettes). Alkyl nitrites are not very stable chemically and should be stored in a cool, dark, dry environment.

Nitrites are inhaled, usually directly from a small bottle. Often these are amber bottles to limit light entry, which can cause decomposition. Some examples are shown in Figure 18.1.

Alkyl nitrites are easily obtainable on the Internet and can be purchased from sex shops, nightclubs and bars in most countries. They are

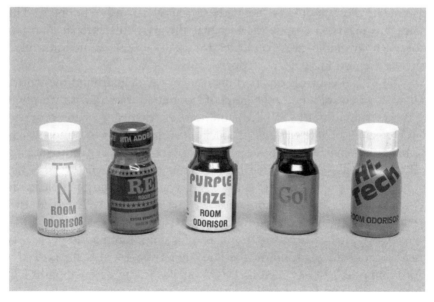

Figure 18.1 A selection of 'poppers' (Photo courtesy of Multimedia Research Partners Ltd).

usually supplied in small thumb-sized bottles and are inexpensive. In the USA, there have been reports of products being adulterated with other chemicals with unknown effects, and there is a need for analysis of commercially available products to assess their purity.[1]

Brand names of nitrite products are often descriptive of the effects sought and examples include 'Stud', 'TNT', 'Locker Room' and 'Purple Haze'.

Effects sought

Rapid deep inhalation produces a sudden intense 'buzz' of excitement. This is often referred to by users as a 'rush' or 'high'. The effect only lasts a few minutes, and is associated with a characteristic warm feeling. Users typically repeat the inhalation at regular intervals to maintain the effect. The 'rush' is probably secondary to the pronounced vasodilatory effects of these drugs. Users may employ alkyl nitrites simply to experience the 'rush'; others use them to loosen inhibition on the dance floor at nightclubs, often in association with other drugs such as ecstasy or LSD (lysergide). Some feel that nitrites may enhance the effects of these other drugs. Certain users believe that nitrites can heighten creativity or the perception of music and some people use alkyl nitrites in a meditative setting.[5–7]

Others use nitrites during intercourse because they claim that nitrites have an aphrodisiac effect, or seem to enhance sexual experience and prolong orgasm. Gay men are particularly likely to use alkyl nitrites, perhaps because these drugs have been claimed to relax the anal muscles during anal intercourse, but they are also widely used by heterosexual men and women.

Adverse effects

Not all users find the euphoria produced by nitrites pleasant.[5–7] In a survey conducted in Virginia, USA, 32 out of a total of 73 who had used the drug found the experience unpleasant.[6] The following effects are common after inhalation of nitrites:

- light-headedness, dizziness, nausea
- flushing of the face, feeling hot
- tachycardia, palpitations
- blurred vision, a feeling of pressure in the eyes, stinging of the eyes

- headache
- inflammation or a 'burning' sensation around the mouth and nose.

The irritant effects of alkyl nitrites are more prevalent after concentrated or prolonged exposure. A facial **dermatitis** has been described.[8] This is a crusted, erythematous reaction of the upper lip, nose and cheeks, sometimes accompanied by a sinusitis-like reaction as well. It resolves within 10 days if there is no further nitrite exposure. Wheezing or inflammation of the eyes can also occur as irritant reactions.

Less-common effects include weakness, cold sweats, ataxia and fainting.

Methaemoglobinaemia, psychosis-like episodes and sudden death have been reported but these are rare. **Methaemoglobinaemia** occurs when the ferrous form of iron in haemoglobin (Fe^{2+}) is oxidised to the ferric form (Fe^{3+}). The ferric form renders haemoglobin incapable of carrying oxygen. The condition can be fatal but for alkyl nitrites severe reactions usually only happen in those who have ingested large quantities, rather than inhaled. However, cases have been attributed to novice users not realising that alkyl nitrites should be inhaled and drinking them instead.[9] Cases of methaemoglobinaemia in those inhaling alkyl nitrites are occasionally reported, and prompt medical management is necessary.[10,11] The symptoms are those of acute anaemia because of the decreased oxygen-carrying capacity of the blood. The effect is reversible either spontaneously over a period of hours as the iron in haemoglobin reverts to the ferrous form or with the assistance of medical intervention (e.g. methylene blue injection), but this particular toxic reaction can persist for considerably longer than the intoxicating effects of alkyl nitrites.

Nitrites may theoretically worsen glaucoma, but the short duration of action should make a clinically significant effect unlikely from a single exposure. Nitrites should be avoided by those with hypotension or heart failure.

The **immune effects** of alkyl nitrites are controversial. It has been suggested that abuse might predispose users, particularly gay men, to developing HIV (human immunodeficiency virus) disease and Kaposi's sarcoma. More specifically, it has been argued that alkyl nitrites could act in one or all of the following ways:[12]

- They might be a marker for high-risk sexual activity, especially anal sex, by increasing libido, loosening inhibitions and relaxing the smooth muscles of the anus.
- These drugs are vasodilators and this property may facilitate virus transmission across mucosal membranes.

- Alkyl nitrites may be metabolised to nitrosamines *in vivo*, which could be carcinogenic and this could in some way precipitate or enable the development of Kaposi's sarcoma.
- Toxic effects upon the immune system could allow viruses and tumour cells to replicate more freely.
- Alkyl nitrites may promote HIV replication in the human body and the growth of Kaposi's sarcoma cells.

However, others have dismissed any association with alkyl nitrites.[1] The case against alkyl nitrites in this situation is not proven. Some of the evidence is contradictory, and much of it is circumstantial, but it would seem prudent for those who are immunosuppressed or at risk for HIV infection to avoid using them.

Alkyl nitrites do not produce dependence, and tolerance is unlikely during the typically episodic use of these drugs, because of their very brief half-lives.

Drug interactions

Sildenafil and related drugs

Given the link that alkyl nitrites have with sexual activity, it is important to note that the manufacturers of sildenafil (Viagra) and related medicines marketed for treatment of impotence, such as vardenafil and tadalafil, advise against the use of alkyl nitrites with their products. This is because the combination may lower blood pressure to cause severe hypotension, even death. Nonetheless this potentially dangerous combination is encountered at street level. A study of 837 gay and bisexual men in San Francisco in 2001 revealed that 18% had used sildenafil with alkyl nitrites at least once.[13]

Pregnancy and breastfeeding

Amyl nitrite has been used to facilitate uterine relaxation in difficult deliveries.[14] In one retrospective study its safety was assessed in 64 women given pre-term caesarean deliveries who were compared to matched controls not given amyl nitrite.[14] The authors concluded that amyl nitrite posed no threat to mother or fetus during this procedure. There are otherwise no studies of alkyl nitrite use or abuse in human pregnancy or breastfeeding.

References

1. Slavin S. Recreational use of amyl nitrite. *Venereology* 2001; 14: 81–82.
2. *Statistics on young people and drug misuse: England, 2003.* Statistical Bulletin 2004/13. London: National Statistics Office and Department of Health, 2004.
3. Aust R, Sharp C, Goulden C. *Prevalence of Drug Use: Key Findings from the 2001/02 British Crime Survey.* Home Office Research Study 182. London: Home Office, 2002.
4. Johnston L D, O'Malley P M, Bachman J G, *et al. Ecstasy Use Falls for Second Year in a Row, Overall Teen Drug Use Drops.* National press release, University of Michigan News and Information Services, Ann Arbor, 19 December 2003.
5. Sigell L T, Kapp F T, Fusaro G A, *et al.* Popping and snorting volatile nitrites: a current fad for getting high. *Am J Psychiatry* 1978; 135: 1216–1218.
6. Schwartz R H, Peary P. Abuse of isobutyl nitrite inhalation (Rush) by adolescents. *Clin Pediatr* 1986; 25: 308–310.
7. Lockwood B. Poppers: volatile nitrite inhalants. *Pharm J* 1996; 257: 154–155.
8. Fisher A A. 'Poppers' or 'snappers' dermatitis in homosexual men. *Cutis* 1984; 34: 118–122.
9. Stambach T, Haire K, Soni N, *et al.* Saturday night blue – a case of near fatal poisoning from the abuse of amyl nitrite. *J Accident Emerg Med* 1997; 14: 339–340.
10. Edwards R J, Ujima J. Extreme methaemaglobinaemia secondary to recreational use of amyl nitrite. *J Accident Emerg Med* 1995; 12: 138–142.
11. Machabert R, Testud F, Descotes J. Methaemagloninaemia due to amyl nitrite inhalation: a case report. *Hum Exp Toxicol* 1994; 13: 313–314.
12. Soderberg L S F. Immunomodulation by nitrite inhalants may predispose abusers to AIDS and Kaposi's sarcoma. *J Neuroimmunol* 1998; 83: 157–161.
13. Chu P L, McFarland W, Gibson S, *et al.* Viagra use in a community-recruited sample of men who have sex with men, San Francisco. *J AIDS* 2003; 33: 191–193.
14. Hendricks S K, Ross B, Colvard M A, *et al.* Amyl nitrite: use as a smooth muscle relaxant in difficult preterm cesarean section. *Am J Perinatol* 1992; 9: 289–292.

19

Smart drugs

It is never wise to try to appear to be more clever than you are. It is sometimes wise to appear slightly less so.
William Whitelaw, The Observer 'Sayings of the Year', 1975

Smart drugs are generally asserted to increase learning ability in healthy people and to induce keener perception, improved memory, sharpened concentration, and even to increase intelligence. Most of those involved in taking them are ambitious, healthy young people who want to increase their mental powers and smart drugs have been the subject of discussion in many popular magazines and newspapers.[1-7] Many of these drugs are also known more formally as 'cognitive enhancers', especially when used clinically in an attempt to improve cognition in humans affected by various medical conditions (e.g. Alzheimer's disease). However, this chapter is concerned with their use in healthy persons not affected by disease-related cognitive impairment. A subgroup of compounds has been referred to as 'nootropics' (especially the pyrrolidone derivatives; see Table 19.1). Nootropics are claimed to improve or activate the natural processes of cognition without the sedative, stimulant or other adverse effects of the traditional psychotropic drugs used medicinally.

Abuse liability

Users might object to smart drugs being referred to as drugs of abuse, and perhaps this is an unfair description. Unlike most classical drugs of abuse, smart drugs are said to facilitate natural mental processes rather than to produce aberrant or novel psychoactive effects. They also do not generally cause dependence or withdrawal reactions. However, smart drugs do share some characteristics with more conventionally defined drugs of abuse:

- They are pharmacologically active substances taken not for a medical condition but to improve personal functioning. Parallels have been drawn between the use of smart drugs to increase mental performance and the use of anabolic steroids to increase physical performance.[8] Both groups of drugs may be taken to enhance social prowess.

- The potential for side-effects is not necessarily appreciated by users and the long-term mental consequences of administration are not known in many cases. Some advocates of smart drugs encourage the unsupervised use of prescription medicines as cognition enhancers. This clearly could be hazardous. Table 19.1 includes some of these.

- There could be important social, safety or financial consequences arising from intense personal use, or widespread population use, of these substances – whether they produce the desired effects or not.

Table 19.1 Examples of compounds that have been advocated as smart drugs

Pyrrolidone derivatives
- Piracetam, pramiracetam, oxiracetam, aniracetam, nebracetam

Nutrients
- Vitamins B_{12} (and other B group vitamins), C and E
- Cycloserine
- Dimethylaminoethanol (DMAE)
- Pyroglutamate, phenylalanine

Acetylcholine 'enhancers'
- Choline, lecithin, inositol
- Donepezil
- Acetyl-L-carnitine (ST200)

Plant-derived products
- Ginseng
- Ginkgo biloba
- Brahmi
- Vincamine, vinpocetine (periwinkle plant)
- Co-dergocrine mesilate (Hydergine, ergot-derived)

Hormones
- Corticotropin (adrenocorticotrophic hormone, ACTH), vasopressin
- Prasterone (dehydroepiandrosterone, DHEA)

Prescription-only medicines (in the UK)
- Selegiline, levodopa, bromocriptine
- Phenytoin
- Ondansetron
- Methylphenidate
- Modafinil
- Nimodipine
- Propranolol
- Procaine
- Meclofenoxate (centrophenoxine)

• The pharmaceutical purity, quality and identity of many of the substances purchased is not regulated and is open to question.

Availability

The examples given in Table 19.1 are not generally controlled by drug misuse legislation and so possession of these substances is not illegal. In the USA, and to a lesser extent in Europe, a range of products is sold in health food outlets and bars with names such as 'memory booster' and 'memory fuel'. These are often merely combinations of simple nutrients. So-called 'smart drinks' are also sold in some clubs, and are advocated as a means of replenishing depleted brain stores of serotonin after using drugs such as LSD (lysergide) and ecstasy: in this way the drinks presumably aim to preserve mental function.

Most of the more pharmacologically active smart drugs are only available by mail order. In many countries, a legal loophole allows members of the public to purchase prescription medicines from overseas suppliers if these are for personal use. This means that individuals can import drugs such as selegiline, propranolol and vasopressin for use without medical supervision. Side-effects in those purchasing prescription medicines have been reported in the medical literature.[9]

Sometimes single drugs are administered; other users take cocktails or mixtures of various products that have alleged synergism. All are taken orally, with the notable exception of vasopressin, which is usually inhaled nasally. Proponents claim that vasopressin has a rapid onset via this route and can thus be taken when required as a quick 'cognitive top-up' for mentally demanding situations.

Development of smart drugs[10]

At first sight, the use of a drug to improve cognition seems feasible. After all, some substances are known to cause memory impairment (e.g. antimuscarinic agents, alcohol and the benzodiazepines). Yet closer examination reveals a more complex situation.

Information about smart drugs has largely arisen from the pharmacological manipulation of learning behaviour in animals and the treatment of dementia/cognitive decline in aged humans and animals. A number of the drugs listed in Table 19.1 are known to improve rodent learning and memory in maze-deciphering and similar experiments; furthermore, some drugs seem to have 'anti-amnesic' effects for both reward behaviour and situations where animals learn to avoid a noxious stimulus.

In addition, over the past two decades many of the substances listed have been studied as possible treatments for the cognitive impairment that accompanies certain forms of dementia, such as Alzheimer's disease. It is widely accepted that cholinergic nerves have an important role in learning behaviour. It is also known that central production of acetylcholine declines with age and this loss may be particularly marked in those with Alzheimer's disease. Consequently, many of the drugs investigated initially were agents that sought to boost cholinergic activity of the brain by acting as precursors to acetylcholine synthesis or by inhibiting the breakdown of this neurotransmitter. Other approaches have sought to increase blood flow to the central nervous system (CNS) by vasodilation, to influence brain metabolism or to increase the activity of other neurotransmitter systems. Often the mode of action is unclear.

Despite extensive investigation, the simple fact is that no drug currently available will substantially reverse the cognitive changes that occur in senile dementia and enable the affected individual to return to a 'normal' pre-dementia life.

Claims made for smart drugs

The supporters of smart drugs can produce an impressive-sounding array of scientific papers to back up their claims. Unfortunately, very few of these studies have involved the target population for smart drugs, i.e. non-demented, healthy and (mostly) young people who want to increase their 'brain power'. A small number of studies have examined the effects of drugs on human learning behaviour outside the dementia setting. For example, in 2002, a small placebo-controlled study in 18 airline pilots suggested that donepezil was able to assist retention of training on complex aviation tasks in a flight simulator.[11] The pilots given donepezil had better recall of training after 1 month of donepezil than the placebo recipients. However, the study was small and the average age of pilots was 52 years.

A high proportion of the research quoted involves the animal studies that have already been alluded to. While much of this work does show that, for example, a particular smart drug will help a rat remember which way to run around a maze, the relevance of this effect to humans is questionable. What does a drug-induced change in animal behaviour really mean in this situation? There is an assumption that changes in animal behaviour in the laboratory can be extrapolated to humans. Yet the human brain is larger and more complex, and human learning or memory can be influenced by a vast array of environmental, personal and social pressures to which laboratory animals cannot be subject. Supporters also assume that the basic neurobiochemical processes of learning/memory are the same in all mammals, which is by no means proven. In addition, animal tests can be difficult to standardise, poorly reproducible and subject to many variables. Can changes in laboratory animals be seriously related to something as intangible as human cognition?

Other evidence cited to support the use of smart drugs in healthy people includes studies of demented patients, as discussed above. These experiments have produced disappointing, often conflicting, results. Where improvement does occur this is frequently limited to small changes in a number of the mental tests and psychometric assessments performed. It is clearly inappropriate to extrapolate the limited improvements seen in tests of demented patients to cognition enhancement in healthy unaffected people. The brain of the demented subject is functioning below the normal standard and would not be expected to respond to drug treatment in the same way as a healthy brain. It is not unreasonable to believe that a drug might improve cognition if there is a disease-related cause for decline. But to imply that these drugs should work in an otherwise healthy brain suggests that the CNS normally functions at suboptimal capacity. This does not seem logical.

Some of the research quoted to support smart drugs has been published in obscure journals where the quality of refereeing might be open to question. Sometimes the studies are poorly designed: using small numbers of participants, giving vague unquantified results and sometimes even involving administration of smart drugs by unrepresentative routes that the general population would not use (e.g. intravenous, intracerebral). Statistical analysis is often dubious. The lack of a consistent mode of action for the different smart drugs – even those with a similar chemical structure – also tends to promote disbelief.

A further complication is that some drugs which are claimed to enhance cognition may actually be removing barriers to memory or intellect rather than boosting mental processes directly – several of the smart drugs have anxiolytic, stimulant, antidepressant, or other psychotropic effects that may help overcome obstacles to cognition.

The final evidence that smart drug advocates produce is the testimonials of users. This is not a form of evidence that stands close scrutiny. For example, it is known that the placebo effect can be particularly marked when psychological/psychiatric conditions are treated,[12] and this might equally apply to attempts to influence other mental processes.

Large placebo-controlled, double-blind trials need to be conducted in healthy young volunteers before the scientific community can evaluate any potential benefits of cognition-enhancing drugs in the target population.

Modes of action[10]

In retrospect, it seems naïve that the early investigators of dementia could have hoped that simply increasing brain levels of acetylcholine would be sufficient to dramatically improve a behaviour as complex as memory and learning. However, a variety of cholinergic enhancers are still used as smart drugs. Choline and lecithin, for example, are converted into acetylcholine by metabolism. Tacrine and velnacrine inhibit the breakdown of acetylcholine but, although widely investigated for the treatment of dementia, they do not appear to have been used commonly as smart drugs. The pyrrolidone derivatives may also enhance the effectiveness of central cholinergic systems, although this group of drugs probably has additional actions via steroids, aldosterone, and glucose metabolism. Their structural similarity to GABA (gamma-aminobutyric acid) might also be relevant.

Certain cognitive enhancers may increase cerebral blood flow by vasodilation (e.g. vinpocetine), facilitate calcium passage across neurones (e.g. nimodipine) or affect neural growth/repair. Drugs that act via specific neurotransmitters are also claimed to have cognition-enhancing effects, e.g. ondansetron (acting via serotonin) and levodopa (dopamine). A range of other neurotransmitter systems may also be implicated, including glutamate, endogenous opioids and beta-adrenoceptors.

Some drugs (e.g. acetyl-L-carnitine) seem able to reduce lipofuscin deposits in the brains of experimental animals. This substance accumulates in the brain with age and may be a cause of neuronal damage. Certain drugs have free radical scavenging properties (e.g. dimethylaminoethanol) or are antioxidants (e.g. vitamin E). As may be expected, many of the smart drugs have a multiplicity of potential pharmacological actions.

Future use of smart drugs[10]

Supporters of smart drugs and associated pharmacotherapy have attempted to link use of these substances with the profitable anti-ageing industry. The condition of age-associated memory impairment (AAMI) has been defined and supported by certain pharmaceutical companies active in the investigation of cognition. This has occurred largely in response to the realisation that drug regulatory authorities are unlikely to allow cognitive enhancers to be marketed without definite treatment goals. This means identifying a condition to be treated in the first place.

If drugs to treat AAMI become available in the future they may become 'lifestyle drugs' for those with or without established AAMI. They may also have military uses. It has been predicted that imposing successful legal controls on the use of a genuinely effective cognitive enhancer would be virtually impossible, and that some form of regulation of this developing industry is needed.[9] The objective of pharmaceutical manufacturers is presumably to launch drugs to treat or prevent the normal (non-dementia) deterioration in memory that naturally accompanies advancing age. But is this a condition which should be treated? Is attempting to change this natural age-related effect the same as, say, fitting a hearing aid or treating maturity-onset diabetes?

If smart drugs are proven to boost memory and intelligence in healthy people, the majority of the population will presumably want to take them. Such a treatment would not be available to everyone: will only the rich in the Western world be able to afford these drugs, rendering them 'elitist'? And who should pay: employers, employees, insurers or governments? Must one take the drug for life to continue to experience the beneficial effects? If so, will long-term treatment affect the neurobiochemical make-up of the brain in other perhaps undesirable ways? Are there disadvantages to being able to remember more?

Alternatively, might smart drugs offer all of us the chance for greater achievements, to release an untapped intellectual resource, perhaps to live to old age without fear of dementia or a deterioration in mental ability? Those selling smart drugs pluck on a notable chord in many people – the desire to be a 'better' person: to perform well in examinations, to obtain a better job, to be more educated. Would any of these objectives be as worthwhile if they were achieved with reduced effort and a tablet, rather than with determined hard work? How far should pharmacological means be used to improve on 'normality'?

Fortunately, we do not have to consider answers to any of these questions yet because there is little evidence that any of the existing smart drugs increases cognition in healthy people in a useful way.

References

1. Heley M. High time to get smart. *Weekend Guardian*, 8–9 June 1991, 14–15.
2. Concar D, Coghlan A. Is there money in lost memories? *New Scientist*, 17 April 1993, 20–22.
3. Rose S. No way to treat the mind. *New Scientist*, 17 April 1993, 23–26.
4. Anonymous. Smart drugs. *Which? Way to Health*, February 1993, 22–25.
5. Geary J. Should we just say no to smart drugs? *Time* 1997; 149: 1–3.
6. Russo E. Seeking smart drugs. *The Scientist* 2002; 16: 27–30.
7. Hall S S. The quest for a smart pill. *Sci Am* 2003; September: 36–45.
8. Canterbury R J, Lloyd E. Smart drugs: implications of student use. *J Primary Prev* 1994; 14: 197–207.
9. Baker L S. 'Smart drugs': a caution to everybody. *Am J Psychiatry* 1996; 153: 844–845.
10. Rose S P R. 'Smart drugs': do they work? Are they ethical? Will they be legal? *Nat Rev Neurosci* 2002; 3: 975–979.
11. Yesavage J A, Mumenthaler M S, Taylor J L, *et al*. Donepezil and flight simulator performance: effects on retention of complex skills. *Neurology* 2002; 59: 123–125.
12. Laporte J R, Figueras A. Placebo effects in psychiatry. *Lancet* 1994; 344: 1206–1209.

20

Substance misuse and the Internet

Knowledge is of two kinds. We know a subject ourselves, or we know where we can find information upon it.
Samuel Johnson (1709–84)

The Internet contains a vast amount of information about substance abuse and it is clearly not possible to cover more than a tiny fraction of the websites available. Selecting which ones to include can only be done in a very subjective way. I have selected about 20 websites that I personally find helpful and, in selecting them, I have tried to reflect a broad range of interests. I have described them as they appeared at the time of writing, although many websites change their appearance and content frequently. There are a lot of country-specific websites containing details of national policies and so forth, but many of these are available via the Virtual Clearinghouse on Alcohol, Tobacco and Other Drugs website (see below) and so are not listed individually below.

General websites

1. National Institute on Drug Abuse
(http://www.nida.nih.gov)

The National Institute on Drug Abuse (NIDA) is a US government organisation. It was established in 1974 and is now part of the US National Institutes of Health, Department of Health and Human Services. The website displays NIDA's mission, which is to 'lead the Nation in bringing the power of science to bear on drug abuse and addiction'. NIDA is a research-based organisation and according to the website supports over 85% of the world's research on the health aspects of drug abuse and dependence.

Basic navigation and content

The home page carries a list of recent publications and announcements, but there is a more extensive list of recently added material that can be accessed by clicking on the 'What's New' section on the navigation bar. The 'Newsroom' on the navigation bar is less useful, mainly carrying details of publicity related to NIDA work. Clicking on 'Publications' on the navigation bar provides access to a list of available publications by series title, but also enables the user to limit their search of the site to publications only.

The home page lists content under three categories: 'Researchers & Health Professionals', 'Parents & Teachers', and 'Students & Young Adults'. The 'Researchers & Health Professionals' section provides links to very comprehensive information about drug abuse trends and statistics in the USA, enables e-subscription to the free journal *Science and Practice Perspectives*, and there is a variety of links related to ongoing and completed research, research funding and so forth. The other sections contain a wide range of teaching and informative materials for members of the public. Helpfully, this is often written for specific drugs and/or aimed at specific sections of the population (e.g. teenagers, women).

The most useful sections of the website are the very comprehensive themed drug abuse pages, which are easily accessed via the dropdown selection under 'Common Drugs of Abuse' on the navigation bar. Each section is devoted to a specific drug of abuse including:

Acid/LSD	Methamphetamine
Alcohol	Nicotine
Cocaine	PCP (Phencyclidine)
Club Drugs	Prescription Medications
Drug Testing	Prevention Research
Heroin	Steroids
Inhalants	Stress and Drug Abuse
Marijuana	Treatment Research
MDMA/Ecstasy	Trends and Statistics

When opened, each of these sections has links to relevant materials on the website. These include Infofacts (short but comprehensive summaries of each drug aimed at members of the public), research reports (overviews of current research knowledge), research monographs (full text research papers), NIDA Notes (summaries of key research papers published in full elsewhere), publications, news items, and therapy manuals.

Good and bad points

The NIDA website is probably the world's single most useful website on drug abuse and dependence for healthcare professionals and the public alike. The content of the website is very extensive, and it is generally easy to find information. There is an accurate and reliable search facility, which is often a good first step in looking for material.

The bad points are minor. It would be helpful for healthcare professionals to have a facility to limit searches to research monographs and NIDA Notes only, and so cut down on the large amount of lay-oriented materials that are often thrown up from searches. There is also only limited information on abuse of plants (e.g. khat) and over-the-counter (OTC) medicines.

2. DrugScope
(http://www.drugscope.org.uk)

DrugScope is a UK organisation based in London, which aims to 'inform policy development and reduce drug-related risk'. It is supported by the UK government and other sources.

Basic navigation and content

DrugScope produces a range of publications aimed at healthcare professionals, teachers and members of the public. Unfortunately many of these publications are not free, and they are not available free-to-view on the website either. Becoming a member of DrugScope is also not free, but enables discounts on publication prices, annual subscription to a regular magazine (six issues) and various other advantages.

There is a regularly updated news section that, although very UK-focused, does include some international items. The two most useful sections of the site are:

Good Practice & Research This includes information under the following headings, although it is not always immediately obvious what each of them means:

Treatment	Availability
Education & Prevention	Official Documents
Criminal Justice	Europe & International
Community & Social Exclusion	

Each one includes a series of FAQs related to the topic in question, and a section called 'Key Issues', which often links to relevant full text documents and reading lists.

Drug Information   Clicking on the 'DrugSearch' option links to a long list of topics, including individual drugs. Each of these topics is then briefly discussed. There are useful sections on subjects that the NIDA website does not include, for example commonly abused plants, adulterants and OTC medicines. The range of topics included is comprehensive, although the information provided is sometimes too brief.

Good points and bad points

The Drug Information section is comprehensive, although it can be lacking in detail. Nonetheless, it at least comprises a helpful introduction to most of the subjects it addresses. The 'Links' section is also helpful and easy to use, but limits its remit almost exclusively to the UK. It is possible to register to receive free email updates on news items and changes to the website. The search facility works well.

The fact that many publications need to be paid for limits the value and impact of both the website and the organisation. There is little detailed clinical information on individual drugs for healthcare professionals. The navigation of the website is not particularly intuitive and it is a website that requires some time and patience in order to get the most from it.

3. World Health Organization
(*http://www.who.int/substance_abuse/en/*)

The World Health Organization (WHO) has been involved in substance abuse since it was founded in 1948. According to its website, WHO's mandate includes:

- Prevention and reduction of the negative health and social consequences of psychoactive substance use.
- Reduction of the demand for non-medical use of psychoactive substances.
- Assessment of psychoactive substances so as to advise the United Nations with regard to their regulatory control.

These activities are coordinated by the WHO Department of Mental Health and Substance Abuse.

Basic navigation and content

On the left-hand side of the substance abuse home page there is a box displaying key contents of the site, which include:

- Terminology and classification – a very useful source of information. Includes an extensive lexicon of alcohol and drug terms, and the full text of the relevant sections of the 10th revision of the International Statistical Classification of Diseases and Related Health Problems (ICD-10).
- Facts and figures – on the global burden of substance abuse.
- Activities – WHO ongoing and completed research related to substance abuse.
- Publications – a collection of detailed full text systematic reviews, advisory publications and summary documents.

Good points and bad points

When the WHO covers a particular subject it is covered well, but topic coverage is patchy in some areas. There is also on occasion a lack of logical internal links within the WHO and other UN sites so that important documents can be missed.

The search engine is effective and, because it is powered by Google, it does tend to retrieve the most useful and popular documents as a priority. However, it is not possible to limit a search to particular sections or topics within the WHO website and because its overall content is very extensive it is important to choose search terms carefully to avoid retrieving too many pages.

4. Virtual Clearinghouse on Alcohol, Tobacco and Other Drugs
(http://www.atod.org/)

This site was created and is maintained by like minded partner organisations on five continents. Its main features are a database of full text policy and practice documents in the field of substance abuse, and a very comprehensive series of links to the national and international organisations that produce them. It is a very helpful site, which saves a great deal of time because it avoids having to search national sites individually. Material contributed by partner organisations must meet a set of criteria to ensure that the Virtual Clearinghouse provides information that is based on the published literature, research, and/or an organisation's recognised policy or program experience. Partners include:

- Australian Drug Foundation http://www.adf.org.au
- Australian Institute of Criminology: Alcohol and Illicit Drugs http://www.aic.gov.au/research/drugs
- Canadian Centre on Substance Abuse http://www.ccsa.ca/
- Drug Misuse Scotland http://www.drugmisuse.isdscotland.org
- European Monitoring Centre for Drugs and Drug Addiction (EMCDDA) http://www.emcdda.eu.int
- United Nations International Drug Control Programme http://www.undcp.org

The larger US organisations are not partners, but the membership is otherwise extremely broad and included nearly 70 in March 2004.

5. US Drug Enforcement Administration
(http://www.usdoj.gov/dea)

The mission of the Drug Enforcement Administration (DEA) is 'to enforce the controlled substances laws and regulations of the United States'. The website has a number of helpful features all accessible via a menu on the left of the screen. The 'News' section gives details of successful law enforcement operations aimed at combating illicit drug production and distribution. There is also a very extensive and instructive photo library. A comprehensive series of summaries about psychotropic drugs that are abused can be found in the 'Drug Information' section and includes prescription medicines (oxycodone, methylphenidate) and plants (khat, salvia), as well as conventional illicit drugs. The 'State Factsheets' section provides access to descriptions of drug usage patterns in each individual US state. The 'Drug Policy' section outlines the main legal controls on illicit drugs within the USA as a whole.

6. Daily Dose
(http://www.dailydose.net)

This website aims 'to provide links to news and reports concerning drug and alcohol misuse (abuse), and drug addiction.' The site is currently sponsored by the Welsh Development Agency and the Wired Initiative, a substance abuse awareness organisation developed at the psychology department of the University of Wales. This is probably the most comprehensive UK-based news service about substance misuse. The website is updated twice a day with news items. Being a UK site there is a lot of

UK-oriented news, but news from other countries (especially the USA) is not neglected. The items are very current and originate from a wide variety of sources. It is possible to subscribe to the news and have it delivered regularly by email, or simply to browse all the items for a particular day or week via the website.

7. Victoria Government (Australia) Drugs Site
(http://www.drugs.vic.gov.au)

This website contains a particularly good series of information bulletins for members of the public on key substances that are abused and also the treatments available (e.g. naltrexone). They are detailed and well written. Under the 'Drugs & their Effects' and 'In your Language' sections there is more general information, which is also in several different languages.

8. National Treatment Agency UK
(http://www.nta.nhs.uk/)

The National Treatment Agency for Substance Abuse (NTA) is a special health authority, created in 2001 to improve the availability, capacity and effectiveness of treatment for drug misuse in England – in other words, to ensure that there is more treatment, better treatment and fairer treatment available to all those who need it. As such it is an infant organisation so its website has rather limited content. The website includes a small amount of useful clinical guidance, but also provides access to *Models of Care*, a document that sets out a national framework for the commissioning of treatment for adult drug misusers in England.

9. Harm Reduction

There are a number of harm reduction organisations, but unfortunately, many of their websites contain little practical information. One of the better websites in this regard is that of the American Harm Reduction Coalition (http://www.harmreduction.org). This website contains useful information leaflets for users, a regular newsletter for practitioners, a practical description of the principles of harm reduction, and a detailed links section. The UK Harm Reduction Alliance website contains information about this organisation's responses to UK issues, a definition of harm reduction, links and a series of discussion lists (http://www.ukhra.org). Note that the extent of harm reduction activities can vary quite considerably between countries for legal, cultural and other reasons; this should be borne in mind when viewing harm reduction sites that do not originate from your own country.

Specific topics

1. World Anti-Doping Agency
(http://www.wada-ama.org/en/t1.asp)

The World Anti-Doping Agency (WADA) is an independent international agency, which sets unified standards for anti-doping work and coordinates the efforts of sports organisations and public authorities. It was established in 1999 and is now based in Montreal, Canada. The agency formulates the world anti-doping code, and is involved in education and research. The website contains the current version of the list of prohibited substances and gives athletes guidance on testing and testing procedures.

2. National Institute on Alcohol Abuse and Alcoholism
(http://www.niaaa.nih.gov)

The National Institute on Alcohol Abuse and Alcoholism (NIAAA) is a US organisation that 'provides leadership in the national effort to reduce alcohol-related problems'. The 'Publications' section holds some valuable resources. *Alcohol Alert* is released quarterly and addresses a key topic based on an evaluation of published literature. Examples include underage drinking, alcohol and the liver, alcohol and HIV/AIDS (human immunodeficiency virus/acquired immunodeficiency syndrome). There are also a number of information leaflets for the public designed to address key issues concerning alcohol and alcoholism (e.g. Drinking and Your Pregnancy). There are educational materials in this section for healthcare professionals as well, and various other reports. The 'Databases' section houses a bibliographic database of published literature concerned with alcohol and alcoholism called ETOH. It contains over 10,000 citations from the 1960s onwards and is invaluable for anyone who is conducting research or who needs a comprehensive literature search in this field. The site also has details of ongoing research into alcohol and alcoholism.

3. International Labour Organization – Substance Abuse and Tobacco in the Workplace Database
(http://www.ccsa.ca/ilo/ilodbdesc.htm)

This database indexes documents concerned with the effects of substance abuse in the workplace. The workplace settings involved are very broad and the documents cover topics related to program planning, policy development, legal issues, statistics, and research.

4. Coffee Science Information Centre
(http://www.cosic.org)

The Coffee Science Information Centre (CoSIC) is a pan-European organisation established in 1990 by ISIC, the Institute for Scientific Information on Coffee, which is based in Switzerland. 'The aim of CoSIC is to provide accurate, balanced and consistent information to all audiences across Europe who have an interest in coffee, caffeine and health. The primary objective is to bring balance to the coffee and health debate.' Detailed, fully referenced assessments of the effects of coffee on key aspects of health are available.

5. WHO Tobacco Free Initiative
(http://www.who.int/tobacco/en/)

Tobacco is the second major cause of death in the world. This WHO website provides facts and strategic support for helping to eradicate the global epidemic of tobacco smoking.

6. Methadone Briefing
(http://www.drugtext.org/library/books/methadone/default.htm)

Still one of the best resources for everything concerned with methadone, this book was published in 1996 but is still valuable. On the first page, the author offers some guidance on major areas of change since the book was originally written, and then the full text of the book can be accessed via the contents on the navigation bar at the top.

7. Volatile Substance Abuse UK
(http://www.sghms.ac.uk/depts/phs/vsamenu.htm)

The UK has, uniquely, established a long-running data series for deaths related to volatile substance abuse since 1971. Annual update reports, published by St George's Hospital Medical School in London, can be found on this website.

User-oriented sites

It is difficult to select a small number of the many thousands of user-oriented websites for inclusion here. However, user-oriented sites are a valuable way to keep in touch with the changing ways in which psychoactive substances are used. Most offer a forum for the sharing of information between users. Some of the material contained on these sites may be misleading, incomplete or incorrect so it would be unwise to rely upon them as a sole source of information.[1] The two websites below are notable for the large amount of material they contain and their comprehensiveness. Both contain a mixture of material in terms of quality.

1. Vaults of Erowid
(http://www.erowid.org)

This is an online library of over 20,000 documents related to psychoactive plants and chemicals from a wide variety of sources. The website states that the 'information found on the site spans the spectrum from solid peer reviewed research to fanciful creative writing.' Clicking on the 'Plants & Drugs' header on the home page leads to an index of psychoactive substances. Each one is covered in varying amounts of detail.

2. The Lycaeum
(http://www.lycaeum.org)

The Lycaeum Entheogen Database (LEDA) can be accessed by clicking on 'Preparations' on the home page. The default page lists mainly naturally occurring products that have been processed in some way. Selecting the heading 'Chemicals' from the left-hand side provides a list of synthetic psychoactive drugs, and the 'Taxonomy' heading leads to a list of naturally occurring substances. All of these are then discussed in some detail.

References

1. Boyer E W, Shannon M, Hibberd P L. Web sites with misinformation about illicit drugs. *N Engl J Med* 2001; 345: 469–471.

Appendix A

Glossary of street terminology

Acid: LSD
Adam: ecstasy
AKA: ecstasy
Amyl: alkyl nitrites
Angel dust: phencyclidine
Backloading or Backtracking: to draw back the plunger of a syringe when injecting, so that blood enters the barrel
Bain: nalbuphine (Nubain)
Barbs: barbiturates
Base: free cocaine base
Bhang: cannabis
Binge: repeated administration of an intoxicating substance several times in a short space of time. Typically applies to cocaine or alcohol
Blasted: under the influence of drugs
Blow: (1) cannabis (2) cocaine (3) to smoke a drug
Blowout: to miss a vein when injecting
Bombed: intoxicated
Bong: home-made smoking apparatus that allows smoke to bubble through water
Bud: cannabis
Bummer: bad trip
Busted: caught using drugs
Buzz: an intense, sudden euphoria that can occur very soon after administering a drug
BZP: benzylpiperazine, trifluoromethylphenylpiperazine and related piperazines
C: cocaine
Calvin Klein: cocaine and ketamine mixture
Cat: methcathinone (not be confused with khat or qat, a psychoactive plant; see Chapter 17)
Chalk: metamfetamine
Charlie: cocaine hydrochloride
Chasing the dragon: the heating of heroin and inhalation of the resultant vapour. Following the plume of smoke with an inhalation device called a toot is 'chasing the dragon's tail'

China white: alpha-methylfentanyl

CK: cocaine-ketamine mixture

Clean: not using, or not in possession of, drugs

Coke: cocaine hydrochloride

Cold turkey: when described as 'doing cold turkey', an individual is undergoing drug withdrawal. The term is most commonly applied to heroin withdrawal

Coming down: the gradual termination of a period of intoxication

Cook: someone who makes illicit drugs, usually amfetamine derivatives

Cooking up: preparing an injection by heating powdered drug with water

Crack: free cocaine base

Crank: metamfetamine

Crap: poor quality drug

Crash: acute post-intoxication dysphoria after abuse of stimulants

Crystal: metamfetamine ('crystals' has also been used to describe amphetamine)

Cutting: the diluting of a powdered drug with another powder that may, or may not, be pharmacologically active

Dike: Diconal

DOM: 3,4-dimethoxymethylamfetamine, an amfetamine derivative

Dope: usually understood to refer to cannabis in the UK. In the USA more often used to describe heroin

Doves: ecstasy tablets, which may have a bird motif

Downers: sedating drugs, usually barbiturates

Draw: cannabis

Dud or **Dummy:** poor quality drug containing little or no active ingredient

Eccies: ecstasy

Ecstasy: 3,4-methylenedioxymethamfetamine, an amfetamine derivative

Eve: 3,4-methylenedioxyethamfetamine or MDEA

Fantasy : gamma hydroxybutyrate

Fix: the administration, and subsequent effects, of a psychoactive substance, usually by injection

Flake: cocaine hydrochloride

Flying or **In flight:** experiencing intoxication

Freebase: homemade cocaine base made from cocaine hydrochloride using alkali

Freebasing: the conversion of cocaine hydrochloride to base cocaine using alkali, followed by vaporisation then inhalation

French blues: diazepam tablets 10 mg

G: gamma hydroxybutyrate

Ganja: cannabis

GBH or **GHB:** gamma hydroxybutyrate

Gear: injection equipment

Georgia Home Boy: gamma hydroxybutyrate

Get off on: experience pleasurable effects from a drug

Glass: metamfetamine

Go-ey: metamfetamine
Grass: cannabis
Grievous Bodily Harm: gamma hydroxybutyrate
H: heroin
Hard stuff: heroin
Hash or **hashish**: cannabis resin
Hash oil: concentrated cannabis resin
Hash plant: cannabis plant
Hemp: cannabis
Herb: cannabis
High: an intense, sudden euphoria that can occur very soon after administering a drug
Hit: (1) a dose of drug (2) a drug purchase
Hitting up: injecting a drug
Horse: heroin
Hot knifing: passing a heated knife through cannabis resin to release vapours that are then inhaled
Huffing: inhaling volatile substances from a plastic bag
Ice: metamfetamine
Jammed up: overdosed
Jellies: temazepam capsules
Joint: home-made cigarettes containing psychoactive drugs. Most often applied to cigarettes containing heroin or cannabis
Junk: heroin
Junkie: regular heroin user
K: ketamine
Kick: pleasurable feeling from taking a drug
Kit: injection equipment
Kit-kat: ketamine
Legal E: benzylpiperazine, trifluoromethylphenylpiperazine and related piperazines
Legal X: benzylpiperazine, trifluoromethylphenylpiperazine and related piperazines
Line: powdered cocaine hydrochloride or amfetamine laid out ready to snort
Liquid ecstasy: gamma hydroxybutyrate
Liquid X: gamma hydroxybutyrate
Lung: flexible plastic smoking apparatus that when squeezed enables smoke held within it to be forcibly ejected
M: ecstasy
Main-lining: the process of injecting
M and Ms: ecstasy
Marijuana or **marihuana**: largely synonymous with cannabis. Usually used at street level to describe the dried flowering heads of the plant
Mary Jane: cannabis

MDA: 3,4-methylenedioxyamfetamine

MDEA: 3,4-methylenedioxyethamfetamine

MDMA: 3,4-methylenedioxymethamfetamine or ecstasy

Meth: metamfetamine

Microdot: dose of LSD in a very small tablet

Moonshine: illicitly distilled concentrated alcoholic drink

Munchies: hunger pangs as a result of intoxication or its after-effects (often applied to cannabis)

Nine ounce block: common size for a large block of hashish

No Pain: nalbuphine (Nubain)

Nuggets: cocaine

OD: overdose

One-4-B – 1,4-butanediol

Outfit: injection equipment

P: metamfetamine

PCP: phencyclidine

Poppers: alkyl nitrites

Pot: cannabis

Puff: cannabis

Pure: metamfetamine

Pusher: an individual who sells drugs

Rave: a party or event where non-stop music and dancing occur

Reefers: home-made cigarettes containing psychoactive drugs. Most often applied to cigarettes containing heroin or cannabis

Roach: butt of a cannabis cigarette

Rock: 'crack' cocaine

Roid rage: violent outbursts of aggression associated with the use of anabolic steroids

Run: repeated administration of an intoxicating substance several times in a short space of time. Typically applies to cocaine

Rush: (1) an intense, sudden euphoria that can occur very soon after administering a drug (2) a generic name for poppers (3) a brand name under which butyl nitrite is sold

Salty water: gamma hydroxybutyrate

Score: to buy drugs

Shit: cannabis

Shooting gallery: place where drugs are commonly injected in a group

Shooting-up: the process of injecting

Sinsemilla: variety of hashish containing particularly high concentration of THC, derived from unfertilised female plants

Skag: heroin

Skagging: taking heroin, usually by vaporisation

Skin popping: injecting drugs subcutaneously

Skunk: cannabis containing a particularly high concentration of THC, due to selective cultivation

Sleepers: sedative drugs

Smack: heroin

Smashed: intoxicated

Smoke: cannabis

Snappers: alkyl nitrites

Snorting: the inhalation of dry powdered drug into the nose

Snow: cocaine hydrochloride

Snowball: mixed injection of cocaine hydrochloride and heroin

Soap: gamma hydroxybutyrate

Spaced out: intoxicated

Special K: ketamine

Speed: amfetamine, but can also be used to describe metamfetamine

Speedball: mixed injection of cocaine hydrochloride and heroin

Spiked: (1) drug or alcoholic drink adulterated with another psychoactive substance (2) injected

Spliff: home-made cigarettes containing psychoactive drugs. Most often applied to cigarettes containing heroin or cannabis

Stacking: the use of more than one anabolic steroid at the same time

Stoned: intoxicated (often with cannabis)

Sulph: amfetamine

Super K: ketamine

Synthetic heroin: illicit fentanyl derivatives

Tab: tablet

Tems: temazepam

TMF: 3-methylfentanyl, a synthetic opioid

Tranx: benzodiazepines, especially temazepam

Trip: an intoxicating experience

Trips: LSD

Uppers: any stimulant drug, but usually amfetamine

Vitamin K: ketamine

Wash: free cocaine base

Washback: process of producing free cocaine base from cocaine hydrochloride using ammonia solution

Wasted: under the influence of drugs

Weed: cannabis

Whiz: amfetamine

Works: injection equipment (i.e. needle and syringe)

Wrap: folded card or paper containing powdered drug such as heroin or amfetamine

Wrecked: intoxicated

XTC: ecstasy

Yaba: metamfetamine tablets

Appendix B

Legal status of drugs in the UK

In the UK, drugs of abuse are controlled by two main pieces of legislation.

1. Misuse of Drugs Act (1971)

This Act classifies drugs into three classes according to the maximum penalty that an offender can expect to receive if he or she contravenes the law. The Act renders possession, export, import, manufacture or supply of any of these drugs illegal except in certain specified circumstances. The lists below comprise examples only and are not exhaustive:

- *Class A drugs*. Cocaine (including crack), ecstasy, LSD (lysergide), mescaline, opium, potent opioids, phencyclidine, psilocin. Injectable forms of drugs in class B.
- *Class B drugs*. Amfetamine, barbiturates, codeine, dihydrocodeine, metamfetamine, methcathinone, methylphenidate.
- *Class C drugs*. Anabolic steroids, benzodiazepines, cannabis, cathine, cathinone, clenbuterol, dextropropoxyphene, diethylpropion, chorionic gonadotrophins and growth hormones.

2. Misuse of Drugs Regulations (updated 2001)

These are principally concerned with regulating the legitimate medical supply and use of potentially abusable substances.

- *Schedule 1 (CD Lic)*. Only those persons specified in the Act or licensed by the Home Office may possess or supply these drugs. None of them can be prescribed. The drugs in this schedule are those deemed likely to have little therapeutic value and so licences are usually only issued for research purposes. The drugs involved include cannabis, cannabinol, cathinone, coca leaf, ecstasy and related drugs, designer opioids derived from fentanyl (but not fentanyl itself), LSD, psilocin, and raw opium.
- *Schedule 2 (CD)*. The Regulations give a long list of exemptions but, in most circumstances, possession of these drugs by a member of the public is only lawful when acting under the directions of a doctor. For those that supply them, the drugs are subject to stringent requirements for storage

and documentation. Examples of drugs affected include amfetamine, cocaine, methylphenidate, most opioids and phencyclidine.

* *Schedule 3 (CD No Reg)*. These are subject to the same regulations as schedule 2 except that the documentation of supply is less rigorous. Barbiturates, buprenorphine, diethylpropion, flunitrazepam, temazepam and cathine are included here. Some schedule 3 drugs are exempt from safe custody requirements.
* *Schedule 4 Part I (CD Benz)*. Comprises mostly benzodiazepines and zolpidem. Part II (CD Anab) contains anabolic steroids, growth hormones, human chorionic gonadotrophin and clenbuterol.
* *Schedule 5 (CD Inv)*. These are preparations containing very small amounts of substances that would otherwise belong to schedule 2 or 3. Examples include codeine linctus, and kaolin and morphine mixture. Suppliers and producers must keep transaction records of their dealings.

Drugs not covered

Certain abused substances are not covered by either of these two pieces of legislation. Examples include alkyl nitrites, many plants (e.g. khat), many OTC medicines (e.g. dextromethorphan), and gamma-hydroxybutyrate.

Index

Please note entries in **bold** type refer to a main section or discussion point, page entries in *italics* refer to figures/tables.